MANUFACTURING HUMANS

MANUFACTURING HUMANS

THE CHALLENGE OF THE NEW REPRODUCTIVE TECHNOLOGIES

D. GARETH JONES

Professor of Anatomy
in the University of Otago, New Zealand

INTER-VARSITY PRESS

INTER-VARSITY PRESS
38 De Montfort Street, Leicester LE1 7GP, England

First published 1987

British Library Cataloguing in Publication Data
Jones, D. Gareth
Manufacturing humans: the challenge of
the new reproductive technologies.
1. Fertilization in vitro, Human—
Religious aspects—Christianity
I. Title
261.5'6   BT708

ISBN 0-85110-771-0

Set in Century Schoolbook

Photoset in Great Britain by
Parker Typesetting Service, Leicester

Printed in Great Britain
at the University Printing House, Oxford

*Inter-Varsity Press is the publishing division of the
Universities and Colleges Christian Fellowship
(formerly the Inter-Varsity Fellowship), a student
movement linking Christian Unions in universities and
colleges throughout the United Kingdom and the Republic
of Ireland, and a member movement of the International
Fellowship of Evangelical Students. For information
about local and national activities write to UCCF,
38 De Montfort Street, Leicester LE1 7GP.*

DEDICATION

To

Barbara and Murray

through whom I have come to appreciate something of
the human face of infertility,

and to

Kathryn, Martyn, Carolyn and Gavyn

who would never have existed had
Beryl and I been infertile.

Contents

PREFACE   ix

1: AN ODYSSEY THROUGH THE NEW REPRODUCTIVE
TECHNOLOGIES   1

*INTRODUCTION – NATURAL WAYS OF PRODUCING A
CHILD:* Natural reproduction; Adultery; Step-parent; Adoption;
Single parent family; Natural reproduction – variations on a theme
– *TECHNOLOGICAL WAYS OF PRODUCING A CHILD:*
Artificial insemination – AIH; Artificial insemination – AID;
Surrogate motherhood (without IVF); Lavage – ovum donation;
Lavage – embryo donation; In vitro fertilization (IVF) – simple
case; IVF – sperm donation; IVF – ovum donation; IVF – embryo
donation; IVF – surrogate motherhood; IVF – surrogate
motherhood and sperm donation; IVF – surrogate motherhood and
ovum donation; IVF – surrogate motherhood, ovum donation and
sperm donation – *MANIPULATION OF THE EMBRYO:*
Research on the embryo; Ectogenesis; Cloning –
TERMINOLOGY FOR THE NEW TECHNOLOGIES

2: RESPONSES TO THE NEW REPRODUCTIVE
TECHNOLOGIES   21

*DEBATE IN THE 1970s – GUIDELINES FORMULATED IN
THE 1980s:* British debate; Australian debate; American debate –
CONTEMPORARY DEBATE AMONG CHRISTIANS: Varieties
of contributions; Responses to the Warnock Committee Report –
THE WIDER DEBATE

3: PERSPECTIVES ON HUMAN LIFE 59

A PLACE TO START – BIBLICAL GUIDELINES ON HUMAN LIFE: Humans as created beings; Humans as God's image; The misuse of human responsibility; Justice and righteousness in human society – *DECIPHERING HUMAN LIFE – PROCREATION AND INFERTILITY:* The desire for children; Childlessness in biblical times; Adoption as a biblical pattern; Adoption in contemporary society – *NATURE OF THE FAMILY:* Biblical perspectives; Sociological perspectives; Implications for contemporary society

4: THE FETUS, MY FELLOW TRAVELLER 94

DEVELOPMENT OF THE EMBRYO AND FETUS – DEVELOPMENT OF THE BRAIN – SPECIFIC ISSUES RAISED IN FETAL DEVELOPMENT: Fertilization; Genetic uniqueness; Pregnancy wastage; Concept of brain birth

5: THE FETUS: MASTER OR SERVANT? 125

PRENATAL HUMAN LIFE – BIBLICAL GUIDELINES – FETUSES AS PERSONS: Clearing the ground; Personhood of the fetus – evangelical contributions: *a.* Fetuses are persons, *b.* Fetuses become persons; Personhood of the fetus – the wider debate: *a.* Fetuses are persons, *b.* Fetuses are non-persons, *c.* Fetuses are potential persons – *MORAL SIGNIFICANCE OF DEVELOPMENTAL ISSUES:* Genetic uniqueness; Pregnancy wastage; Emergence of a functioning brain – *FETUSES IN A HUMAN CONTEXT:* Fetuses under threat; Innocence and conflict

6: FREEDOM TO BRING LIFE INTO EXISTENCE? 168

ARTIFICIAL INSEMINATION BY DONOR (AID): General arguments; Ethical analysis – *IN VITRO FERTILIZATION (IVF) – SIMPLE CASE:* General considerations; Ethical assessment – *IN VITRO FERTILIZATION – SPARE EMBRYOS AND DONATIONS:* Spare embryos; Gamete donations – *SURROGATE MOTHERHOOD:* General considerations; Ethical assessment

7: FREEDOM TO MANIPULATE HUMAN LIFE? 208

INTRODUCTION – FETAL RESEARCH: Types of research and guidelines; Queries raised by the guidelines; Ethical assessment – *RESEARCH ON HUMAN EMBRYOS:* General considerations; Ethical assessment: *a.* Relationship between research on IVF-produced embryos and on fetuses, *b*. Status of IVF embryos, *c*. Therapeutic and non-therapeutic research on embryos, *d*. IVF, spontaneous abortion, and research, *e*. Ambivalence of embryo research

8: CERTAINTIES AND QUANDARIES   240

CHRISTIANS AND TECHNOLOGY – CHRISTIANS AND PUBLIC POLICY – RECOMMENDATIONS FOR SOCIETY: AID; IVF – simple case; IVF – spare embryos; IVF – gamete donations; Surrogate motherhood; Research on human embryos – *REFLECTIONS ON CHRISTIAN ATTITUDES:* Accepting uncertainties; Establishing certainties; Advice to a Christian couple

EPILOGUE   265

Chorion biopsy; IVF-related techniques; Embryonic biopsy; Trans-species fertilization; Mass production and culture of human embryonic material

GLOSSARY	270
NOTES ON CHAPTERS	279
ADDENDUM	298
INDEX OF SCRIPTURE REFERENCES AND NAMES	300
INDEX OF NAMES	302
SUBJECT INDEX	303

Preface

This book is intended as a follow-up to my earlier book, *Brave New People* (published originally in 1984). Many may wonder whether another book in the area of ethical issues at the commencement of life is warranted, especially by an author who has already written in the area (and who in doing so found himself at the centre of a momentous storm in the United States).

At the time of finalizing *Brave New People* in the latter part of 1983 I was aware of the speed with which the new reproductive technologies were moving. I was also aware that if I delayed in having that book published, there would be little available on the burgeoning reproductive technologies written from the perspective of an evangelical Christian. As it turned out, the publication of *Brave New People* in mid-1984 proved timely, since the ethical debate on these technologies burst into prominence at that time. It is no exaggeration to say that there has, since then, been an explosion of interest and concern on all sides. So dramatic has this been that it has proved exceedingly difficult to keep up with the torrent of literature. What is particularly significant is that rapid developments have not only taken place in laboratories and clinics. Developments have been as frenetic in ethical and theological circles as they have been in scientific circles, and they have involved church synods and social questions committees, legal bodies, a host of clubs and organizations, and women's magazines.

There is no getting away from IVF and its kin. Anyone who

shows no interest in these issues is simply turning away from one of the most revolutionary developments confronting mankind. It is no longer simply a matter of finding a solution to some forms of infertility, although this is still its *raison d'être*. Rather, we are confronted with philosophical and theological matters of profound importance. As we come face to face with the meaning of prenatal human life, we are forced to ask searching questions about ourselves, who we are, and what the meaning of our own existence is. It is impossible to discuss what we should or should not do to the prenatal version of ourselves, without also looking at what we – as postnatal humans – are.

It is for these reasons that the influence of the new reproductive technologies has spread far beyond laboratories and clinics. It is also for these reasons that discussions about these technologies are proving divisive. They are threatening value systems and accepted beliefs; they are forcing us to ask questions we have not previously had to ask.

Manufacturing Humans takes up where *Brave New People* left off. In many respects the scope of *Manufacturing Humans* is much narrower than that of *Brave New People*. I have addressed myself to the concerns that have arisen since mid-1984, and I have specifically avoided covering the same ground as that covered in *Brave New People*. I am very much aware that a great deal of what I have written is tentative, and will need to be revised in the light of further thinking. While some would see this as a criticism of my position, I do not agree. We have to start somewhere, and I am aiming to provide my readers with a starting point. I shall be delighted if what I have written is taken seriously, even if some wish to dispute the directions my thinking takes, and perhaps disagree with many of my conclusions. Above all, I hope that this book, along with *Brave New People*, will be accepted as part of the dialogue that is so essential if we are to cope with the challenges facing us at the commencement of human life.

I am greatly indebted to many people. First, I wish to express my indebtedness to those who so vigorously criticized my treatment of therapeutic abortion in *Brave New People*. While those who did this in the United States forced the original edition off the American market (although a revised edition was subsequently published there), their criticisms resulted in my having to look very seriously at the status of the fetus. This served as the stimulus for a detailed treatment of this crucial topic and that, in turn, ushered in this present book. I would also like to thank those organizations who have invited me to speak on these topics, and who have encouraged me to keep on thinking and writing in this hazardous area. In particular I am indebted to the Christian Medical Fellowship of Australia, the Christian Brethren Research Fellowship of New Zealand, and the Faculty of Medicine of the University of Otago. I should like to thank Robbie McPhee who has turned my very rough sketches into the diagrams that appear in the following pages, and Lesley Davies for her efficient secretarial assistance. I also wish to acknowledge my indebtedness to Dr David Green of the Department of Pharmacology, University of Otago, for the idea behind the 'tables' in chapter 1.

Above all, however, I am indebted to Barbara Telfer. Not only has she done the word processing in her usual meticulous fashion, but she has edited my writing, raised numerous queries, and found references galore. Without her assistance this book would never have been completed in the four-months of 'spare-time' work allotted to it.

D. Gareth Jones

1

An Odyssey Through the New Reproductive Technologies

Introduction

As little as ten years ago it was possible to write about *in vitro**
fertilization as some forbidding spectre on the horizon. The
unreality of the procedure was accentuated by use of the misleading description 'test-tube babies'. Today, the situation is
quite different. Almost everyone, it seems, is familiar with the
process, and more and more people are at ease with its abbreviation, 'IVF'. Nevertheless, familiarity does not ensure an
understanding of the technique, nor of the multitude of social
and ethical issues surrounding it. Neither dare we limit any
consideration of IVF to the technique in its present form. This
is undoubtedly just the beginning of many extensions of it, all
of which will demand consideration in their own right.

IVF** is the first illustration we have had of our ability to
'manufacture' other human beings. My use of an industrial
term is deliberate, because the fertilization of human ova in
the laboratory is more akin to factory production than to a
human and sexual activity. Its goal is the production of
embryos which, if required, will be placed into a human uterus
for further development. This uterus may or may not belong to

*There is a glossary of technical terms on page 270.
**As acronyms and abbreviations proliferate, some duplication is
inevitable; and it may prevent some uncertainty if I clarify at the
outset that in this book, the abbreviation IVF is never used except to
represent '*in vitro* fertilization', and AID is never used except to
represent 'artificial insemination by donor'.

the woman from whom the ova[1] originally came. If not immediately required, the embryos may be frozen for subsequent use, used in a research project, or discarded.

Inevitably, the element of human control in the treatment and use of the embryos is paramount. What is more, the control is of a technical nature. Admittedly, the type of control being exerted at present has, as its goal, the alleviation of infertility and the production of a child for a couple who would otherwise be childless. In many ways this is a commendable use of human expertise, and it is not one to be harshly decried by those who have experienced little difficulty in having children by natural means.

Nevertheless, no matter how sympathetic one may be about IVF in general, one aspect of technical control should not be overlooked. Once human embryos have been made accessible in this way, they have been made available for a vast range of therapeutic and research purposes. They represent a fascinating world of dividing cells, developing tissues, and nascent organ systems. They are the embodiment of ever-increasing organizational patterns and of emerging complexity, and above all, these processes – so important to an understanding of early development – can all be observed in the human being (as opposed to laboratory animals).

IVF's value as a means around infertility for some of the many infertile couples in our communities is but the tip of the iceberg of the potential it holds out for manipulating human embryos. This is not of necessity a condemnation of IVF, but it is a reminder that we are dealing with a phenomenon of momentous proportions. The grandiose dreams of visionaries about altering the human constitution and making new kinds of human beings may finally become reality. IVF makes it all possible, although hopefully most of the science fiction nightmares will never come to pass.

In this chapter I want to pursue the technical possibilities opened up by IVF. These are best illustrated by viewing them in the context of the whole gamut of ways available to us of producing a child. What is perhaps surprising is that we already employ a large number of ways of doing this, quite apart from any sophisticated technical procedures. In our undue fascination with scientific expertise, it is very easy to overlook the adaptability of natural reproduction. Therefore it is to natural reproduction and its many offshoots that we need to turn first.

Natural Ways of Producing a Child

1. Natural Reproduction
Consider the following table:

Biological Parents:	$X_1 + Y_1$
Fertilization:	Natural insemination into X_1
Gestation:	X_1
Social Parents:	$X_1 + Y_1$

X_1 and Y_1 are the couple in whom we are interested. I shall refer to them as a married couple, with X_1 as the wife and Y_1 as the husband. In the next section (Technological ways of producing a child) they will have an infertility problem. For the moment, however, they have no problem. The gametes (ovum and sperm) come from X_1 and Y_1 themselves, making X_1 and Y_1 the biological parents. Fertilization occurs by natural insemination of sperm into X_1, who then carries the fetus to term. In other words, gestation takes place in X_1. Additionally, they rear the child themselves, so that their influence extends throughout gestation and also through the years of childhood. The two people concerned, X_1 and Y_1, are therefore the social parents as well as the biological parents.

The scheme outlined here is the epitome of natural, sexual reproduction. Not only this, but it takes place within the confines of a relationship in which the man and woman are ideally committed to each other, having a stable, ongoing relationship. The consequences of this are that it has the potential of enabling the child to be nurtured within an environment in which there is no doubt about the identity of the parents nor of their relationship to the child.

2. Adultery

Biological Parents:	$X_1 + Y_2$
Fertilization:	Natural insemination into X_1
Gestation:	X_1
Social Parents:	$X_1 + Y_1$

In this particular example of pregnancy resulting from adultery the sperm comes from a male third party, Y_2. The wife in the couple with which we are concerned (X_1) carries the fetus to term, and it is this couple, X_1 and Y_1, who serve as the social parents. From this it is evident that X_1 is both the biological

and social mother, whereas the biological father, Y_2 (the third
party) has nothing to do with the bringing-up of the child. The
social father, Y_1, is not related biologically to the child.

The end result biologically is the same as with two technological methods of producing a child, namely, AID (number 2
in the following section) and IVF accompanied by sperm donation (number 7 in the following section). The major differences,
in strict biological terms, are with the methods of fertilization –
natural, or artificial insemination and IVF respectively. Accompanying these differences, at least between natural insemination on the one hand and artificial insemination or IVF on the
other, is a moral gulf of immense proportions.

In practice, of course, the social situation may be far more
complex than the simple arrangement proposed above. The
social parents indicated above (X_1 and Y_1) may not remain
together for long; another individual (X_2 or Y_3) may intrude, so
that the child will, in practice, experience more than three
parents. But more of this in the following examples.

What we need to bear in mind is that human history is replete
with families in which one of the social parents is not a biological parent. This observation neither justifies nor condemns
this particular arrangement, but it is a salutary reminder that
mixed genetic parentage is not the creation of biological tech-
nocrats.

3. Step-parent

One does not have to look to adultery as the sole pre-
technological example of mixed genetic parentage. A family
situation involving step-parents is another example. In this
instance, a child conceived by one couple is raised for some part
of its childhood by another couple of which only the husband or
wife is related biologically to the child.

Biological Parents: $X_1 + Y_1$
Fertilization: Natural insemination into X_1
Gestation: X_1
Social Parents: $X_1 + Y_2$

In this instance, X_1 is the biological mother of the child, and Y_1
is the biological father in the first marriage. On the death of Y_1
or on the break-up of the original marriage, Y_1 entirely or partly
ceases to be involved in the rearing of the child. If X_1 remarries,
another man (Y_2) takes over the role of social father to the child.

The child in this illustration has three parents. The complicating factor here is that the child may actually know, and have to deal with, three parents. Even if the biological father (Y_1) dies, the child may have known this person as his or her 'father' for a number of years. On acquiring a social father (Y_2) later on, the child will have to cope quite literally with two 'fathers'. This may be even more obvious when re-marriage follows divorce, since under these circumstances the child may have to relate to the two 'fathers' simultaneously.

An equivalent illustration is provided by the complementary step-parent situation, in which it is the 'mother' who changes. In this instance we have:

Biological Parents: $X_1 + Y_1$
Fertilization: Natural insemination into X_1
Gestation: X_1
Social Parents: $X_2 + Y_1$

Even if the demands on the child differ when there are two 'mothers' rather than two 'fathers', the overriding principle is the same. An important point in the context of the new reproductive technologies is that the presence of two 'fathers' or two 'mothers' is a much more complex situation than that introduced by a number of the technological procedures emanating from IVF.

4. Adoption

Biological Parents: $X_2 + Y_2$
Fertilization: Natural insemination into X_2
Gestation: X_2
Social Parents: $X_1 + Y_1$

The issue in this instance is not mixed genetic parentage, but a complete divorce between the biological parents and the social parents. The child has four parents, although only the social parents are responsible for the child's upbringing. In most cases, however, the child will be aware that the social parents are not his or her biological parents, and in early adulthood it may be possible to become acquainted with the biological parents or, more commonly, the biological mother.

Of all the 'manipulative' procedures in the reproductive area, adoption has acquired the greatest degree of social acceptance. This is in spite of the major gulf it necessitates between biological and social parenthood. It can only be concluded that, until recent years, this gulf has been seen as being less detrimental to the child than a single-parent upbringing. What principally concerns us from the point of view of the new reproductive technologies is the acceptance of the concept of social parentage denoted by adoption.

A variation on adoption is fostering, with its overtones of temporary relationships with a succession of social parents.

5. *Single Parent Family*

Biological Parents: $X_1 + Y_1$
Fertilization: Natural insemination into X_1
Gestation: X_1
Social Parents: X_1 (or Y_1)

This is a re-enactment of the situation previously encountered (in number 3 this section) except that the parent lost through death or divorce is not replaced. The result is the one-parent family rather than the two- (or even, in practice, three-) parent family. The child is brought up by just one parent, although on many occasions grandparents, relatives or friends may be intimately involved in the child's development.

6. *Natural Reproduction – Variations on a Theme*
It is not my purpose to attempt to sketch all the varieties of natural reproduction in which humans have indulged. Nevertheless, some are relevant to my discussion in later chapters dealing with the limits society may or may not wish to impose on the application of the new reproductive technologies.

Several illustrations are found in the Old Testament. For instance, in Genesis 16:1–15 Abram had had no children by Sarai, his wife. She suggested that this might be rectified by Abram sleeping with Hagar, her maidservant. The result was the birth of a son, Ishmael. In similar vein, Jacob had children by Bilhah, the servant of one of his wives, Rachel, and also by Zilpah, the servant of Leah, his other wife. (Gn. 30:1–13).

This pattern may be expressed as follows:

Biological Parents: $X_2 + Y_1$
Fertilization: Natural insemination into X_2
Gestation: X_2
Social Parents: $X_2 + Y_1$

In the case of Abram, he is represented by Y_1 and Hagar by X_2. Sarai his wife, X_1, does not feature in the reproductive process or, one imagines, in the parenting role. In spite of this, Abram is provided with a son and an heir.

A totally different arrangement has been provided in much more recent times by those families in which the children have been brought up by 'nannies', or away from home in boarding schools. Under these circumstances we have the following:

Biological Parents: $X_1 + Y_1$
Fertilization: Natural insemination into X_1
Gestation: X_1
Social Parents: $(X_1 + Y_1); X_2; Z$

In this illustration the biological parents are, to some extent, the social parents, although this is only partially the case. Considerable responsibility for parenting also falls to the nanny, X_2, or to the staff of the school (Z). Examples of these arrangements can be found in many diverse locations, and they occur for a wide variety of reasons. Children of the English Royal Family are frequently brought up in this way, as are the children of many missionary families.

A much more extreme example of this type of arrangement is provided by orphans brought up in institutions rather than in a family environment. Here the lack of both social and biological parents during the formative years of childhood may have devastating consequences for the social and psychological adjustment of the developing child. These effects are, however, quite different from those envisaged as stemming from the new reproductive technologies.

Further patterns encountered in present-day society include those in which a child experiences a succession of 'fathers', or in which the social parents are of the same sex. The fact that such patterns exist in society in no sense legitimizes them. Neither do they justify the deliberate creation of children by technological means for single parents, couples of the same sex, or for any others outside stable heterosexual family relationships. On the other hand, it would be short-sighted to ignore their present existence. These patterns may prove a potent influence upon societies at large, as regards the directions in which they may wish the new reproductive technologies to develop.

Technological Ways of Producing a Child

1. Artificial Insemination – AIH

Biological Parents: $X_1 + Y_1$
Fertilization: Artificial insemination into X_1
Gestation: X_1
Social Parents: $X_1 + Y_1$

The overall processes here are exactly the same as with natural reproduction, except that sperm from the husband (Y_1) is artificially deposited in the uterus of the wife (X_1). Gestation occurs in X_1, and our couple, X_1 and Y_1, are the social parents as well as the biological parents. No aspect of the marital relationship is breached in this instance, unless it is considered that the intrusion of an artificial element does this.

2. Artificial Insemination – AID

Biological Parents: $X_1 + Y_2$
Fertilization: Artificial insemination into X_1
Gestation: X_1
Social Parents: $X_1 + Y_1$

In this case, the sperm comes from an anonymous donor, Y_2, and is artificially inseminated into the wife, X_1. Gestation occurs normally in X_1. The husband, Y_1, contributes nothing and so is not the biological father, although he is the social father. The mother is both the biological and social mother. Here a third party has been introduced into the reproductive process itself. The resulting child will have three parents, because only the mother is both a biological and a social parent. In practice, however, society has attempted to reduce this to two parents – the social parents – since the anonymity of the biological father, Y_2, has been assiduously protected.

3. Surrogate Motherhood (without IVF)

Biological Parents: $X_2 + Y_1$
Fertilization: Natural or artificial insemination into X_2
Gestation: X_2
Social Parents: $X_1 + Y_1$

The wife of our couple is infertile and is also incapable of carrying the child throughout gestation. She is replaced for both these functions by another woman, X_2, who is insemi-nated with the sperm of the husband, Y_1. X_2 carries the child to term, and then hands over the child to the social parents X_1 and Y_1. The novel features of this arrangement are that con-ception of the child in a third party is intentional, on the understanding that the third party's involvement will be con-fined to the period of gestation. A radical separation has been introduced therefore, between child-bearing and child-rearing, a separation that has been deliberately brought about. The legal nightmare of surrogate motherhood is well known, while the intrusion of money into the arrangement raises numerous issues about 'buying a child'.

While I have included this form of surrogacy, sometimes referred to as 'partial surrogacy', in the technological category, this is only the case when artificial insemination is employed. This is usually the case with surrogacy, although not always. Strictly speaking, therefore, when intercourse takes place between the commissioning father, Y_1, and the surrogate mother, X_2, the surrogacy belongs to the natural reproduction category.

4. Lavage – Ovum Donation

Biological Parents: $X_2 + Y_1$
Fertilization: Natural or artificial insemination into X_2
Gestation: X_1
Social Parents: $X_1 + Y_1$

In this case, the wife X_1 is infertile, and so another woman, X_2, is inseminated with the husband's sperm. Three or four days after fertilization, before the start of implantation, the donor's uterus is flushed out (lavage) and the embryo is retrieved and transferred to the uterus of the infertile woman, X_1. If the embryo implants successfully, the recipient carries the preg-nancy to term. The major difference between this procedure and one utilizing IVF is that the donor of the ovum does not have to undergo a general anaesthetic and laparoscopy for ovum retrieval. A disadvantage is that, if the flushing out procedure is unsuccessful, the donor may become pregnant (which is certainly not the desired outcome).

5. Lavage – Embryo Donation

Biological Parents: $X_2 + Y_2$
Fertilization: Natural or artificial insemination into X_2
Gestation: X_1
Social Parents: $X_1 + Y_1$

This is the same as in 4, except that in this instance both social
parents X_1 and Y_1 are infertile. The ovum donor, X_2, is therefore inseminated with sperm which is also from a donor, Y_2.
The embryo which is transferred to the wife in our couple (X_1)
is entirely the result of gamete donation. This is, therefore, a
form of *prenatal adoption*, the difference between this and child
adoption being that the adoptive individual has been brought
into existence to serve the needs of the adopting (social)
parents, and that the social parents experience the pregnancy
and childbirth. The resulting child has four parents, two biological parents and two social parents, each of which has been
knowingly involved in the production of a four-parent child.

6. In Vitro Fertilization (IVF) – Simple Case

Biological Parents: $X_1 + Y_1$
Fertilization: IVF
Gestation: X_1
Social Parents: $X_1 + Y_1$

This is IVF in its standard or simple form. The biological
parents are the social parents, and gestation occurs in the wife,
X_1. In all these respects it is identical to natural reproduction.
The one crucial divergence from natural reproduction is, of
course, the manner of the fertilization which occurs in the
laboratory under controlled scientific conditions. An event that
has traditionally taken place in the darkness and mystery of
the woman's reproductive tracts can now be followed step by
step by a laboratory technician using a dissecting microscope.
What is more, it is this accessibility of the gametes and resulting embryo that constitutes the basis of control, manipulation
and experimentation.

Before a woman's ova can be obtained for IVF, however, in
many programmes hormonal stimulation of her ovaries is
used, while a general anaesthetic is required to enable laparoscopy to be carried out to retrieve ova suitable for fertilization.
In many IVF programmes surplus embryos will be frozen, and

this should entail serious thought about the range of uses to which these embryos might be put if they are not all required to establish a subsequent pregnancy. Our couple (X_1 and Y_1) will therefore have to be prepared to face a demanding range of clinical procedures on the wife, as well as serious ethical considerations regarding the ultimate fate of any embryos not required by them. In the future, ova will almost definitely be followed by ultrasound, thereby dispensing with the need for general anaesthesia (see Epilogue, p.265).

7. IVF – Sperm Donation

Biological Parents: $X_1 + Y_2$
Fertilization: IVF
Gestation: X_1
Social Parents: $X_1 + Y_1$

The husband, Y_1, is infertile and so a sperm donor, Y_2, is used. Although the wife, X_1, produces ova, these have not been successfully fertilized by the sperm from Y_2 following artificial insemination. Despite this, fertilization does occur following IVF. The resulting embryo is implanted in X_1, and pregnancy occurs in a straightforward manner.

8. IVF – Ovum Donation

Biological Parents: $X_2 + Y_1$
Fertilization: IVF
Gestation: X_1
Social Parents: $X_1 + Y_1$

As in the case of lavage and ovum donation (number 4 above), the wife (X_1) is infertile but is capable of carrying a fetus to term. An ovum is donated by another woman (X_2) and this is fertilized in the laboratory by the husband's sperm. The resulting embryo is placed into X_1, in whom gestation takes place. The child has three parents, since the biological mother differs from the social mother. This is the converse of AID, although the emphasis placed on the anonymity of the donor in AID cannot be maintained to the same extent in ovum donation. This is because the menstrual cycles of the two women, X_1 and X_2, have to be synchronized, a requirement that will continue in force until it is clinically commonplace to freeze and thaw ova.[2]

9. IVF – Embryo Donation

Biological Parents:	$X_2 + Y_2$
Fertilization:	IVF
Gestation:	X_1
Social Parents:	$X_1 + Y_1$

Both members of our couple, X_1 and Y_1, are infertile, although the wife is capable of sustaining a pregnancy. An embryo which, under present circumstances, would be a spare embryo from another couple on an IVF programme, is placed in X_1 and gestation proceeds. This embryo may or may not have been frozen, although it may become increasingly common to use previously frozen embryos. Since the biological and social parents are different, this is another example of prenatal adoption. One difference between prenatal adoption in this instance and that associated with lavage (see number 5 above) is that the embryo has probably not been specifically produced to meet the needs of the prospective social parents. The embryo is surplus to the needs of another couple, and was brought into existence for them rather than for the adoptive parents. In this regard, it has a great deal in common with conventional adoption.

10. IVF – Surrogate Motherhood

Biological Parents:	$X_1 + Y_1$
Fertilization:	IVF
Gestation:	X_2
Social Parents:	$X_1 + Y_1$

This has similarities to the category of surrogate motherhood already considered (number 3 above), although the introduction of IVF makes surrogacy a far more radical procedure. This stems from the possibility opened up by the transferring of an embryo (rather than semen) to the surrogate mother, who will then serve solely as an incubator for the couple's embryo. This is the situation depicted above, and it is sometimes described as 'full surrogacy'. The major difference between partial and full surrogacy is that in partial surrogacy the surrogate mother is the genetic mother of the child, whereas in full surrogacy she has no genetic relationship to the child. The implications of this difference could be very considerable from the child's point of view.

Apart from this consideration, which has received little attention up to the present, the major justification for using IVF would be subfertility on the husband's side. IVF may lead to fertilization, even if artificial insemination has proved unsuccessful. As with surrogate motherhood without IVF (number 3 above), the essential prerequisite for surrogacy is the wife's inability to sustain a pregnancy.

11. IVF – Surrogate Motherhood and Sperm Donation

Biological Parents: $X_1 + Y_2$
Fertilization: IVF
Gestation: X_2
Social Parents: $X_1 + Y_1$

This is a further development of the IVF and surrogate motherhood combination, brought about by the infertility of the husband, Y_1. This can be bypassed by the use of a sperm donor, Y_2. Once fertilization has been effected in the laboratory, the fetus is carried to term in a surrogate mother, X_2. In this instance, the wife, X_1, is only involved in producing the child via the ovum. Her husband, Y_1, has no involvement at all. This arrangement (like those below) is a further example of full surrogacy.

12. IVF – Surrogate Motherhood and Ovum Donation

Biological Parents: $X_2 + Y_1$
Fertilization: IVF
Gestation: X_3
Social Parents: $X_1 + Y_1$

The social mother, that is, the wife of the couple with whom we are concerned (X_1) is infertile, and is also incapable of sustaining a pregnancy. There are therefore two problems to be overcome in this case, and they are solved by using two different women. The first of these is X_2, who provides the ovum; she is therefore the donor. Fertilization occurs by IVF, and the child is carried by the second woman, X_3, who is the surrogate mother. Obviously, two women would not be required if the ovum donor was also the surrogate mother (as in number 3 above). IVF makes possible the separation of the donor and the surrogacy roles. The social father, Y_1, is also the biological father.

13. IVF – Surrogate Motherhood, Ovum Donation and Sperm Donation

Biological Parents: $X_2 + Y_2$
Fertilization: IVF
Gestation: X_3
Social Parents: $X_1 + Y_1$

This is the same as number 12 above, except that the husband in the couple (Y_1) is also infertile. Both social parents therefore, are infertile, added to which the wife is incapable of sustaining a pregnancy. The resulting child in this instance has five parents.

Manipulation of the Embryo
Considerable discussion surrounds the means becoming available to us of manipulating the embryo or of controlling the development of the embryo and fetus during gestation. In this section I want to illustrate how these procedures may affect the relationship between the embryo or fetus and the biological or social parents.

1. Research on the Embryo

Biological Parents: $X_1 + Y_1$
Fertilization: IVF
Gestation: none
Social Parents: none

Debate about research on human embryos centres on embryos created in the laboratory by IVF. They are, therefore, pre-implantation embryos (less than 14 days after fertilization) that exist outside a woman's body. Moreover, they have never existed in any environment other than a laboratory one. Such embryos can be produced in a number of ways. I shall mention just two of these at this juncture.

The embryos may be superfluous to the needs of a couple in a clinical IVF programme. These are the 'spare' or 'superfluous' embryos about which we hear a great deal. In the illustration above, they are depicted as coming from the married couple, X_1 and Y_1, on whom I have been focusing. They are embryos which have resulted from the fertilization of X_1's ova by sperm from Y_1; for one reason or another this couple has no use for one or more of these embryos, and they have given permission for them to be used in a research programme.

An alternative source of embryos is donation. In this instance, both the ovum and sperm have been donated by two individuals, the sole intention being to produce an embryo for use in a research programme. In these circumstances, the biological parents could be represented by X_2 and Y_3, since in all probability they would be unknown to each other.

I shall deal in detail with the issues raised by such research in chapter 7. What needs to be stressed in the present chapter is that, as illustrated above, the embryo will never be transferred to a woman's uterus. There is, therefore, no gestation and obviously there are no social parents. All embryos on which research has been conducted are doomed to a brief existence in the laboratory (a maximum of 14 days according to most present guidelines; see chapter 2).

Once consent is given for an embryo to be used for research purposes, the biological parents have relinquished their claim to be parents. The embryo, under most current guidelines, will never be transferred to a woman's uterus for further development. Its existence has, to all intents and purposes, already come to an end. An embryo in a research programme has no parents and no future.

2. Ectogenesis

This refers to the maintenance of the embryo, and later the fetus, in an artificial environment in the laboratory for the whole of the gestation period. Ectogenesis will dispose of the role of a woman and her uterus in the development and maturation of the fetus. While this is not an imminent possibility, it behoves us to look at its repercussions for parenthood.

Biological Parents: $X_1 + Y_1$
Fertilization: IVF
Gestation: E
Social Parents: $X_1 + Y_1$

This outline clearly demonstrates that there is no parenting role for either X_1 or Y_1 at any stage throughout gestation. There is no pregnancy in the conventional sense, since no human being is pregnant. Once the fetus has developed sufficiently and is capable of an 'extra-uterine' existence, ectogenesis (E) has come to an end and the social parents, who may or may not be the same individuals as the biological parents, can take over. Just as there is no gestation in human terms, neither is there 'birth' in a biological sense.

Of the arrangements I have already considered the one most akin to ectogenesis is the IVF-surrogate motherhood combination (number 10 in the previous section). The difference, of course, is that the human surrogate in that instance (X_2) has been replaced by a non-human artificial environment (E) in this model. In discussing ectogenesis, therefore, it may prove helpful to start from a consideration of IVF-surrogate motherhood.

3. *Cloning*

This is asexual reproduction, with the result that the new individual is derived from a single parent and is genetically identical to that parent. Sperm are no longer required, and so there is no fertilization as in natural sexual reproduction.[3] In terms of the schema I have been employing in this chapter, cloning can be sketched as follows.

Biological Parents: ovum from X_1; nucleus from X_1, Y_1, X_2 or Y_2
Fertilization: none
Gestation: X_1
Social Parents: $X_1 + Y_1$

There is only one biological parent, and I have given a number of possibilities. X_1 provides an ovum; this is unfertilized, and its nucleus is removed in the laboratory. This is then replaced with the nucleus of a specialized body cell (for example, from the mucosa on the inside of the mouth) from either X_1 herself, or from her husband, Y_1, or from other individuals, X_2 or Y_2. The unfertilized ovum from X_1, with its new nucleus, proceeds to divide and differentiate *as if it had been fertilized*. In order to do this, it must be placed in the uterus of X_1 (exactly as in the most straightforward type of IVF), and gestation takes place as normal. The critical feature of cloning is that the resulting child is genetically identical to the individual who contributed the body cell nucleus, whether it was X_1, Y_1, X_2 or Y_2. In other words, the child and the person donating the nucleus are identical twins belonging to different generations.

Cloning is a futuristic technique, and it should not be regarded otherwise. It is quite different from any other procedure considered in this chapter, because of its asexual nature and consequent lack of the genetic recombinations and reshuffling which are so much a part of sexual reproduction. It deviates from natural reproduction far more radically than any other procedure one is likely to consider, and yet gestation is straightforward and the environment provided by the social parents could be remarkably conventional.

Cloning highlights a fact that should have come to the fore by this stage: that the wide variety of forms of both natural reproduction and the new reproductive technologies challenges conventional reproductive patterns at different points. In some it is the discontinuity between biological and social parents, in others it is the lack of stability of the social parents; for yet others, it is the nature of the fertilization process, or the person in whom gestation takes place. Any assessment of these procedures needs to take this diversity into account, and it also needs to balance the advantages and disadvantages of the procedure being considered. This is no easy task, and we should not expect any ready agreement on these issues even by those with an essentially similar theological base. But more of this in the next chapter.

Terminology for the New Technologies
Any new area of discussion introduces a new language, and this is often a source of confusion. At the beginning of a new development, the ideal is to introduce terminology that is clear and consistent. Unfortunately, this may be more difficult to achieve than one imagines, and 'lay terms' may be difficult or even impossible to dislodge.

I am referring in this book to the 'new reproductive technologies'. They will of course not always be new, and so this adjective will disappear in time. However, they will always remain technological procedures, no matter how sophisticated or how readily available and accepted they become within society. An almost equivalent term is the 'new birth technologies'. Some people use the general term 'artificial reproduction'. This is quite correct and is useful, since it describes all techniques by which conception is brought about by artificial means, that is, other than by sexual intercourse. For many years the term 'artificial insemination' has been used, emphasizing the technological aspect of the procedure. It would be unfortunate, however, if the artificial aspect of this technology were to be emphasized in derogatory or even condemnatory ways.

By far the most crucial new technique in the whole domain of reproductive technology is *in vitro* fertilization. In the Introduction to this chapter I dismissed the popular term 'test-tube babies'. The fertilization involved in the technique is not carried out in a test tube, and it is nine months before a baby emerges. I am relieved that, even in the public mind, 'test-tube babies' are gradually receding into the mists of history.

The term '*in vitro* fertilization' means fertilization 'in glass'. The expression '*in vitro*' is a technical one and is used routinely in biological experimentation. It refers to the growth of cells and tissues in media in the laboratory (*in vitro*), as opposed to their growth in the body (*in vivo*). The term simply refers to the fertilization of an ovum by a sperm in appropriate media in a laboratory. It denotes a procedure, and does not even specify which species of animal is involved. These are deficiencies, since it tends to focus on a process rather than on the people involved, or on the resulting child. Despite this, it is an accurate description of the procedures, and it can be very conveniently abbreviated to IVF. As long as the reasons for the use of this term are borne strictly in mind, and as long as it is viewed rigorously within a human context, it has much to commend it. What is more, the term IVF has gained very wide acceptance within the general community and also in scientific circles.

Some have argued against the use of the term IVF, and have proposed instead 'external human fertilization'.[4] There can be no doubt of the accuracy of this term; it also focuses attention on the human nature of the fertilization and on its location outside the body (external). The contrast with internal (natural) human fertilization is clear. Nevertheless, the word 'external' is a vague description of the nature of the fertilization, and tends to be a distraction. It is also worth remarking that the term 'external human fertilization' has not been readily accepted. For these reasons, I prefer to retain the term IVF.

Frequently, the term 'IVF' is employed to cover two related procedures: the fertilization itself, and the transfer of the resulting embryo to the uterus of a woman. This is 'embryo transfer', which is sometimes abbreviated to ET. Strictly speaking, therefore, 'IVF' by itself should be distinguished from 'IVF accompanied by ET'. In practice, however, this is not always done. It is also possible to distinguish between *embryo transfer* (when the embryo is transferred to the uterus of a woman other than the one who produced the ovum) and *embryo replacement* (when the embryo is placed in the uterus of the woman from whom the ovum was obtained). While there are indeed these two categories of women receiving the embryo, the designation 'embryo *replacement*' is not completely accurate. It is also safer, when describing the procedures, to specify precisely who is going to receive the embryo. I am not convinced, therefore, that the term 'embryo transfer' should be confined to just one of the categories.

In the schemes outlined in the previous sections I have drawn a distinction between the 'biological' parents and the 'social' parents. This is a relatively simple distinction. I have also specified the woman in whom the gestation of the fetus occurs. It is possible to be more explicit than this by describing the mother and father roles separately.[5] The mother role can then be subdivided into the *genetic* mother (the woman producing the ovum), the *carrying* mother (the woman in whose uterus the fetus implants and matures), and the *nurturing* mother (the woman caring for the baby after birth). The term '*complete* mother' is also used to describe a woman who undertakes all three roles. Equivalent subdivisions of the father role are *genetic* father (the man providing the sperm), *nurturing* father (the man caring for the child following birth) and *complete* father (who performs both roles in relation to any individual fetus/child). It is also possible to specify combinations of roles, such as genetic-carrying mother or genetic-nurturing mother. While these distinctions are useful ones in delineating roles within reproduction, I shall use them only when there is need to be very specific. On other occasions I shall content myself with the biological-social distinction within parenting.

Surrogate motherhood refers, as I have already indicated, to a woman who carries a fetus to term for another woman (or couple). In the traditional surrogate arrangement the surrogate mother is also the genetic mother of the child (genetic-carrying mother). In combination with IVF, however, the surrogate mother may not be the genetic mother. If an embryo is transferred to the surrogate mother she may simply serve as the carrying mother, leaving the other woman as the genetic-nurturing mother. Of course, other combinations of roles are also possible. The issue at stake, though, is whether the genetic-carrying or the carrying-mother (the surrogate mother in conventional terminology) should be the one described as the surrogate mother. Why not characterize the nurturing mother (the wife of the couple desiring the child) as the surrogate mother? Is she any more the 'real' mother simply because it is she who wants the child and has instigated the proceedings to produce a child? Is 'nurturing' more important than 'carrying' a child?

My point in raising these questions in this chapter is not to attempt to answer them here, but to reveal the extraordinary complexity of the issues raised by manipulative reproductive technology. Many of our assumptions are being challenged in a most fundamental manner, and it is just as well for us to begin to face up to this before proceeding any further. In spite of these comments, I shall have to continue using the surrogate motherhood designation in the usual way – otherwise, confusion galore will reign.

I have already alluded to the use of the terms 'full' and 'partial surrogacy'[6], 'full surrogacy' denoting the use of IVF (the surrogate is the carrying mother alone) and 'partial surrogacy' the case where natural intercourse or artificial insemination is used (the surrogate is the genetic-carrying mother). It must be observed, however, that this is an entirely arbitrary designation. It appears to suggest that the less the surrogate does, the more complete is her role. Underlying this use of the terms 'full' and 'partial' is the assumption that the greater our dependence on artificial reproduction, the more complete it is. This, I contend, is an assumption that needs to be challenged.

2

Responses to the New Reproductive Technologies

Debate in the 1970s

The deluge of statements on IVF and allied procedures over the past two to three years should not be allowed to obscure the debate that went on in the 1970s. While some of that debate may appear outdated in today's terms, it set the scene for much of the subsequent serious discussion. It is perhaps surprising that one of the prime exponents of the ethical debate, Professor Paul Ramsey of Princeton University, wrote his seminal book on genetic control, *Fabricated Man*, in 1970.[1] In this and other writings, Ramsey contended for a conservative position on IVF and indeed on any manipulations of the embryo and fetus.

Ramsey, writing before the successful application of IVF in humans, argued that: 'The decisive moral verdict must be that we cannot rightfully *get to know* how to do this [IVF] without conducting unethical experiments upon the unborn who must be the "mishaps" (the dead and retarded ones) through whom we learn how.'[2] Underlying this objection is Ramsey's concern for the fetus and, in particular, that it should not be exposed to any harm not beneficial to its own existence. Coupled with this is the further objection that a hypothetical or unborn child is being submitted to a dangerous procedure. Ramsey has expressed this issue in a variety of ways: the possibility of damage to the IVF fetus cannot, by definition, be completely excluded. When mishaps occur they must, Ramsey envisages, be discarded. What is even more serious, these hazards are being imposed non-therapeutically on the child-to-be without its consent. As this fetus has been artificially conceived, the risks to which it is exposed are man-made and, therefore, need not have arisen in the first place. For Ramsey, therefore, the 'treatment' of infertility by directing attention at the fetus rather than the mother changes the essence of intervention in the reproductive process.

Even the plight of an infertile couple does not, from Ramsey's perspective, justify IVF, since 'it is not a proper goal of medicine to enable women to have children . . . *by any means* – means which *may* bring hazard from the procedure, *any* additional hazard, upon the child not yet conceived'.[3] The emphasis here is on the possibility of harm to the fetus, harm which is not of benefit to the fetus itself and which need not have arisen if IVF had not been undertaken. Even a small risk of grave induced injury is a morally unacceptable risk, rendering unethical all forms of experimentation connected with IVF.[4]

Closely associated in Ramsey's thinking with fetal harm is the related issue of fetal consent. A fetus cannot consent to the procedures of IVF; therefore, IVF should not be undertaken. Unconvincing as the consent argument may be in its own right, Ramsey never strays far from his basic premise that the treatment of infertility should be by direct surgical therapy and not by IVF. The fetus, therefore, should never be subject to the possibility of harm or placed in the impossible situation of giving its consent to a procedure designed to bring it into existence. For Ramsey, IVF takes us into the realm of biological manufacture, and out of the domain of medical ethics. This is because it is being used to meet human *desires* rather than treat human *maladies*.

Ramsey's analysis of IVF leads him to view it as a technological artifice; it is 'reproduction' as opposed to 'procreation'; it is artificial rather than natural. He is opposed to what he sees as the scientific ethic, in which scientists will manage everything and do whatever can be done. In his view this leads inevitably to the destruction of human values and human meaning.

Another significant commentator on bioethical issues is the American ethicist, Leon Kass. He, again, has consistently advocated the view that natural reproduction is superior to anything artificial. 'There are', he writes, 'more and less human ways of bringing a child into the world . . . the laboratory production of human beings is no longer *human* procreation, . . . making babies in laboratories – even 'perfect' babies – means a degradation of parenthood.'[5] For him, therefore, IVF debiologizes procreation, marriage and the family. '*Human* procreation is begetting. It is a more complete human activity precisely because it engages us bodily and spiritually, as well as rationally. . . . What is new is nothing more radical than the divorce of the generation of new life from human sexuality and ultimately from the confines of the human body.'[6]

Many of Kass's emphases are very similar to those of Ramsey, including that of fetal consent to non-therapeutic research. Kass, for instance, writes: 'One cannot ethically choose for [a hypothetical child] the unknown hazards he must face and simultaneously choose to give him life in which to face them.'[7]

The end-result for Kass, as expressed in his writings in the early 1970s, was that it would be foolish to acquire and use these powers. Writing later, in 1979, after the birth of the first child by IVF, Kass again stresses that what is at stake is the idea of the humanness of our human life, the meaning of our sexual being, and our relation to ancestors and descendants.[8] In this 1979 essay, however, Kass treats very seriously the issues raised by ongoing research and clinical work, and he concludes that the early embryo is to be treated as a pre-viable fetus, and is to be given respect for what it is, now and prospectively. He opposes most research on human embryos, except for some observational and non-invasive experiments. In terms of clinical IVF, he adopts the position that any risks to the fetus should be equivalent to, or less than, the risks imposed by normal procreation. To insist on more rigorous standards, he argues, is 'a denial of equal treatment to infertile couples contemplating *in vitro* assistance'.[9]

Kass's move towards accepting the legitimacy of IVF under certain circumstances is rigidly circumscribed by the principle of having a child of one's own. For him, IVF is legitimate when it enables a married couple to have 'a child who is flesh of their separate flesh made one'. When used to move outside this relationship, IVF will – he believes – serve to confound and complicate parentage and lineage.

Another way of emphasizing the importance of the family was developed by Richard McCormick, a Roman Catholic theologian, in some of his earlier writings. He argued that the transfer of procreation to the laboratory undermines the justification and support which biological parenthood gives to the monogamous marriage. He considered that it is in the family that we learn to become persons, experiencing the basic form of human love and caring, and learning to take possession of our capacity to relate to one another in love.[10] To undermine the family, therefore, would be to compromise the ordinary conditions of our growth as persons.

Dr. Robert Edwards, the Cambridge University physiologist responsible for much of the pioneering work in developing IVF as a clinical procedure, has been actively engaged since around 1970 in the ethical debate surrounding it. Indeed, in British circles he attempted to stimulate debate on the ethical issues long before such debate became fashionable, and at a time when Christian groups appeared to have little interest in such matters.

Since this early stage in the debate, Edwards has consistently put forward the view that research is to be guided by the needs of infertile patients and the well-being of any resulting children. Writing in 1972, he stated: 'We believe it essential that doctors and scientists are free to pursue research into aspects of knowledge that could contribute to the well-being of humanity provided the rights of the patients, including those of the fetus, are safeguarded as far as possible.'[11] He saw no objection to 'selecting against afflicted blastocysts', that is, discarding those with genetic abnormalities, since this course of action he believed (and still believes) is preferable to either aborting affected fetuses or producing handicapped children. In line with this, he has for many years argued that 'the rights of blastocysts must be subordinated to the general good of society', a position he has defended by reference to prevailing liberal attitudes on abortion.

Limited as the debate on the new reproductive technologies was in the first half of the 1970s, it incorporated most facets of the much more recent debate. It also had the advantage of being conducted in a non-emotive atmosphere. The pity was, though, that relatively few people were interested in the debate at that time, since it was considered at best to be dealing with erudite theoretical matters, or at worst sensational science fictional nightmares.

For myself, writing in 1974, I laid stress on the importance of further animal experimentation, conceding however that when clinical trials were inaugurated with a substantial chance of success, the needs of the couples concerned and the welfare of their children should be regarded as paramount. I accepted that, compared with these needs, 'blastocysts and even much later stages of fetal growth must be viewed as of secondary importance'.[12] I stipulated that all IVF procedures should be confined to the family situation, and I accepted that by allowing IVF I was 'allowing inroads into the control man is exerting over his reproduction and hence over himself'. I accepted control of this order, on the grounds that God has given to human beings responsibility for exerting authority over our environment and ourselves.

Also writing in 1974 Bernard Ramm, an American evangelical theologian, attempted to set forth a preliminary ethical evaluation of biogenetic engineering.[13] Accepting the complexities of the task, he recognized four alternative ethical systems: person-centred medical ethics, utilitarian medical ethics, utopian or futurologist medical ethics, and the humanitarian ethics of scientists. He considered that the person-centred approach was the most viable one for most Christians, the emphasis here being that 'each patient is a person before he is a patient and when he becomes a patient he is still first a person'. The person must be respected, because he or she is a unique centre of values. Ramm conceded, however, that Christians suffer from pluralism as much as does society, and they lack an all-embracing evangelical Christian synthesis. Not only this; like many others within society, Christians are coming to the conviction that the supreme norm in ethics is not the sheer fact of life but, in some senses, the quality of life. A question from which it is becoming increasingly difficult to escape, therefore, is – in Ramm's words – 'What is human life intended to be?'

Ramm's perceptiveness may not have endeared him to many groups of Christians, and yet he unequivocally stresses basic Christian contentions. He writes: 'Man treads not only a pathway of physical evolution, growth and improvement but he also treads a spiritual pathway which is governed by far different rules than the former.' Even disease need not be seen as necessarily damaging spiritual self-fulfilment.

Guidelines Formulated in the 1980s

1. British Debate
Although IVF procedures were developed initially in the United Kingdom by Robert Edwards and Patrick Steptoe[14],

and although Edwards attempted to stimulate debate on these developments among a wider public, remarkably little happened until various professional bodies began issuing guidelines in 1982. These accepted the legitimacy of IVF, and concentrated instead on the acceptability or otherwise of laboratory experimentation using human embryos.

In November 1982 the Medical Research Council's (MRC) guidelines[15] contended that 'scientifically sound research involving experiments on the processes and products of IVF between human gametes is ethically acceptable' on condition that any resulting embryo is not returned to the uterus, and that the research is directly relevant to clinical problems such as contraception and the treatment of infertility and inherited diseases. The guidelines also allowed for the specific fertilizing of human ova *in vitro*, so that the resulting embryo can be used in a research programme. They also allowed for the use in research of embryos no longer required for therapeutic purposes, provided that the informed consent of the donating couple is obtained. The MRC proposals specified that human embryos should not be cultured *in vitro* beyond the implantation stage (14 days after fertilization); neither should they be stored for unspecified research usage. A particularly contentious proposal in these guidelines was the support given for studies on interspecies fertilization, on the ground that such studies could provide information on the penetration capacity and chromosome complement of sperm from subfertile males. In this case, embryos should not be allowed to develop beyond the early cleavage stage.

Another medical body to issue guidelines in the early 1980s was the Royal College of Obstetricians and Gynaecologists (RCOG) which, with the Royal Society's guidelines, set the scene for later developments. Both these bodies argued that the implantation stage is too soon in human development to be taken as an end-point for research. The RCOG specified 17 days after fertilization, since this corresponds in their view to the early development of the nervous system. The Royal Society allowed a degree of flexibility, leaving the decision to local ethics committees. Underlying this flexibility is the premise that the value of the information potentially obtainable from this research is to be the primary consideration when deciding how long the embryos are to be maintained. The research possibilities envisaged in the Royal Society's guidelines include investigations into the teratogenic effects of drugs and viruses, studies of metabolism and gene expression in early development, and the genetic manipulation of embryos.

The guidelines formulated by the British Medical Association (BMA)[16] were somewhat more conservative than some of the above. They approved observations on spare embryos, in order 'to ensure that effectiveness of *in vitro* fertilisation and embryo replacement and transfer treatments are maximised and risks minimised'. The report hoped that such observations would provide information to optimize the *in vitro* nutrient media for IVF. The guidelines stipulated, however, that observations should normally be completed within five to ten days of fertilization, and always within 14 days. The BMA's recommendations refrained from using the word 'experiment', although they probably would allow observations aimed at quality control of embryos – but not those involved in the testing of hypotheses. Embryos manipulated in any way must not, according to these guidelines, be replaced in a woman's uterus. In more general terms, the BMA guidelines recommended that IVF procedures should be confined to a few special centres in the United Kingdom, and that all attempts to secure pregnancies by these means and their outcome should be recorded. Emphasis was placed on the need to assess the stability of the family relationship of couples undertaking IVF. Approval was given for the use of donated sperm and donated ova, and for the storage of embryos (for up to 12 months). Surrogate motherhood and cloning were found to be ethically unacceptable.

All these guidelines served merely as a forerunner to the most extensive and authoritative report issued in' Britain, the Warnock Committee Report published in July 1984[17]. This report stemmed from an Inquiry set up by the British Government, under the chairmanship of Dame Mary Warnock, to report into human fertilization and embryology. It was established in July 1982 with the following terms of reference:

> To consider recent and potential developments in medicine and science related to human fertilisation and embryology; to consider what policies and safeguards should be applied, including consideration of the social, ethical and legal implications of these developments; and to make recommendations.

The techniques discussed are: artificial insemination, *in vitro* fertilization, ovum donation, embryo donation, and surrogacy. In addition, consideration is also given to the freezing and storage of human semen, ova and embryos; research on human embryos; and some future developments in research. Both abortion and contraception were considered to fall outside the Committee's terms of reference.

The basic tenets of the Report's recommendations were that:
- infertility is a condition meriting treatment;
- access to treatment should not be based exclusively on the legal status of marriage;
- it is better for children to be born into a two-parent family, with both father and mother;
- any third party donating gametes for infertility treatment should be unknown to the couple.

The Inquiry saw little need for formal regulation of AIH, although it considered that it should be administered by a medical practitioner. Grave misgivings were expressed, however, regarding posthumous AIH.

The Inquiry came out in favour of the availability of AID, with AID services subject to certain licensing arrangements. The child born of such insemination should in law be treated as the legitimate child of its mother and her husband, with the husband being registered as the father (perhaps with the words 'by donation' added after the man's name). Donors should be screened and medically examined. Although accepting the principle of donor anonymity, the Inquiry recommended that, on reaching the age of 18, the AID child should have access to basic information about the donor's ethnic origin and genetic health. The Committee recommended that any one donor should be allowed to father a maximum of ten children.

Following a discussion of the major arguments generally employed against IVF, the Committee concluded that IVF should be available, subject to the same type of licensing and inspection recommended with regard to AID. Like AID, it should be available within the National Health Service, possibly in specialized units. Further, in the Committee's estimation, IVF as a technique has passed the research stage and can now be regarded as an established form of treatment for infertility.

The legitimacy of *ovum donation* was accepted because, it is argued, it would be illogical not to accept it, seeing that both AID and IVF had been accepted. The only stipulation was that the donor should be properly counselled and made fully aware of the risks. The anonymity of the donor was again stressed. Since ovum donation results in the genetic mother (donor) being a different person from the carrying mother, the Inquiry recommended that the carrying mother should be regarded in law as the mother of the child.

Embryo donation was considered the least satisfactory form of donation, although (with the exception of the lavage technique) it was accepted as a treatment for infertility.

Surrogacy appears to have provided the Inquiry with one of its most difficult problems. Its failure to agree was manifested by a statement of dissent by two of its members. The conclusion was reached that surrogacy for convenience alone is 'totally ethically unacceptable'. This was based on the danger of exploitation of one human being by another. The Inquiry's major concern, therefore, was with the commercial exploitation of surrogacy, and the recommendation was made that legislation be introduced to render criminal the creation or operation of 'surrogacy agencies'.

The Inquiry had no objection to the freezing of semen and embryos, subject to automatic five-yearly reviews of semen and ovum deposits ('ovum' is referred to in the Inquiry's Report, although I imagine it is 'embryo' they have in mind). Where a person dies during the storage period, the right of use or disposal of his or her gametes should pass to the storage authority. The storage of embryos should be for a maximum period of ten years. The Inquiry also advocated that legislation be enacted to ensure that there is no right of ownership in a human embryo.

The Inquiry agreed that the embryo of the human species ought to have a special status, and that no one should undertake research on human embryos if the same purposes could be achieved by the use of other animals. The recommendation was made that human embryos should be afforded some protection in law, although this protection may be waived and research on human embryos allowed under license (three members dissented from this recommendation). The time limit set for research was 14 days after fertilization, and no embryo on which research has been carried out is to be transferred to a woman. Three members dissented to the proposal that human embryos should be used in research.

Embryos used for research purposes may, according to the Inquiry, be 'spare' embryos, embryos brought into existence specifically for research purposes, or embryos resulting from other research. Restrictions regarding research should be imposed by a licensing body. There was considerable disagreement over the proposal that embryos should be specifically produced for research purposes, with four members in disagreement (in addition to the three members who disagreed with any research on embryos).

The Committee, in its consideration of future developments, approved of trans-species fertilization as part of a recognized programme for alleviating infertility or diagnosing subfertility. Any resultant hybrid should, in the Committee's view, be terminated at the two-cell stage. The Committee felt that the routine testing of drugs on human embryos was unacceptable (due principally to the large numbers of embryos required), although it was prepared to allow such testing on a 'very small scale'. The gestation of human embryos in the uterus of another species for gestation should, according to the Committee, be a criminal offence. Other futuristic techniques were discounted.

The exhaustive nature of this Report is obvious even from the selections I have referred to above. Any serious look at society's response to these bioethical issues has to take these views into account. However, the Report is not satisfactory for those who wish to know *why* the Committee came down in one way or another. There is repeatedly a gulf between, on the one hand, the pros and cons on an issue, and on the other, 'The Inquiry's view'. This is of little help for those who are looking for ethical guidance on these matters, and it is this that has led to the intense, and at times acrimonious, debate within British society. Many facets of this debate will emerge within subsequent sections and chapters of this book.

2. Australian Debate

Much of the debate in Australia has taken place in the state of Victoria, since the major developments in IVF have been carried out in that state, in Melbourne. In order to tackle the host of issues precipitated by those developments, the Victorian Government set up a committee to consider the social, ethical and legal issues arising from IVF. The chairman was Professor Louis Waller, the Victorian Law Reform Commissioner.

The Committee produced an *Interim Report* in September 1982.[18] In this it concentrated on the most common situation in which IVF was employed in Victoria, namely, that involving a husband and wife supplying their own genetic material for the production of an embryo to be inserted into the wife's uterus with the goal of having a child of their own. The Committee considered that this form of IVF was acceptable to the Victorian community, and should be recognized in those terms.

More specifically, it considered that there should be a campaign to educate the public regarding infertility, and that there should be legislation to authorize certain hospitals as centres in which IVF programmes may be conducted. The terms of authorization should provide that:

a.   before a couple is admitted to an IVF programme they must have undertaken all other medical procedures relevant to overcoming their infertility during a period in excess of 12 months;

b.   the IVF programme is limited to cases in which the gametes are obtained from husband and wife, and the embryos are transferred into the uterus of the wife;

c.   appropriate counselling is undertaken before, during and following admission to an IVF programme.

In this *Interim Report* certain issues were not considered, including freezing and thawing of embryos, the use of donor ova and donor sperm, surrogate motherhood, and the fertilization of embryos specifically for research purposes. Basic to the report was a desire to put forward recommendations that would be approved of by the community in Victoria.

This *Interim Report* was followed in August 1983 by a report on donor gametes in IVF.[19] This second report again assessed its recommendations in terms of what practices it considered would have substantial support within the Victorian community. It also commented that participation is a matter of free choice for the couple, thereby allowing for divergences of practice in contentious areas. In this report the Waller Committee recommended that the use of donor sperm, donor ova and donor embryos in IVF should be permitted; counselling should precede, accompany, and follow participation in donor gamete IVF programmes; donors should also receive comprehensive information and counselling about the implications of gamete donation; known donors could be used where both partners request it; and non-identifying information about the sperm or ovum donor should be offered to the recipient.

A substantial list of further recommendations touched on various facets of consent procedures, the authorization of hospitals dealing with donor gametes, and stipulations concerning the couples eligible to receive donor gametes and the donors providing gametes.

The third and final report of the Waller Committee appeared in August 1984 and dealt with the freezing of embryos in IVF programmes.[20] The Committee concluded that the freezing of embryos should be permitted, under certain conditions including: authorization of the hospitals where a cryopreservation programme is to be conducted, prohibition of the storage of large numbers of frozen embryos, agreement of the couple concerned for freezing of their embryos, prohibition of the couple from selling or casually disposing of embryos, making a decision regarding disposition of the embryo before the storage procedure is initiated, and limitation of long-term storage of embryos to five years in the first instance.

This final report also considered the question of research on embryos. It concluded that such research should be limited to the excess embryos produced by patients in an IVF programme. Any research should be carried out immediately, in a current project, and the embryo should not be allowed to develop beyond 14 days after fertilization. The Committee also decided that no surrogacy arrangements should be allowed as part of an IVF programme.

In the light of the recommendations of these three reports by the Waller Committee, the Infertility (Medical Procedures) Act 1984 was assented to in November 1984 by the Victorian Parliament.[21] This Act covers IVF with no donors, with male donors, with female donors, and with male and female donors. It also covers the keeping of records by approved hospitals, the disclosure of non-identifying information to donors and patients, conscientious objection to participation in treatment, and surrogate motherhood. The Act specifies that couples involved in IVF procedures, or a woman receiving a donation in an IVF procedure, are to be married.

Although committees are working on guidelines for IVF in other Australian states, the only Federal body to have touched on these issues is the National Health and Medical Research Council (NH & MRC).[22] In a report issued in October 1983, the NH & MRC worked from the premise that IVF is a justifiable means of treating infertility. Each centre offering an IVF programme should have all aspects of its programme approved by an institutional ethics committee, and a register should be kept of all attempts made at securing pregnancies by these techniques. Treatment of infertility should be carried out within 'an accepted family relationship', although ovum donation is accepted as part of treatment within this relationship. The storage of human embryos 'may carry biological and social risks', and therefore should be restricted to early, undifferentiated embryos. Research with 'sperm, ova or fertilized ova' is accepted up to the time of implantation. Both surrogacy and cloning are found to be ethically unacceptable. The NH & MRC report specifically refers to those who conscientiously object to any IVF programmes, and considers that they 'should not be obliged to participate in [such] projects . . ., nor should they be put at a disadvantage because of their objection'.

3. *American Debate*

The Ethics Advisory Board of the Department of Health, Education and Welfare (DHEW) in a 1979 report,[23] concluded that research involving human IVF is 'acceptable from an ethical standpoint'. By this it meant that the research is 'ethically defensible but still legitimately controverted', rather than that it is 'clearly ethically right'. The basis of this conclusion was that, while the human embryo is entitled to profound respect, this does not necessarily encompass the full legal and moral rights attributed to persons. It concluded that some embryo loss associated with attempts to assist otherwise infertile couples to bear children using IVF be regarded as ethically acceptable. Throughout its report, however, the Board stressed the need to support more animal research in order to assess the risks to both mother and offspring associated with IVF.

In supporting human IVF research without embryo transfer, the Board concluded that the research should be designed primarily 'to establish the safety and efficacy of embryo transfer, and to obtain important scientific information toward that end not reasonably obtainable by other means'. No embryos should be sustained beyond 14 days after fertilization. With human research involving embryo transfer, gametes should be obtained from lawfully married couples. In these two situations, the Board emphasized the importance of animal research and of well-controlled clinical trials respectively.

The Board conceded that potentially valuable information about reproductive biology, and the aetiology of birth defects, may also be revealed through human IVF research without embryo transfer. It made no judgment about the ethical acceptability of such research, unrelated as it is to the safety and efficacy of procedures for overcoming infertility.

Contemporary Debate among Christians

Prior to the focusing of the debate on the new reproductive technologies in the 1980s, many Christians were reticent to tackle the specifics of issues such as AID and IVF. Apart from writers such as Ramsey, McCormick and Häring, remarkably few attempts were made by Christians to analyse bioethical issues, other than abortion, in a detailed manner. While some attention was paid throughout the 1970s to genetics and genetic engineering, issues emanating from the new reproductive technologies were either ignored or treated at the level of general principles.[24]

1. Varieties of Contributions

With the advent of the 1980s Christians began to realize that 'the age of genetics has arrived'. J. Kirby Anderson, in developing this theme in his book *Genetic Engineering*,[25] looked carefully at a wide range of issues in genetic engineering, artificial reproduction, and genetic manipulation. His aim was to delineate a perspective on these areas for Christians. In his section on IVF he concluded:

> Although IVF provides a means by which to help infertile couples, it is fraught with many scientific, social, ethical, and theological problems. . . . There are options other than IVF for infertile couples; therefore IVF seems an inappropriate technology for medical science at this time.

Anderson's assessment of IVF leant heavily on the approaches of Paul Ramsey and Leon Kass. He emphasized what he saw as scientific problems, such as the possibility of fetal abnormalities, and the great loss of fetal life. In the ethical area his concerns revolved around the slippery slope argument, the conflict between means and ends, and the place of reproductive technology in society. These concerns led him to fear the 'immoral consequences' of IVF, including its use outside the marriage bond, in surrogacy arrangements, and in attempts to improve the genetic fitness of mankind, in the development of 'genetic supermarkets', and in the mixing of genetic material.

Anderson showed his concern that 'the sanctity of human life is not trampled underfoot in the mad rush for new reproductive technologies', and he feared that IVF 'will affect future generations in a profound way'. In concluding that IVF is an inappropriate technology for medical science, since it does not 'cure any disease or improve the health of the mother', he opted instead for tuboplasty (surgical repair of the woman's tubes); adoption; a technique known as low tubal ovum transfer (to bypass a blockage in the woman's uterine tube); or for a couple to remain childless.

The theological considerations which undergirded these ethical concerns were: the effects of IVF on the sanctity of human life (loss of fetal life in IVF procedures); a biblical view of marriage (IVF separates the physical dimensions of sexual intercourse from the emotional and spiritual ones); and a biblical view of technology (should humans be involved in genetic manipulations that could affect future generations adversely?). It is clear from this brief summary that Anderson's stance is a conservative one, both socially and ethically. While he raises many valid considerations, he is pessimistic about the ways in which biomedical technology will be applied. His assessment therefore depends as much upon a moderately anti-technology stance (although some of the alternatives to IVF advocated by him rely on very sophisticated technology) and on a fear of the misuse of technology, as it does on positive ethical and theological principles. It is also viewed within a framework of extreme applications, so that surrogate motherhood rears its head as frequently as does the simple case of IVF.

While Anderson's treatment of IVF was from an American background, that of Daniel Overduin and John Fleming[26] was from an Australian one. Overduin, a Lutheran pastor and theologian, and Fleming, an Anglican parish priest, in their book *Life in a Test-Tube*, presented a broad sweep of human procreation and human life. In tackling the questions raised by contemporary bioethics, they took as their basis *rule ethics*, with their fundamental concepts of: the sanctity of human life, the principle of double effect, the principle of totality, the distinction between ordinary and extraordinary treatment, the principle of justice, and the necessary involvement of socio-moral policy-making institutions in society.

Overduin and Fleming recognize two fundamental objections to IVF. The first is that 'IVF involves the foreseen loss of
human embryos due to the intervention of human hands'.
These embryos, they argue, have been lost in developing IVF
as a successful procedure, are being lost in 'the development of
IVF for a surrogate mother', and are being continually lost in
each application of IVF. The second objection is that IVF
involves separating the initiative and procreative aspects of
intercourse. This they see as in opposition to what they consider the primary purpose of the sexual relationship, namely,
the begetting of children. For these authors, once IVF is seen
as a means of aiding and abetting nature, there can be no
objection to surrogate motherhood, cloning, or the complete
gestation of the fetus in an artificial womb. Not surprisingly
then, they argue that IVF is unacceptable even when the
sperm and ovum are taken from a married couple.

The root problem for Overduin and Fleming is that any foray
into reproductive technology is in opposition to 'natural law'.
The simple case of IVF therefore, is to be condemned along
with AIH, AID, ovum or embryo donation, surrogate motherhood, and cloning. They write: 'Once we begin to accept that
human life can be destroyed and experimented with, it is
difficult to place restraints on those involved. It also means
that justice will be increasingly violated as the horizons of the
new biomedical technology are expanded'. For them, any tam-
pering with human procreation is to dehumanize love, marriage, a loving sexual relationship, and the begetting of
children. The deleterious consequences of IVF (and AID) are
inescapable, since they involve 'the destruction of human persons and the violation of the ethical integrity of natural marriage'. This may seem an extreme conclusion and yet it follows
from their premise that scientific insights and developments
must be subject to ethical insight. Since the latter is based on
rule ethics and natural law, grave misgivings are inevitable
when confronted by the techniques of IVF. The 'reality of
moral evil' overrides any good (such as the provision of a child
for an infertile married couple) that may result.

This position has been clearly recognized by James B.
Nelson and Jo Anne Smith Rohricht[27] who comment: 'Theologians and ethicists have dealt more with the threat, perhaps,
than with the promise. This is in character with religious
thinking over the centuries, since one important function of

religion and its institutions is the conservation of basic values'. They continue by noting that, in the case of reproductive technology, this may provide 'a needed balance to the technology/research orientation of the physicians and scientists who dominate the new medicine and its developmental research'.

In their own assessment of IVF and AID, Nelson and Rohricht stress an ethic of responsibility. They accept that human technological pride may become an uncontrollable monster; and it could prove that the fearful are correct. This is a possibility. On the other hand, they argue, there is no necessary and fated reason why this must be so. They write: 'God gives us the awesome human freedom to use our technology both to destroy and to enrich human life. In the process of using medical technology responsibly, we are called upon to make particular decisions about particular techniques'. They add: 'AID and IVF are not morally comparable . . . to a multitude of personal-life-threatening scientific technologies already within our powers to employ'.

Their conclusions are that IVF as a *procedure* is a viable moral alternative for a married couple, although gamete donation raises a variety of additional and morally relevant, complications. However, they recognize that there may be certain circumstances under which the employment of ovum or sperm donation may be a responsible use of medical technology towards divinely intended human ends. They reach the same conclusion in the case of AID. When it comes to *public policy* however, they conclude that IVF is an inappropriate priority. This is because many persons in the United States (the context in which Nelson and Rohricht are writing) are without adequate medical care.

Paul D. Simmons,[28] in his analysis of bioethical decision-making relating to birth and death, does not draw specific practical conclusions on either IVF or AID. Nevertheless, he probes perceptively concepts such as procreation, infertility and parenting within a biblical framework. For Simmons, infertility is a theological issue; since the intention of God in creation and redemption is frustrated. God's intention is that people should be able to experience the powers of procreation, and to engage in the procreation of life. This is, he argues, the special gift and the promise of the creator. For him therefore, and in terms of Old Testament examples, creative options can be employed to bypass the frustration of infertility. This principle does not establish the moral acceptability of biotechnical reproductive procedures, but it does open the way for them.

Simmons argues against the view that infertility is a reflection of God's will, since the providence of God cannot be inferred 'from just anything that takes place in nature'. We cannot conclude that God makes some women infertile any more than that he directly causes people to be born blind (Jn. 9:1–5). We are therefore to take advantage of the information and abilities provided by medicine, and to live in the realization that God in Christ has demonstrated that his nature is one of love (1 Jn. 4:7).

He further contends that human medicine bridges the gap between the world of the natural and the artificial. Many 'natural' processes, such as infant mortality and haemophilia, are inimical to human well-being, and contradict the intention of God that people should be healthy. In the same way, infertility is natural, and 'is also inimical to human well-being and thus contrary to God's intention'.

A rather different approach is adopted by Oliver O'Donovan, Regius Professor of Moral and Pastoral Theology in the University of Oxford. Writing from an evangelical perspective,[29] his overall message appears to be that technical inroads into the processes of bringing children into the world are fraught with danger. This is the realm of what he describes as *artifice*, which he always contrasts with nature. Indeed he seems wedded to the natural order, so that anything that disrupts this order will probably prove unacceptable. Not surprisingly, he argues that the connections between sexual union, procreation, pregnancy, and a relationship with the ensuing child are not to be broken. To do so is, as the title of a book of his (*Begotten or Made?*) suggests, to 'make' children rather than to 'beget' them, and making is a technological process rather than a human/natural one.

This leads him to the view that 'when we start making human beings we necessarily stop loving them; ... that which is made rather than begotten becomes *something* that we have at our disposal, not *someone* with whom we can engage in brotherly fellowship' (italics mine). O'Donovan also confesses: 'I do not know how to think of an IVF child except ... as the *creature* of the doctors who assisted at her conception'.

The end-result for O'Donovan is that he comes down against AID and IVF. His arguments appear to drive him to a rejection of most technology associated with conception. He goes to some lengths to justify adoption, while rejecting artificial insemination, although in doing so he virtually converts adoption into fostering.

O'Donovan's opposition to technology is based on his view of the 'rightness' of the natural order, and of his low regard for human decision-making. He appears to believe that we have no way of saying 'no' to any particular technological development, so that it is preferable to steer clear of technology altogether.

O'Donovan's ideas are salutary reminders that biomedical technology could well become out of control (he would probably argue that it is already out of control). The dividing line between the good and evil uses to which these techniques are put is a fine one, and it is this tension that leads to the diversity of responses, of Christians, to IVF and its associated procedures.

This diversity has been highlighted yet again by the contributors to a book: *Making Babies*,[30] published on behalf of the Social Responsibilities Commission of the Anglican Church of Australia. The Commission itself, over the years 1982 and 1983, issued a number of statements. On IVF, it concluded: 'We consider that the use of the procedure of IVF may be ethically acceptable, in the case of childless married couples who cannot have children by other means.' Among the accompanying guidelines were: it should be available only to married couples, the number of embryos fertilized should be restricted to the number required to accomplish a successful pregnancy, professional counselling should be provided before and after participation in an IVF programme, there should be no abortion of an abnormal child as a matter of course, and experimentation beyond IVF should not be permitted. Subsequently, the Commission called for a limit on the freezing of embryos, stipulating that the minimum number possible should be frozen (if this is to take place at all), and these should be implanted in the uterus of the biological mother. In relation to AID the Commission concluded that: 'AID is inconsistent with Christian moral tradition and [we] cannot therefore recommend it'. However, in terms of public policy, it recognized that AID has been operating for some years and in this context suggested a number of guidelines. These included: AID should be available only to married couples; AID children should be told of their true origins, because deception is damaging to both parents and the child; and professional counselling should be made available before, during and after the AID process.

The contributors to *Making Babies* varied from one who recognized nothing inherently immoral about IVF technology and who also supported the development of genetic engineering techniques aimed at preventing and treating genetically determined diseases, to one who rejected IVF on the ground that it involves a radical disregard for human embryonic life. Most of the other contributors adopted a more accommodating response, accepting IVF under certain conditions and with well-defined stipulations. Perhaps the major accomplishment of *Making Babies* was to take discussion of IVF out of the debating chamber and to set it within the context of practical Christian concern. This is well illustrated by the chapters underlining family issues and pastoral care dimensions. This attempt to view IVF alongside AID and adoption, and to ask how society should be directing and providing counselling for couples facing IVF and how it should be responding to children produced by IVF, is a much needed emphasis within contemporary society. And this is an area where far more Christian attention needs to be directed. Perhaps this is only possible, however, within a country (such as Australia) where IVF is already accepted as a normal part of medical treatment for at least some infertile couples.

2. *Responses to the Warnock Committee Report*

It is a long way from some of the attitudes to which I have just alluded, to some aspects of the debate in the United Kingdom following the publication of the Warnock Committee Report in July 1984. Although reactions in British society have varied from complete acceptance to complete rejection of the Report, with some even viewing it as a relatively conservative and restrictive document,[31] the predominant response within evangelical circles has been to see it as a dangerously liberal approach to the new reproductive technologies. It is therefore, to these negative reactions that I shall turn first.

The Very Rev. Professor Thomas Torrance, formerly Professor of Christian Dogmatics at the University of Edinburgh, produced an impassioned retort to the Warnock Committee Report.[32] The emotional intensity of his response undoubtedly mirrors that of many others who have had little previous contact with the ethical dilemmas posed by contemporary biomedicine. Torrance writes:

> The application of modern scientific technology to human reproduction has thrown up an issue of the utmost gravity. ... What is at stake is nothing less than the future of the human race, but what is also at stake is the integrity of the scientific and moral conscience. In experimentation with human foetuses, in the manipulation of human embryos, in test-tube fertilisation, in the cross-fertilisation of human with non-human species, in surrogate motherhood, medical science has brought us to an ultimate boundary beyond which a civilised and God-fearing society committed to the sanctity of marriage and the structure of the human family, *may not go.*

Torrance writes that the Warnock Committee Report outraged his conscience at a deeper level than almost anything else in recent years.

The fundamental principle for Torrance is that no human being should be treated as a means to an end, and this includes the human embryo, no matter how early in development. As a result he regards it as morally indefensible to bestow upon the alleviation of infertility a higher right than that accorded to the gamete or embryo. The act of choosing between embryos, or the destruction of embryos, is regarded as an utterly abhorrent form of exploitation. Torrance writes: 'All experimentation on human embryos ... is experimentation on human beings, and all the more reprehensible since it is manipulation and exploitation of human beings at their weakest, when their claims on our protection are morally strongest.' Any pragmatic justification of technological interference in the natural processes of reproduction is described as 'reprehensibly deceptive' and 'utterly wrong'. Basic to these responses are Torrance's Christian convictions that: humans have been made in the image of God, the incarnation of Jesus gave to the human embryo a sacred inviolable status, the embryo is a person, and we may never treat other human beings (at any stage of their existence) as means to an end.

Torrance's impassioned plea reminds us of the dangers of uncontrolled utilitarianism. However, choices frequently have to be made between patients within modern medicine, let alone between human embryos. And for Christians these choices have to be directed by Christian concerns. It is also difficult to believe that gametes are more important than the medical concerns of infertile (or fertile) couples, or that the Christian principles from which Torrance works encompass a respect for gametes. Nevertheless, Torrance's fears are important ones and should not be disregarded by those over-enamoured of technological expertise.

CARE (Christian Action Research and Education) Trust, in a detailed critique of the Warnock Committee Report,[33] concluded that although help should be given to the infertile, and while research into genetic defects and hereditary diseases is an important field of human investigation, the law must assert the inviolability of all human beings from the time of fertilization and the fully human status of every embryo whatever its origin. To this end, CARE Trust advocates legal changes to protect human embryos from deliberate mutilation and destruction, to preserve the centrality of the family in society, to guard against the commercialization of human procreation, and to prevent the fragmentation of motherhood, fatherhood and childhood. The Trust also concludes that 'every child has a right to be born the true child of a married couple'. In order to bring this about, it is advocated that any kind of embryo research, freezing, storage, sale, purchase, or disposal of a human embryo should become a criminal offence. It is also advocated that AID, surrogate motherhood, sex selection, trans-species fertilization and human cloning should all be forbidden by law. CARE, perhaps surprisingly, sees no objection to either AIH or IVF within marriage; in the latter case, as long as the gametes are those of the husband and wife.

The principles for public policy which were considered appropriate in the CARE Trust retort to Warnock are: the equal protection of all innocent human life, the protection of marriage and the family, and the retention of the traditional ethical commitments of the medical profession (utmost respect for human life, belief that the interests of the patient are paramount, informed consent). The Trust also viewed with concern the implications for society of a shift in attitudes and behaviour resulting from a move from natural procreation towards the manufacture of human offspring, while it called for a willingness to subject scientific developments to radical scrutiny, and if necessary call a halt to them.

In dealing with infertility, CARE Trust argues that it is not a malfunction, and that it is still an uncharted area. As such, 'it seems particularly unwise to legitimize . . . . controversial practices'.

The central contention of the position put forward by CARE Trust is that the human embryo is a human being, deserving of full human status from the moment of fertilization. With this in mind, it is not surprising that the destruction of any embryo is described by terms such as killing, torture under licence, assault, murder, and slavery. The human embryo is a 'citizen', and it should be treated as such until it is proved 'beyond any doubt whatsoever' that it is other than this. Similarly it is assumed that the embryo (even prior to 17 days gestation) can feel pain ('some form of primitive sentience') and can suffer. It is up to those unconvinced by this assumption 'to demonstrate conclusively that such sentience does not exist'.

An anti-technology stance emerges when it is stated that the technological production of children is 'inevitably dehumanising'. The new reproductive technologies (including IVF) 'are all acts of mastery belonging to the category of manufacture'; all of them (including AIH) 'treat human individuals as subjects of technological domination' and so are hostile to a truly human view of the human individual.

The end result of this critique is a total rejection of practically all technological inroads into reproduction. Rejection of reproductive technology is regarded as essential for the protection of our true humanity. The only exception appears to be 'simple' surgery for the treatment of infertility. The dilemma for the infertile is succinctly expressed in these words: 'Barrenness should drive us to prayer for relief, but not to the procreation scientists.' Surprisingly, it is also stated that we should be prepared to welcome new techniques offering help to the infertile and also research programmes investigating genetic disorders and inherited diseases; we are not told, however, whether or under what circumstances it will be legitimate for Christians to utilize these technical developments.

The Christian Medical Fellowship (CMF) of the United Kingdom, in its submission,[34] concentrated on specific points in the Warnock Committee Report. Emphasis was placed on the family as the basic unit for society, and consequently the stance was adopted that AID and IVF should be available only within marriage (defined as a stable heterosexual relationship, whether registered or 'common law'). Counselling should take

on a wider dimension, incorporating a moral dimension. The
Fellowship additionally considered that a clause should be
added exempting anyone with a conscientious objection from
participating in any treatment involving artificial insemination or IVF. On the question of research on the human
embryo there was a divergence of opinion within the CMF
group, although some believed that research should never be
permited (unless to the benefit of the embryo itself), holding
that this violates individual human dignity. There was agreement, however, that if such research is permitted in society it
should be allowed only when it can clearly be shown to be of
value in advancing the understanding of problems of pregnancy failure, such as infertility, spontaneous abortion, and
serious congenital abnormality. No research should be conducted on embryos specifically brought into existence for research
purposes. In place of a 14-day limit on experiments, it was
suggested that there should be specific time limits, appropriate
to the solution of the specific problems being investigated.
Under no circumstances however, must this exceed the first
evidence of cerebral activity.

The tenor of this submission is quite different from that of
the two previous ones I have outlined. To some extent, this
may reflect the nature of the CMF, in that it represents the
views of a large cross-section of Christian doctors (although
distinctively evangelical in its theological affirmations). It is
not the mouthpiece of a pressure group with distinctive views
on specific issues, such as the status of the embryo or abortion.
This is clearly and helpfully brought out in successive issues of
the CMF journal, *In the Service of Medicine.* In one, the case is
put for a moratorium on embryo research, whereas in the next
one an alternative viewpoint is expressed, advocating the use
of spare embryos by learning as much as possible from them,
since this may serve as a means of helping other women.[35]
Justification for the latter position was put forward in terms of
the principle that to know to do good and to refrain from doing
it, is sin. Alongside this is the view that spare embryos outside
a woman's body are not living fetuses, since they have no host
in which to implant and develop further.

The last two responses to the Warnock Committee Report
with which I shall deal are from Church bodies. The first is the
statement of the Board of Social Responsibility of the Church
of Scotland, included in the Board's report to the 1985 General

Assembly.[36] While accepting AIH and IVF (without superovulation), the Board rejected AID, on the ground that it is an unwarranted intrusion of a third party in the marriage relationship. In similar vein, the Board rejected ovum and embryo donations in IVF programmes, considering them to be invalid techniques. Due to its belief in the inviolability of the human fetus, the Board rejected the production of spare embryos, or research (of any description) on embryos. Further, the Board called for an 'immediate moratorium on all experimental works which are not a part of treatment designed to improve the life prognosis of and benefit to each and every individual human embryo so exposed'.

Interestingly, the Board accepted the storage of embryos, although only in order to facilitate conception. Any excess embryos 'should be destroyed after couples indicate that they have no wish for additional children', and in cases where the marriage relationship ends. Surrogacy, it considered, is demeaning to both mother and child, and should be made illegal. While affirming its belief in marriage as the relationship in which human sexuality is to be fulfilled, and while rejecting AID as an option for Christian couples, the Board recognized that the technique is established within society as a help for the infertile. It was prepared therefore, to recommend legal changes to regularize AID and to protect the resulting child. The Board also raised a number of items for discussion within the Church, including the need for pastoral concern for childless couples, and the priority that should be accorded medical assistance to the childless, and infertility research and treatment. It is interesting to note the contrasts between these recommendations and those of CARE Trust. Both start from much the same view of the human embryo, and yet the Church of Scotland report accepts AIH and IVF (in its most straightforward form), the storage of embryos (although, confusingly, it objects to superovulation) and the destruction of excess embryos. It is also prepared to face up to the social reality of AID, though disagreeing ethically with it. The CARE Trust position appears to reject all these possibilities, although it inconsistently approves of AIH and some IVF. It has to be concluded, therefore, that even when the same theological base is used as a starting point, the manner in which these principles are applied may differ, and divergent recommendations may result.

The Board for Social Responsibility of the General Synod of the Church of England has produced a specific response to the Warnock Committee Report,[37] as well as a report of a Working Party on human fertilization and embryology.[38] In its response to Warnock, the Board supported all the recommendations of the Report, except for embryo donation and the production of embryos for research purposes. The Board also suggested ways in which the Warnock Committee Report might be strengthened; namely, there should be provision for statutory counselling services for couples who have had children by AID and IVF, the sale of semen by 'donors' should be stopped forthwith, and research should be undertaken on the special needs of children born through AID or IVF.

A feature of the Board's response was the division of opinion among its members on many of its conclusions. In referring to this, it was stated that: 'We make no apology for the range of ethical judgement among our members on these issues. They stem from different theological viewpoints and different ethical stances ...' The conclusion of the response is also noteworthy, and deserves to be quoted at length:

> Some of our reasoning may seem to some people to be radical in the light of past thought and practice before the new technologies had become possible. We wish to affirm however the large area of common ground among us all on which our reasoning is based. We take our stand on our convictions about the nature of human life in the image of God and our duty to respect it. We are united in our conviction about the importance of marriage and the family and our need to uphold and support them. We are united in our commitment to ensure that informed and sympathetic pastoral help is offered to those who suffer from childlessness or infertility.

In the light of these affirmations, it has to be asked why the conclusions arrived at in this instance are diametrically different from those of some of the other individuals and Christian groups we have already considered. The reasons, it seems, revolve around the status of the embryo, and also around the response to changes in scientific thought and experience.

The majority of members of the Board for Social Responsibility considered that, until the embryo has reached the first 14 days of its existence, it is not entitled to the same respect and protection as an embryo implanted in the uterus. It is also argued that, while an embryo should be treated with respect, its life is not so sacrosanct that it should be accorded the same status we afford 'human beings'. One consequence of this view, as understood by the members of the Board, was to allow spare embryos to be used for research purposes.

While the well-being of the family is emphasized, it is also concluded that a couple may hold in good conscience the conviction that the semen of a third party introduces nothing alien into the marriage relationship and does not adulterate it as physical union would. The exclusiveness of the marital relationship concerns the physical relationship between husband and wife, and not the giving and reception of semen. The inevitable outcome of this view is that AID and ovum donation are not regarded as a threat to marriage and the family. Although it might be expected that embryo donation would also be accepted on this basis, there was division of opinion among the members of the Board. And so, while the response sets forth arguments that would open the way to embryo donation, including the blessings that come from a right use of medical technology and the legitimacy of fashioning nature for our own good ends, this recommendation of the Warnock Committee was not accepted. The opposing arguments which led to this rejection centred on the dangers of treating the child resulting from embryo donation simply as a *product* rather than a full human being. They also highlighted the point that the technological interference implict in embryo donation extends well beyond the remedying of a natural defect, and this in itself is to be condemned.

The detailed reasoning behind these conclusions is contained in the Working Party's report: *Personal Origins*.[39] This provides a valuable insight into the theological perspectives of the members of the Board, and the conflicting principles in a number of important areas. Whether we agree or disagree with the conclusions of the Board, the theological concepts set forth are extremely helpful and need to be set alongside those outlined previously. What emerges is that Christians of varying traditions are grappling with very similar biblical and ethical concepts, although both the emphases and some of the interpretations differ quite considerably. It behoves us, however, to avoid undue dogmatism, and to look instead at the *practical* outcome of our principles as they affect infertile couples, the children produced using the new reproductive technologies, marriage and the family, society, and the value we (and others) place on prenatal and postnatal human life.

Among the issues discussed in *Personal Origins* are human dominion, the status of the human embryo, marriage and the family, conclusions for practice, and questions concerning pastoral care. In its treatment of the status of the human embryo, two schools of Christian thought were highlighted, the one taking its point of reference from the continuity of the individual subject, and the other with its emphasis on the attributes that must be possessed by a developing embryo before it can be called a person. The Working Party recognized 'in both these approaches the possibility of a scientifically judicious and theologically responsible set of convictions'. The two approaches pay careful attention to the scientific evidence, although their interpretations focus on different features of the evidence (the genetic evidence over against the neurological evidence). Both approaches are committed to achieving a biblical understanding of humanity and to applying it to contemporary questions. Here again though, the two approaches highlight different elements in the biblical conception of humanity (individual existence as rooted in the calling of God, *e.g.* Lk. 1:41–44, over against the human being as a subject of consciousness, *e.g.* Gn. 1:26). The members of the Working Party also recognize that both approaches have a proper claim to continuity with elements of Christian tradition, either the recognition of a decisive moment of beginning, or that such a moment belonged not at the start of the embryo's physical development but some way into it.

Considerable as some of these differences are, especially since they have led in different philosophical directions, there is some important common ground. And this is that both schools of Christian thought

> ... acknowledge that the human status of the unborn child is something which must be discerned, quite apart from our wishes or our decisions, as a reality which simply commands our recognition as of a right. However difficult it may be to decide whether the early embryo is, or is not, a human being, in the most important sense of the term, the question to be resolved is still about whether something is or is not the case ...

The Wider Debate

If there are divergences of opinion within Christian circles, the divergences within society at large are even greater. In this section I shall look at a few recent contributions to the reproductive technology debate. Although these contributions include some by Christian writers, I have placed them in this section since they have not been written from an explicitly Christian point of view.

The first contribution is from a professedly conservative standpoint, and is that of the American ethicist, Hans Tiefel.[40] Tiefel's assessment of IVF leads him to conclude that both clinical and non-clinical IVF are morally unjustifiable; the former is rejected because it entails possible and even likely risks to offspring, and the latter because it treats the earliest forms of human life as having less than human standing. The consequences for Tiefel are that alternative solutions should be sought for female infertility, while research on human embryos should be limited to therapeutic projects.

Tiefel's objection to IVF as a procedure, therefore, revolves around the possibility of harm that may befall the child. To Tiefel there is a major gulf between 'offspring who are actually on the way', and 'the would-be child that is not yet conceived'. He writes 'Our responsibilities to living offspring, before and after birth, should not be undercut by the risks they face. But offspring who are concepts rather than conceptions may not claim that immunity. We literally do not owe them a living.' For Tiefel, the possibility of any damage at all to an IVF child would appear to proscribe its use. He concludes by arguing that no-one has the moral right to endanger a child while there is yet the option of whether the child shall come into existence. It is this, he claims, that makes IVF *unnatural* 'in the sense of being possibly harmful to human beings'.

Tiefel's stress on attempting to avoid injury to the IVF embryo and fetus is commendable. However, his arguments also appear to make immoral many instances of natural fertilization, such as conceiving a child in a society where malnutrition is endemic, or where there is a family history of a genetic abnormality, or where the woman smokes or drinks alcohol or even takes certain forms of medication during the pregnancy. Tiefel's argument comes down, in the end, to the unnaturalness of IVF.

The status of the embryo is critical for Tiefel in his assessment of research on human embryos. For him, the embryo is 'indeed someone', and the need for consistency leads him to argue that if *any* embryos count as human beings, *all* do. In essence his position can be summed up as follows: 'The minimal rights we should share with even the earliest versions of ourselves are the rights not to be used merely as a means to the ends of others and not to be killed.' More specifically, this leads him to conclude that this kind of respect 'excludes dissection and other scientifically promising but fatal designs'. Hence his rejection of all forms of non-therapeutic research on embryos.

In an analysis of the ethical aspects of the new reproductive techniques by a Working Party for the Council for Science and Society in the United Kingdom,[41] the principal conclusions have much in common with those of the Warnock Committee Report. I shall not reiterate them here. What is of particular interest is the discussion of the social issues raised by the new techniques. Considerable stress is laid upon whether procedures such as AID and IVF are of overall social benefit. In all these techniques, the Working Party considers that it is the child's interests that should be regarded as paramount, since it is the child who has to endure any problems during the whole of his or her life. Counselling of the would-be parents is, therefore, recognized as being of major significance. It is further recommended that would-be parents should be advised to remain childless rather than bring children into being by means that will deprive them of knowledge of their genetic father, or of continued contact with their carrying mother. Openness within the family is regarded as essential, leading to the conclusion that the parents of AID children should divulge at a fairly early age the nature of their conception.

Serious questions are asked about the effects of artificial reproduction on marriages and particularly on those arrangements where there is secrecy and deception. Since the rules behind normal marriage arrangements avoid confusion in the child, the Working Party is concerned that the children resulting from artificial reproduction arrangements should not be *confused* by the techniques that have led to their coming-to-be. It is argued:

> To make one donation either of semen or of oocyte is to take certain social risks, but to compound them by making two donations, of both semen and oocyte, is to increase such risks very considerably. This is what takes place when a donated

oocyte is fertilized *in vitro* with donated semen and the embryo implanted in the wife's uterus. It has to be asked if this practice is not likely to leave a child in great confusion.

In the light of this consideration, it is concluded that at least one parent should be a 'complete parent'.

From this point, the Working Party questions the role of the medical profession in artificial reproduction. It is concluded that what is provided is not a treatment, but a service. This, in turn, is a piece of social engineering designed to meet the desire of a couple for a child. Where donated gametes are involved, the end result may be potentially detrimental to society. A related aspect of this issue is where the donation is to a single person, rather than to a couple. The Working Party considers that AID to single women will increase the social problems of child-care and welfare, and it sees the encouragement of lesbian families as a threat to normal family life.

In 1981 Clifford Grobstein reviewed a number of scientific and social issues raised by IVF in his book: *From Chance to Purpose*.[42] In this he was responding to the welter of debate initiated by the hearings on the reproductive technologies conducted by the Ethics Advisory Board of the DHEW.[43] Of especial concern in the current context are the general queries he raises about artificial reproduction in its broadest sense. He contends that there is something special about the choices now before us, since they have been self-created through deliberate scientific effort. The options before us are numerous, and raise profound questions. Do we await passively each new potential application and decide upon it on its individual merits? Or do we anticipate developments in order to formulate a general policy to guide us when each issue arises? If we aim for a policy, will it be to influence particular applications, or to formulate which purposes are legitimate and which are illegitimate?

Grobstein accepts that we can go in either direction. Underlying these contrasting strategies however, is a deeper issue: Can anything now done make any real difference; is the advance of technology inexorable? And has technology become a destroyer rather than a servant? Grobstein seems unwilling to accept such inevitability. While recognizing the heavy burdens placed on us by technology, including artificial reproductive technology, he presses forwards seeking ways in which we can have a say in our transformation: *who* will be doing the transforming, for what *purpose*, and with what probable *consequence?*

To this end, Grobstein suggests various mechanisms for policy formulation and also various principles to be included in what he describes as a future-operative tradition. These include: a clear statement that the objective is to *preserve* and not change humanity; the giving of the highest priority to correcting and eliminating of the most obvious *defects* (genetic and developmental abnormalities); an acceptance that intervention should *never* be practised with the intention of reducing or limiting individual human potential, and an acceptance that interventions to satisfy individual needs or preferences without direct alteration of human attributes (for example, sex selection) must be assessed in terms of collective purposes and possible consequences.

Basic to Grobstein's view of IVF is his view of the human embryo. What matters is not the beginning of human life itself, but the manifestation of *self*. He contends that, until eight weeks of gestation, the human embryo lacks the two essential aspects of personhood; affective recognizability by other people, and internal conscious awareness. Anything before this is a *preperson*, even a *preembryo*.[44] In IVF, therefore, it is not existing persons that are being manipulated, so it is impossible to violate the rights of persons in this procedure. Since further development of the embryo (and therefore, using Grobstein's terminology, the emergence of persons) is impossible without implantation in a woman's uterus, preimplanted embryos have no special status. Grobstein comments 'The capability of producing a person under appropriate circumstances should not be confused with the realization of that capability.'

Grobstein's views have proved influential, especially among scientists. Although many would not go as far as Grobstein, and although Grobstein suggests possibilities rather than probabilities, his approach is an attractive one for many who refuse to ascribe complete protectability to the embryo from the moment of fertilization. I shall return to his dependence upon biological and behavioural developmental landmarks in assessing the value to be ascribed to embryos and fetuses, when I consider the concept of brain birth in chapters 4 and 5.

A *utilitarian* approach to the new reproductive technologies is clearly illustrated by Professor Peter Singer, Director of the Centre for Human Bioethics at Monash University in Australia. In *The Reproduction Revolution*,[45] he and Deane Wells justify every possible application of these technologies, including surrogate motherhood. Their approach is to consider the objections raised by others to IVF and its various extensions; these they dismiss to their own satisfaction, leaving them free to conclude that all these procedures are legitimate. In this way, they justify IVF plus all forms of gamete donation.

Singer and Wells argue that IVF is analogous to other forms of medical treatment. Since medical treatment should be made available to all those in need of it (irrespective of social class, religion, life-style or moral character), and since the need for IVF can be established by the strength of the desire for children, it follows that anyone who could provide an IVF child with a good home should be able to have a child by IVF. In this way, Singer and Wells lay the foundation for allowing anyone (married and unmarried couples, infertile and fertile couples, single women and lesbian couples) to benefit from IVF facilities. The premise from which they work is that the purpose of restricting IVF to married couples is to provide children with a good home. They then argue that they know of no empirical research which demonstrates that married couples provide children with a better home environment than unmarried couples in a long-standing relationship. From here they jump to single-parent families, on the grounds that it cannot be shown that *every* single-parent family could not provide a child with a good home. Consequently, single-parent families *as a class* cannot be excluded from IVF.

Subtle as this form of argumentation is, it takes no account of any ethical norms other than utilitarian ones, and it closes its eyes to sociological evidence. It also overlooks the obvious point that IVF and its associated techniques are involved in producing children in quite a different way from anything previously known within society. The possible implications of this for the resulting children are ignored by Singer and Wells.

The same lack of any concern for the implications of a new technique for society are shown in the discussion on donor sperm and ova. Even if some of these children (as with AID children) suffer as a consequence of their mode of conception, we are reassured that they

> . . . will not suffer to the point at which they would rather not have been born. . . . If their lives remain well worth living despite the psychological difficulties, and if AID satisfies the

deep desire of the couple for a child, then it is difficult to see how AID could be condemned on the grounds of its possible consequences for child or parents.

In view of this rationalization, it is not difficult to appreciate that no counter-arguments from a *human* standpoint will deter Singer and Wells from advocating any and every application technology makes feasible.

When discussing the status of prenatal human life, Singer and Wells frame their case within the context of a very strong pro-life position. Their readers are therefore confronted with just two alternatives – the authors' very liberal viewpoint, and a very conservative viewpoint. In this way Singer and Wells are able to dismiss all opposing viewpoints simply by dismissing a strongly conservative one.

They use as the basis for their position the premise that it is not wrong to destroy either the ovum or the sperm *before* they have united. From this, they argue that there is no moral obligation to preserve the life of the embryo *after* the ovum and sperm have united. Their argument consists of a number of strands.

The first is that the very early embryo cannot feel pain or be conscious in any way. Such an embryo, they conclude, is *totally* different from a later embryo that has a brain and can feel pain. They suggest 'that the embryo be treated as a thing, rather than a person, until the point at which there is some brain function'. They are not sure when the brain actually develops, although they assume it could not be before the end of the sixth week of gestation. They accept the permissibility of research on the embryo, although it should stop 'as soon as the embryo reaches the stage at which it may be conscious'.

From this it follows that, since the attribution of a right to life depends on the possession of capacities distinctive of most human beings (their own assumption), human life does not exist from fertilization. This is an assertion made by the authors; they do not argue it through. The result is that in their argument the early embryo is not entitled to any special moral status.

Even the potential of an early embryo is to no avail. They consider that everything that can be said about the potential of the embryo can also be said about the potential of the ovum and sperm when separate *but considered jointly*. This, how-ever, does not give to the ovum and sperm as isolated entities the same moral status as the embryo. If they are indeed considered to have the same status, despite their differences, the argument used by Singer and Wells for the different moral status of the early embryo and later fetus falls.

When they turn to surrogacy, Singer and Wells do not argue for it but assume its validity, and instead devote most of their attention to the legal requirements of surrogacy. For them, altruism is a crucial sentiment. They write: 'To prevent the expression of human altruism, where that altruism could be harnessed to the increase of human happiness, just because of the abuses that would occur where profit and not love became the motive, would be to throw the baby out with the bath water.' Once again, little attention is paid to the consequences of surrogacy, for either the surrogate or the child. In this way they see full surrogacy (involving IVF, where the surrogate is not the genetic mother) as preferable to partial surrogacy. Children resulting from full surrogacy may feel uncomfortable about it, but 'they can put the whole episode firmly in the past, and say that what they are *now* has not been affected by what happened then'. Such prognostications are interesting, but they are a far cry from the 'empirical data' Singer and Wells conveniently use to support their case in some other instances. There is for example no discussion of bonding, nor why a woman should want to be involved in full surrogacy.

Although I am not dealing specifically with ectogenesis in this book, the arguments put forward by Singer and Wells in its favour deserve to be mentioned, since they epitomize much of the authors' approach to assisted reproduction. Their reasons in favour of ectogenesis are: to help couples have a child, to create a source of spare parts needed to replace diseased organs, to eliminate the wastage of embryonic life now caused by abortion, to eliminate the present inequality in the division of reproductive labour, and to reduce the possessiveness of natural mothers. Realizing that ectogenically produced children may develop abnormally, Singer and Wells advocate working up to ectogenesis very gradually. The reasoning behind this ardent desire to see ectogenesis as a feasible proposition appears to be a manipulative one, especially as a means of providing a source of embryonic material for surgical use. Their logic even leads them in the end to consider growing embryos, with the intention of destroying selected brain regions as a means of eliminating the capacity for consciousness. We may well recoil in horror at such science fiction nightmares, and yet they are seriously put forward by Singer and Wells as one of the logical end results of their utilitarian system.

A radically different approach to that of the technologically-centred approach of Singer and Wells is provided by (secular) feminist critiques of the new reproductive technologies.[46] While it would be misleading to suggest that there is one feminist perspective, the range of responses which come under the heading of feminist have a number of characteristics in common.

Feminists regard themselves as pro-choice, supporting the right of women to choose in all areas of their lives – to choose pregnancy or abortion, to choose alternative medical treatments or none at all, to choose their lifestyle with or without a partner, with a man or a woman. The aim is to live life as self-determined, full human beings. It is within this context that feminist literature concentrates on reproductive issues such as abortion, ultrasound procedures, amniocentesis, sex preselection prior to birth (and even prior to fertilization), cloning, ectogenesis, surrogate motherhood, AID and its availability to lesbians and single heterosexual women, 'egg farming', and of course IVF.

Underlying all these issues is the question of choice. Who controls these technologies, and who has access to them? A typical feminist answer to this question is that biological technology is in the hands of men, so that the reproductive revolution will turn out to be a new form of enslavement for women. Infertile women are seen as being used by the medical profession in order to gain funding for research which is not necessarily intended to help the infertile person. In even more sinister tones, men are viewed as attempting to control pregnancy, childbirth and motherhood – the last of women's powers. When this is accomplished, women will be made obsolete, permanently unemployed and disposable. What is fundamentally amiss is that women are not in a position where they can control their own bodies.

IVF, while not seen as being as grotesque as some of the more extreme reproductive techniques, is regarded as an illustration of the medicalization of women, which will produce further debilitation of women's bodies and spirits. The use of this technology, it is claimed, fails to account for the whole context in which a woman may choose a particular reproductive technology. In more picturesque language it has been claimed 'With the advent of the new reproductive technologies, the myth of patriarchal creation is re-fabricated. Once more, man fashions woman in his own image.'[47] The same writer asks: 'Why do such technologies eminently reinforce the biomedical 'fact' that a woman's reproductive system is pathological and requires an enormous amount of biointervention? Why do these techniques reduce the totality of a woman's being to that which is medically manipulatable?' The danger with these technologies lies, not in the technologies themselves, but in the patriarchal and anti-feminist society in which they are applied.

Implicit within some of these criticisms of the new reproductive technologies is a profound concern at the toll imposed by medical technologies. Within a feminist perspective, however, this is allied to the power given to physicians to exert authority and control over the ways women experience birth and child-rearing. It is in these terms that IVF is often condemned, since it is seen as an illustration of women relinquishing control over their own reproduction, as well as exposing themselves to indignities and the possible side-effects of the technology.

Pregnancy itself may be regarded as a conflict of rights between a woman and her fetus. The woman's freedom of choice has, under normal circumstances, led to the pregnancy and therefore to the fetus. When reproductive technology is required to bring the pregnancy about, and when this is seen as being a male-dominated enterprise, conflict ensues. Feminist writers are, however, ambivalent about certain freedoms in this area, notably about the role of surrogate mothers and about providing ovum and embryo donations ('egg farming'). Here, again, competing freedoms come into conflict, especially against the background of a patriarchal medical technocracy.

Perhaps the supreme contemporary expression of feminism in the reproductive area is donor insemination for lesbians and single heterosexual women. This is regarded by some feminists as representing a new reproductive choice, one that can remain in the control of women. While some writers are well aware that the children resulting from such arrangements are not to be the subjects of a social experiment, it is also argued that: 'we should . . . take joy in the fact that we have broken new ground. We have created new and important life choices for many people. We have taken back a little more of what is rightly ours – the chance to make decisions about how we will live our lives.'[48]

The perspectives presented by feminist writers do not provide a coherent picture. Nevertheless, they demonstrate in general terms what a woman-centred approach may amount to. Whatever we wish to make of it, it is a totally different world from that of most other perspectives, according to which either the status of the fetus is of crucial concern, or the development of technology to improve the quality of life and the happiness of society is dominant. Somehow, we are going to have to make our way through this maze of conflicting assertions and beliefs in the following chapters.

3

Perspectives on Human Life

A Place to Start

In approaching questions concerned with the nature of human existence and the meaning of human life, it is important to reveal the framework within which one intends to operate. This is not to limit the scope of the debate, since we all have some framework or other for our thinking. For instance, the framework may be a religious one or a non-religious one; it may be Kantian or utilitarian; it may depend on some form of supernatural revelation, or it may have a secular humanist base. Within any of these frameworks there is room for immense diversity, while between them there is sometimes considerable overlap. From this, two points become evident: on the one hand, our starting point will exert a great deal of influence on our viewpoints and attitudes regarding specific ethical issues; on the other hand, agreement on general principles may not of necessity lead to agreement on the way in which these principles are interpreted in specific instances. While it is essential to outline the basic principles on which one's arguments are based, it would be unwise to overlook the major gulf between those principles and the contemporary world in which they have to be applied.

The framework within which I am writing is that of evangelical Christianity, with its dependence upon the revelation of God in the Bible. It is to the Bible that I look for principles to govern and direct our view of human life, since I consider that God's revelation in the pages of the Bible is authoritative in bioethics, just as it is in any other area of life. Having said this, however, we have to ask what we mean by this statement. In what sense is the Bible authoritative in bioethics? What sort of answers do we expect to find in the Bible?

To these questions a number of answers may be given. One approach uses the Bible as a source of moral rules.[1] According to this approach, moral dilemmas can be sorted out by discovering an appropriate moral rule, such as the rule against the taking of human life, and against committing adultery. Such rules are absolute, and quite naturally are generally regarded as rigid and fixed. To deviate from an absolute stance on *these* ethical issues is to depart from the Bible as one's sole authority in matters of conduct. Even within this approach however, there may be difficulties. This is because rules sometimes come into conflict, for example, when one life has to be taken in order to save another life – as in abortion to preserve the mother's life, or as in some instances of self-defence. The conflict in such cases is over the application of the rule, but whenever this occurs a decision has to be made on which rule to adhere to. Such conflicts are not new, and Christian tradition has conceived of many rules as having exceptions. It should not surprise us, therefore, that when we turn to contemporary bioethical questions, we have to face conflicts of this sort. Not only this, but it should also be obvious that there are no ready-made rules in the Bible for some of the questions confronting us in this area (such as IVF or embryo donation). How do we then respond as Christians? One course of action is to take a rule formulated for another culture and context and apply it in what seems an appropriate way to our own, quite different, set of circumstances. Alternatively, we admit that the Bible is silent in this instance and from this conclude that it provides no direction at all. Although the first course of action sounds straightforward, there is inevitably room for divergence of opinion over the manner in which rules are applied.

A second approach to the nature of biblical authority for contemporary issues is to recognize in the Bible sets of *moral principles*. An example of such principles is the dignity and worth of every individual before God. According to this approach, the general principles in the Bible are applicable for all times. What we have to do is to seek to understand their meaning and relevance, and then apply them to the specific problems with which we have to contend. It is up to us to use our judgment, discrimination and intelligence; and then, in faith and in obedience to the dictates of the Holy Spirit, to make decisions in the concrete circumstances of which we are a part.

A third approach stresses the response in faith which the believer is to make to the living presence of God. This has been termed the *relational or response approach*. The critical aspect of this approach is our response to God and his leading. Rules or principles assume secondary importance, as the existential emphasis comes to the fore. The chief concern is with what God is doing now, and therefore, with the manner in which he wants us to respond and live, rather than with commands or directives he has given in the past.

These are important theological issues, and I am not qualified to probe deeply into them. I raise them, though, to show their significance for decision-making in complex bioethical matters. My own approach is to acknowledge that the biblical writers enunciate certain basic rules, especially those enshrined in the Ten Commandments. Nevertheless, these in their stark simplicity will not provide us with specific direction in a host of contemporary situations. This does not mean that they have been abrogated, but that they need to be fleshed out by more specific moral principles. There may be times when dealing with the extremes of human life – at the very beginning and at the very end – when it is not clear how the moral rule against the taking of human life can best be applied. It is then that the moral principle of the dignity of each individual human being may be of considerable assistance in determining what is the most ethical course of action to take in this circumstance. Moral principles permeate the Bible; and it is these that I shall attempt to uncover in the following pages.

Once we have some idea of the biblical principles, however, we have to apply them; and it is at this point that we need Christ as our authority. In Jesus Christ we recognize the perfect synthesis of justice and forgiveness, responsibility and understanding, commitment and love. The outworking of all the rules and principles of the Bible must be in the context of our own Christ-centred relationship with other people. We must convey to others the life of the risen Christ, rather than a harsh unyielding legalism. We are to be firm, and we are not to yield on our own standards, but our stance needs to be one

infused with the concern for wholeness in human life so elo-
quently shown by the incarnate Son of God.

Another way of expressing this is along the following lines:
always do that which generates or maintains love relationships with God and man.[2] More specifically, the love referred to
here is *agape*. This means meeting the other person's proper
needs and desires, whether these be biological, psychological or
spiritual. Such agape relationships cross the boundaries of
family and culture, although they find their fullest expression
within the family, especially between a man and his wife and
between both of them and their child(ren).

I am well aware that the position I am adopting will be
interpreted by some Christians as a 'woolly' one, in which far
too much decision-making is left to the judgment and discern-
ment of the individual or the doctor. My response is that this is
what I find in the New Testament. As we examine the
attitudes of Jesus Christ towards such 'hard-and-fast' issues as
the observance of the Sabbath Day, divorce, and adultery, we
find an intriguing mixture of unequivocal principles, concern
for human and individual well-being when surrounded by the
unyielding legalism of others, and standards far in excess of
those expected by even the religious leaders of his day. The
totally revolutionary attitudes of Jesus cannot be neatly
encased within a few absolute regulations, such as 'observing
the Sabbath Day to keep it holy', even though he had no
intention of decrying such a regulation. His concern was with
the impact of a particular principle on people, so that it would
benefit people (as it was intended to do) rather than become a
meaningless burden for them.[3]

It is within this context that I shall examine IVF, AID,
surrogate motherhood, and the many other new reproductive
technologies. In my view, the tenor of the New Testament
forces me to enquire how these procedures will benefit the lives
of *people*. In order to do this, I shall have to ask a range of
searching questions: Of what importance are children to married couples? To what lengths should couples go in order to
acquire children? What is the family and what are its bounds?
Under what family circumstances do young children prosper?
What is the relationship between the unborn human (embryo
and fetus) and children and adults, and do we treat them in
precisely the same way, or not?

Even the simple act of spelling out questions such as these

highlights the nature of the problem confronting us. While the Bible will provide us with very important guidelines on some of these matters, it will not provide us with black-and-white answers on many of the specific situations we meet today. Neither should we expect it to do so. Just as it did not provide our forebears with answers to some of their queries (Should a woman in labour be given an anaesthetic? Should babies be vaccinated?), we will not find in its pages a statement as to whether IVF should be used to provide an infertile couple with a child, nor whether women in an IVF programme should be superovulated.

To expect specific answers from the Bible to such questions is to misunderstand the meaning of the biblical revelation. It is also to ask the wrong sorts of questions. What the Bible provides is a true understanding of the human condition in relation to God's purposes for us as individuals and in community. In doing this we are given an accurate and utterly reliable insight into the value bestowed by God upon human existence, the dignity of individual human beings, and the ways in which we should treat each other.

These are principles of inestimable significance, constituting as they do the bedrock upon which any Christian ethical system has to be based. It is to these and related principles therefore, that I shall turn in the remainder of this chapter.

Biblical Guidelines on Human Life

Humans as Created Beings

The status of human beings in a Christian context is grounded in the biblical teaching on creation, since it is in this teaching that we begin to appreciate the *raison d'être* of human existence.[4] According to the biblical writers, human beings have been created by God (Gn. 1:26, 27; 2:7). We are not as we are for no apparent reason; we are not the end-product of random, purposeless processes. Rather, we have been brought into existence by the deliberate actions of God, the creator of all that is. In speaking like this, the Christian is making a philosophical statement; our concern is not with observable physical and biological processes, nor is it with the precise scientifically-describable mechanisms by which we acquired our present bodies and brains. What we are asserting is that, no matter what processes have been at work at the scientific level of analysis, we owe our existence and meaning ultimately to God. It is God who is at the centre of life, not some impersonal force or purposeless vacuum. We, both individually and collectively, have meaning because a personal God has created us.

It should not surprise us then, to learn that Christians recognize an absolute distinction between God, the creator, and those whom he has created, human beings. This is a distinction between God, who is the source of all that exists, and ourselves in our complete dependence upon the sustaining energy and purposes of God for our very existence. Christians acknowledge that everything comes from God, including all that we are or are ever likely to become.

It is this exalted distinction between God and everything he has made, including human beings, that characterizes the whole biblical ethos. God is self-existent and almighty; we, on the other hand, are dependent on God and we need God if we are to express our true humanity. Our creation, by and for God, implies that it is never possible for us to rise to a position where we will no longer be subject to him. Since we are creatures in God's universe, we will never outgrow our need of God's support and direction. No matter how technologically sophisticated we may become, we will remain beings whose ideals and ambitions can be fulfilled only as they conform to the goals set by the one who gives us life.

A Christian framework recognizes that human beings are limited because we are creatures in a God-ordered and God-sustained world. We must operate within a particular natural and social framework, not because this is an arbitrary limitation, but because it is one that is inherent within the Creator-creature relationship. We are not gods and we shall never be able to transcend our creatureliness. We will never become something radically different from what we now are as human beings.

It is totally misleading therefore, to think that we, as humans, can become or even have become creators in the way in which God is Creator. To alter our environment in quite dramatic ways, or to change ourselves by manipulating our genes, is quite different from bringing into being something that did not previously exist and that could never have existed apart from our actions. That is creation in the true sense of the word, and we are not creators in that sense. Nevertheless, we are far from nothing. It would be quite wrong to denigrate what we are, or to downgrade the immensity of our present abilities. They are considerable, and they reflect what we are as God's creatures.

The point we need to realize is that our abilities, great as they are, have severe limitations. There is much we *can* control and yet there is far more we *cannot* control. The crucial issue, which is often overlooked, is that what we cannot control will, in the foreseeable future and perhaps always, remain elusive. It is the short-term scientific achievements that are controllable, leaving the long-term ones beyond our reach. Perhaps this is a fundamental limitation built into our human finiteness. We are created beings who will never be in a position where we can step beyond the bounds of our creatureliness. What we find is that we cannot change the groundrules of the universe; we can only understand them and to some degree direct them. This is precisely what the scientific enterprise allows us to do; this is where its power lies, and this is a vital sphere in which we should be exercising our responsibility as God's creatures.

Our creatureliness also points to another important facet of human existence, and this is that we are an integral part of the natural world. As such, we are subject to the demands, delights and difficulties of all the interrelationships that make up the natural order. As human beings we cannot act as though the physical world does not matter, nor as if we ourselves are not physical beings. There can be no question, then, that human life is a biological phenomenon; but is it nothing more than a biological phenomenon? Does it not also involve a relationship to God and his purposes, and does it not also take account of our relationships with one another?

As we turn to the biblical writers, it is difficult to escape from one underlying theme; that human life is invariably seen by these writers as constituting a unity.[5] For them, a human being cannot be isolated into a series of individual, more-or-less independent units. There may be references to body, soul and spirit, or to body and soul, or to flesh and spirit, but these are not regarded as isolated segments of the human individual. They are all integral components of what it means to be human; one is as important as the others. This is not all, though. Just as various aspects of the individual human being cannot be viewed in isolation from each other, neither can any human being be viewed in isolation from God. A supreme characteristic of humanness, beyond the narrowly biological, is our potential for responding to the overtures of God. That potential implies that we are beings stemming from the purposes of God, and beings who achieve significance and freedom within the designs of God. We are, however, not just individuals standing before God; we are people living in community. This is where we are to live out our God-relatedness and where we are to put into practice our response to God. Just as we need God, we also need each other, whether this be in families, social groups, churches, cultures, or whole societies.

Human beings are both biological and spiritual beings; not one or the other, nor one more than the other, but both. We cannot separate these two facets of what we are. Strictly speaking, we are biological-spiritual beings. We cannot, therefore, go the way of the gnostics and regard matter as inherently evil; neither can we go the way of the hedonists and regard matter and present satisfactions as our only significant concerns. Material concerns need to be seen in terms of spiritual issues, and spiritual concerns need to be seen in terms of material considerations.

The emphasis in the Old Testament is consistently on the whole life of a person, never on the body as the material element and a soul as the spiritual element. Closely related to this is another element of Hebraic thought to which I have already referred, and this is that the relationships of the individual are indispensable – to others in the human community, and also to God. This capacity for forming personal relationships (or rudiments of it) is present in all human beings. It is a capacity which needs to be actualized if human life in all its fullness is to be experienced.

In the New Testament the concept of the person is more difficult to unravel because of its use of the Greek language and its dependence upon certain Greek modes of thought. The emphasis, however, is on the quality of the life of a person in relation to God and to other human beings. In order to unravel some of the New Testament teaching on human life, I want to follow J. Robert Nelson in his book *Human Life*,[6] by considering three New Testament words.

The first of these, *bios*, was used principally in the New Testament to denote bare subsistence, survival, and the means of keeping alive (Mk. 12:44; Lk. 15:12–30; 1 Tim. 2:2), although on some occasions it was equated with the lusts of the flesh (1 Pet. 4:2) or with the pride of life (1 Jn. 2:16). This aspect of human life has something in common with biological life and its basic necessities and drives.

The second word, *psuchē*, meant far more than psyche, soul or mind. Indeed, it appears to have had three major connotations. The first describes a human being's vital functioning, that is, life as opposed to death. Jesus urged his followers not to be unduly anxious about their *psuchē*-life (Mt. 6:25). In its second sense *psuchē* describes aspects of a person's inner life, such as the mind, will and emotions. Jesus told his followers to love God with all their *psuchē* – heart, strength and mind (Mt. 22:37; Mk. 12:30; Lk. 10:27). Third, *psuchē* is also human life transcending present reality: 'Whoever would save his *psuchē* will lose it, and whoever loses his *psuchē* for my sake and the gospel's will save it' (Mt. 10:39; 16:25–26; Mk. 8:35–36; Lk. 9:24–25). This is life transcending time and mortality through faith in God's grace and power.

The third word, *zōē*, is life in full abundance, the life that only Christ can give (Jn. 10:10). This is life with an eternal quality, and it is inseparable from faith in Jesus Christ.

These various facets of human life are not three distinct kinds of life, but they are three dimensions of the quality of one human life. They underline the intrinsic value of human life, in whatever condition it may present itself, for no other reason than that it is from God. All human life has worth, no matter how privileged or demeaned it may be by society's standards. Nevertheless, these three words do point to different levels of the realization of life's potential, levels that may be dependent upon the stage of biological development it has reached, the richness or paucity of the relationships established with other human beings, and the closeness or otherwise of a living relationship with God. All human life is not the same, although it always has a derived worth – derived from the value bestowed upon it by God. As we shall see in later chapters, this will not solve all our problems in the ethical domain. What it does provide us with is an important base from which to work.

Humans as God's Image
In order to fill out aspects of the previous discussion, we need to move on to another crucial biblical emphasis, namely that human beings have been created in the image and likeness of

God (Gn. 1:26, 27; 5:1; 9:6; 1 Cor. 11:7; Col. 3:10; Jas. 3:9). The picture suggested by this statement is of God as the original and human beings as copies of that original in at least certain respects (though not in all respects, since God does not have a body). This analogy tells us that human beings have many God-like attributes. This is a startling affirmation, because it appears to break down the barrier between God, our Creator, and we ourselves in our created form. This is not so, because the distinction remains. But what does come through is that God, in making us, gave us something of himself. He imparted to us some of his own characteristics. We are like God, in that we are persons who can relate to our world, to other human beings, and also to God. We make choices and act upon them; we have values and value systems; we are aware of ourselves and of others; and we are held responsible for our actions. In a nutshell, we are aware of God and we are capable of freely-willed responses to his call. We have some of the personal features of a personal God.

As we turn to the Genesis account of the creation of mankind, we find that God treated Adam as a being in his own image, capable of deciding issues morally and rationally (Gn. 2:16,17). There is no hint in the Bible of God treating human beings in any other way, even when it would lead them into grave strife. The moral responsibility characteristic of humans is an echo of the moral responsibility of God, enshrining as it does the capacity of acting wisely and in love. We are to act as responsible beings under God, because we are like God.

In biblical terms, we have been given responsibility under God to rule wisely over the remainder of God's creation (Gn. 1:26, 28; 2:19; Ps. 8:6–8). We have been placed in control of everything else he made, and also over the weaker and dependent members of our own species. We have been given immense responsibility under God, which involves the onerous privilege of making decisions and choices affecting other human beings, other species and the environment.

We find this difficult territory, since responsibility frightens us. Our temptation is to shun responsibility, either by erecting a plethora of laws and regulations to minimize the necessity of decision-making, or to act as if there were no restrictions at all. Either way, we shield ourselves from hard decisions, and we neglect one of the crucial means by which we exercise our likeness to God. We dare not underestimate God's high view of human beings, but neither dare we make ourselves into something we are not. It would be dangerous in the extreme to conclude that we actually are gods. In some ways we are quite unlike God, because we are limited, finite beings who are totally dependent upon God for life and existence. Despite this, we are sufficiently like him to have a personal relationship with him and he with us.

We must also strive resolutely against placing human competence and human aspirations at the centre of our existence. Whenever this is done, we leave no room for a view of human dignity centred on our relationship to God. It is at this point that some of the dangers of an immensely powerful biomedical technology become evident. Since the success of this technology has been gained through human brilliance and initiative, its continued success demands further human effort. All too easily, we come to adopt a humanistic outlook; technology alone matters and technology is a product of the human mind. Technology becomes an end in itself and its pragmatic success is so impressive that it comes to replace God as the centre of our daily lives. This is an issue to which I shall have to return in later sections, since divergent views on the role of technology in human reproduction are leading to mutually exclusive opinions on its ethical acceptability in this area.

Our creation in God's image begins to assume an even greater significance once we realize that the Son of God assumed human identity. In doing this, he revealed the image of God in human form, as Jesus – the carpenter's son and the inhabitant of a small country in the Middle East. In Jesus we see God incarnate, God in truly human form – real God and real man – and yet, still an ordinary human being. Perhaps that should be re-phrased – an *extraordinary* human being, 'extraordinary' because this is what all human beings are in the sight of God. Jesus, the God-man, has bestowed upon the human race an unequalled value.

The message of the New Testament gospels and letters is that God's concern for mankind was such that Jesus Christ, his Son, not only took on human form but also gave his life on behalf of mankind. This is the ultimate in self-giving and, quite apart from its theological significance, it denotes the value placed by God on human well-being.

From this it follows that both the creation and redemption of mankind demonstrate that human life is precious to God. We are accountable to him for our own lives and, where we are responsible for another human life, we are accountable to God for that life. To undervalue human life is to fail to take seriously the work of God. In particular, it negates the incarnation and Christ's commitment to humanity in becoming one with God's creation; it adopts values quite different from those of Christ, for whom human life merited the loss of his own life.

The value of human life in God's sight leads to the concept of the dignity of human beings. This dignity, as we have just seen, stems from our creation by God and is revealed supremely in the redemption made possible by Christ. It rests not on what human beings can accomplish in material or social terms, but on the fact of God's love. Consequently, human dignity is always based on what individuals *are* in the sight of God and never on what they can *do* for society, for mankind, or even for God. Those who are of no functional value to society have dignity; they are important in the sight and purposes of God.

From this it has been argued that, if individuals have a dignity bestowed upon them by God, they are to be treated as ends in themselves. That is, they are of value for what they are now, and also for what they may become in the future. As a result, individuals are never to be valued simply because of their possible or probable value to another individual or to an organization. To treat people in this way is to treat them as nothing more than means to an end, and therefore as the property of another. The end result of such a view is to deny that individual human beings have a worth and dignity of their own. We shall have to work out in the chapters that follow just how far this principle takes us.

The Misuse of Human Responsibility

There is one further biblical principle that I have not, as yet, specifically dealt with. This revolves around the all-too-frequent observation that the actions and motives of humans are polluted. In biblical terms, we no longer reflect God's perfect moral character, because Adam and Eve misused their freedom and sought power and knowledge independent of God (Gn. 3:6). Human beings throughout history have acted in the same way. We do not always exercise authority wisely, our intellectual and moral capabilities are frequently defective, we seek to live apart from God and to become gods in our own right. All too frequently we exploit the weak and dis-advantaged, and we constantly love ourselves at the expense of others.

Our lives are confused and we are characterized by mixed motives. We are filled with fear in the face of an uncertain future, since we have no hope or faith. We long for good things, and yet so often we pervert that which is good. Envy, jealousy, suspicion and lovelessness repeatedly intrude into our rela-tionships, debasing them and alienating us from one another. We are anomalies in God's creation, because although we are like him we want to live as though he does not exist. We have become like God in a wrong sense: we 'know good and evil' (Gn. 3:22). We are capable of both; in most situations both are present, and too often we fail to distinguish the one from the other.

So it is hardly surprising that we generally misuse the possi-bilities opened up by biomedical technology. The good and evil uses to which technology can be put are intermingled. In some instances, we cannot have the one without the other, while in others we find it difficult to know in which direction we should go. The technology itself opens the way to a wide diversity of possibilities, all of which will probably be utilized by some group or society. The benefits and hazards of biomedical tech-nology exist alongside one another, reflecting the wonder and the tragedy of human life, with its God-likeness and its rebel-lion against God's authority. David Atkinson has argued, in the light of Genesis 9:1–7, that the existence[7] of conflicting moral claims is a symptom of the fallenness of this world order. He writes: 'There may be some situations in which we cannot act in a way that is wholly good and wholly free from guilt.' A consequence of this is that we may need to work within a hierarchy of moral claims, according to which we evaluate lesser evils and greater goods.

To expect too much of biomedical technology is to under-estimate the effects of human sin and rebellion, and to ignore the limitations of a created being. Although technology in this and other spheres has made an immense contribution to human welfare, it has not altered the basic human condition. The extent to which it is used for good or evil depends upon the motives and aspirations of human beings, and these remind us of the creatureliness and fallenness of mankind.

Justice and Righteousness in Human Society

In considering our status as created beings, one of the features to emerge was the importance of our interrelatedness with others in the human community. Human life, therefore, needs to be seen in social as well as individual terms. From this viewpoint, it must be asked whether there are any principles, at the social level, that are crucial for the furtherance of human welfare. Of all the possibilities, justice and righteousness appear to stand out as of critical significance.

Time and again throughout the Old Testament we are brought face to face with the lack of justice within society, and God's forthright condemnation of this state of affairs.[8] In Amos's time, for instance, the injustice within Israelite society was an essential ingredient of the people's rebellion against God. Bribery, inequitable land and property deals, oppression, dishonesty, crime and violence characterized that society (Am. 2:6,7; 3:9,10; 5:7–20). So deeply rooted were these evils that nothing less than a moral reformation of the whole society was required. 'Seek good and not evil, that you may live. . . . Hate evil and love good; enthrone justice in the courts' was Amos's plea to them. These people were very religious, even if their religion was far from pure, yet it made little difference to their social attitudes. Significantly, Amos cites their social misdemeanours as the first reason for God's condemnation of them (Am. 3:9–4:5). God is concerned for social justice, and he is concerned that his own people put justice above everything else within society. The Israelites, by turning justice upside down, brought righteousness to the ground (Am. 5:7).

Much earlier in the history of the Jews, the concept of social justice was written into their way of life. In Leviticus, the Jews received these instructions: 'You shall not pervert justice, either by favouring the poor or by subservience to the great. You shall judge your fellow-countrymen with strict justice' (Lv. 19:15). A person must be treated as a human being, and this demands scrupulous justice.

Justice is not an abstract concept to be viewed idealistically. It is a basic ingredient of equitable societies and of an equitable world. If societies are not equitable, justice is at a premium, because lack of justice is closely associated with greed. This is something that surfaces repeatedly in the Old Testament. Jeremiah wrote: 'Think of your father: he ate and drank, dealt justly and fairly, all went well with him. He dispensed justice to the lowly and poor; did not this show he knew me? says the Lord. But you have no eyes, no thought for anything but gain' (Je. 22:13–17). The gain referred to is 'greedy wrong-doing'. It is unjust and stems from personal desire and ambition (Ex. 18:21; Hab. 2:9–11). Where this exists, there can be no justice, righteousness or social stability.

Social justice therefore, is as much a matter of personal life-style as of legal ordinances. Where some individuals live self-indulgent, greedy, unjust lives, others will lose out and be unjustly treated. Where injustice serves the greed of some individuals it leads to the deprivation of others.

Jesus came to demonstrate the reality and nature of justice, since nothing less is consonant with either human dignity or the character of God. We are to love our neighbours as ourselves. Jesus linked this obligation with our duty to love God with all our heart, soul, mind and strength (Mk. 12:28–34; Lk. 10:25–28). Love therefore, is the essence of the moral law (Mt. 22:40).

There can be no escape from the principle of self-effacing love. If this is the governing principle in our response to our enemies (Mt. 5:43; Lk. 6:27–31; *cf.* Rom. 12:20) – the extreme situation at the individual level – it must also be the principle by which Christians respond to groups of individuals with whom they have no natural affinity.

This love was underlined by the leaders of the early church. To John it was axiomatic that the Christian exemplified the love of Christ in his relationships with those around him. And so, if people have enough to live on they must, as followers of Christ, help others who are in need (1 Jn. 3:16–18). To ignore the plight of needy fellow human beings is to withhold from them the love of God. It is to refuse to do good, which in Christian terms is sin (Jas. 4:17). This responsibility of love is a fundamental requirement of Christian living.

Although these principles of justice and self-effacing love are generally applied to situations of material and physical need, they are equally applicable in matters of health and of physical and psychological well-being. They are not, therefore, so far removed from the issues being discussed in this book as might appear at first glance. Consequently, they provide an important perspective on human life.

Deciphering Human Life

With these principles as background, the next task is to examine what elements within them are of assistance in approaching the issues emanating from the reproductive revolution. Inevitably, this involves some interpretation of the general principles. Nevertheless, there is no avoiding this, if the principles are to be applied to the contemporary questions confronting us.

1. *Human life, for each one of us, is on loan from God.*[9] It is a gift from God, and its intrinsic value should never be viewed as primarily biological. Its value is derived from God, and is to be seen as coming from him and as being for his use. Life belongs only to God, so that Paul could write: 'You are not your own; you were bought at a price. Therefore honour God with your body' (1 Cor. 6:19,20). The value of human life cannot be isolated from its relationship to God. Hence, in assessing how to deal with difficult ethical questions in the realm of bioethics, we must always work within that framework rather than view each human life in abstract absolute terms. If the term 'intrinsic' is used, it should be in the context of a life-derived-from God, not as a life-in-isolation-of God

2. *The wholeness of human beings implies that their biological-spiritual unity must be treated with seriousness.* It also means that the biological aspect of human life cannot be subdivided into discrete genetic and environmental components. Consequently, human life cannot be defined solely in terms of its genetic uniqueness, any more than it can be defined only in environmental, social or spiritual terms. If this is true, it follows that the individuality of human beings derives not only from their genetic uniqueness, but also from the myriad environmental and spiritual factors essential for healthy personal development. Individuality is lost when there is no scope for growth and fulfilment as a being in one's own right, and when the opportunity to become oneself is denied or frustrated. What is of critical importance, therefore, is human *value*, rather than the mere *existence* of human life in its barest essentials. This applies through all stages of human existence from the earliest beginnings of human life in the uterus, to the end of (earthly) human existence in extreme old age. A corollary of this is that, although human value can be lost (as in a

long-term persistent vegetative state), there is never a time
when technologically unassisted human life has no human
value at all.

3. *Human life should always be characterized by the potential
   to transcend what one is at present.* For the individual this
   entails the potential to become more fully human in all
   aspects of one's life – in matters of health and culture, in
   family life, in the nature of one's employment, and in obedience to God's revelation and specific directives. It also
   implies that we are to assist and encourage others, so that
   they have the opportunity, under God, of realizing their
   potential. Potentiality, in these terms, applies with equal
   force to prenatal and postnatal life. Its emphases may vary
   at different stages of biological development, and the way in
   which it is applied will differ between societies. Nevertheless, it is less than Christian to live as though all that
   matters is the existence of human life regardless of its
   quality. Such an attitude leads to mediocrity in our own
   lives and to a gross neglect of the welfare and aspirations of
   others. Our life in mutually responsible community with
   other persons demands that we view others as God's image-
   bearers, and that we serve and honour them. This is the life
   of self-sacrifice to which God has called all who acknowledge and worship him.

4. *The quality of an individual's life is important.* It is unfortunate that the term 'quality of life' in bioethics has, in the
   eyes of some, become confined to the biological or medical
   quality of life. This I reject, since it reduces human existence to physical dimensions alone, which is a complete
   antithesis of the biblical picture of human life. Equally
   unfortunate is the backlash this has entailed, so that for
   others 'quality of life' is virtually a term of abuse. This I also
   reject, since for quite different reasons it fails to grasp the
   wholeness of the biblical view of human life. When life is
   defined in the various ways suggested previously by the
   words *bios*, *psuchē*, and *zōē*, the quality of life in this broad
   sense is seen to be an essential attribute of a Christian
   perspective on human life. The goal for the lives of
   individual human beings is an adequate physical existence
   and a satisfactory day-to-day experience of family and
   social obligations, work, recreation, moral responsibility,
   and a whole range of challenges and expectations. It also

incorporates spiritual experience, the service of God and one's fellow human beings, and interaction with other humans in love, forgiveness and hope.

It follows that any available technology should be used to contribute to the richest possible life for the individual and for the enhancement of family life. Technologies, therefore, should cause us grave concern if they devalue the individual and his or her relationships. Conversely, and in terms of medical priorities, technologies should be positively encouraged if they hold out the possibility of enriching the life (or future life) of that person, and of those closely related to him or her.

5. *The undervaluing of human life may take many forms.* It may certainly stem from the widescale destruction of fetal life for superficial reasons. But it may also be the result of the irresponsible creation of new life – within marriage or outside it, in bed or in the laboratory. It may stem from pregnant women smoking, or drinking alcohol, from unjust social or commercial practices, from an inequitable distribution of resources within our society or between societies, and from gross inequality of opportunity within a society.

Tragically, human life is easily wasted, and all instances of such waste – whatever the motives – are an implicit denial that human life is precious to God. Wastage of human life is all around us. Millions of people are killed in wars, in automobile accidents, in earthquakes and famines, by other people in murders or by themselves in suicides, and by smoking cigarettes and drinking alcohol. Malnutrition has killed countless human beings, as have epidemics of infectious diseases, while the loss of prenatal human life through spontaneous and induced abortion outstrips all other forms of human wastage put together. The widespread loss of human life in these ways leads to a debasement of human existence, which is seen as being readily expended and of little value. This, in turn, engenders a callousness towards human life. So much of this wastage is, theoretically at least, preventable. And yet, we have learnt to live with it and accept it as a 'normal' part of human society. Even if appalled by a murder, we accept road deaths with little questioning of their futility. They, along with all other forms of pointless human wastage, are destructive of hope and question the value placed upon human life by God.

6. *Although all human life has value and worth, choices some-times have to be made between one human life and another, or one group of humans has to be favoured above another group.* Any such choices are invidious, and we should aim to ensure that, as far as possible, our social and economic systems do not precipitate these dilemmas with their overtones of injustice, exploitation and consequent despair. In the final analysis, however, our world is a sinful one, and it is this fact that forms the basis of the ethical ambiguity, the moral imperfection and the errors of judgment with which we have to contend. Much as we might wish that all human life were of absolute value, in practice as well as in theory, this does not appear to be the case. Is it possible to argue that the lives of any particular groups of humans should be regarded as inviolate? If this is done, on the grounds that the weak are entitled to the strongest protection, we may find that it fails to do justice to the overall challenge presented by the Christian imperative to value and enrich all human life. For instance, to argue in this way with respect to fetuses, infants or the demented, would mean *always* putting their interests above those of other interested parties, regardless of the consequences for these other parties. This is to go beyond the biblical imperative that these (and other defenceless) groups are to be given very considerable protection.

7. *Choosing between the lives of different human beings is a reflection of our responsibility as human beings under God.* Such responsibility has, of course, many more ramifications than this particular one alone. Our technological prowess has brought within our control an important area of our own potential as human beings. This is an extension of the God-given mandate to subdue the earth and bring it within our control. We are responsible, therefore, both for ourselves and others as human beings, and for nature in general and the human species in particular.

Our responsibility, therefore, soon uncovers the difficult relationship between the individual and the species.[10] In alleviating the suffering of one individual, or allowing into existence an individual who would otherwise not have lived, we may be altering the genetic balance of the species. These are two different levels of concern which, in the biomedical sphere, correspond to the family doctor's concerns with the individual, and the biomedical scientist's concerns with

society. Technological developments need to be viewed with
these different levels in mind, since they highlight different
ways in which our technological abilities may be applied.
What they emphasize is the short-term and long-term uses
of these abilities, the short-term revolving around the treatment of individual patients and the long-term their cumulative, and often unforeseen, effects on whole populations.
Human responsibility may well lie in balancing the advantages and disadvantages of our technological prowess.

Technology, in these terms, has possibilities for the good
of human life, and it is appropriate that we, as created
beings, should fulfil our God-given directive to utilize it in
ways that will further human welfare. Choices are implicit
in this, between one application of a technological development and an alternative application; between one
individual who could benefit from a particular procedure
and another individual who has to lose out because of a lack
of resources; between children in one country who benefit
from expensive medical care, and children in another
country for whom even the most basic of medical resources
are unavailable. However complex some of these choices,
they are nevertheless choices that individuals or societies
are making repeatedly – either deliberately or without
thinking.[11]

For some Christians, however, the only choice appears to
be the rejection of technology. For some, technology is a
philosophy to be criticized.[12] Biblical responsibility would
then amount to a critical reflection of the values inherent in
a technological culture since these, it is argued, are anathema to the Christian gospel and inhibit freedom of
thought and open discussion. The 'technological good' and
the control implicit in this are to be challenged and rejected.

Such a rejection of technology is not an inevitable outcome of the general biblical principles I have just considered. I am not convinced that anti-technological stances
are as biblical as some of their protagonists claim. It may be
better to distinguish between *technology*, as the application
of scientific developments, and *technocracy*, as the overall
organization and perhaps philosophical direction of a technological culture. In these terms, my concern with
reproductive developments is with technology. While I concede that, even at this level, technology cannot and should

not be considered philosophically neutral, I also contend that it is possible to analyse individual technological developments without becoming embroiled in the debate on technocracy. The question which has to be considered is whether it is feasible for Christians (and others) to utilize certain technological achievements without committing themselves philosophically and theologically to the values inherent in a technological culture (whatever these values may be). It is also pertinent to point out that developments in reproductive technology are just one illustration of a host of technological developments, neither more nor less forebidding than many others.

The perspective which I believe emerges from the biblical teaching on human life is that our technological expertise is one of the riches bestowed upon us by God, and as such is to be employed wisely and responsibly. We are to be thankful for these riches, but we are also to realize the responsibility bestowed upon us to be faithful in our stewardship of such abundant resources. We are never to confuse these riches with faith. If we do, we confuse the creature with the Creator, and the difference between inordinate dependence upon human expertise and worshipful dependence upon God.

Here we have something of the freedom to be responsible or irresponsible. Whatever abilities we have can be used wisely or unwisely, and the more powerful those abilities the greater the consequences for good or evil. In this we reflect all over again the choice made in the Garden of Eden. We know good and evil, and therein lies our constant dilemma and our never-ending temptation.

Procreation and Infertility

The 'Brave New World' of reproductive technology has its roots in one of the most fundamental of all longings – the desire for a child. It is not the desire for power or glory or even a perfect body, but the much humbler longing for progeny. There are, of course, additional elements and we would be unwise to downgrade these. Nevertheless, the drive behind much of the work in reproductive technology is the problem of infertility. It behoves us therefore, as we seek Christian directions for our bioethical thinking, to pay sufficient attention to both the place and importance of infertility in almost every aspect of this debate.

The Desire for Children

The desire for children stems from our creation as male and female, that is, as sexual beings. An essential component of God's creation of man was the duality of man, male and female (Gn. 1:27), both of whom bear the image of God. Not surprisingly, therefore, the biblical concept of personhood is very closely related to sexuality, which fulfils several fundamental needs in human beings, including the need for companionship and intimacy and also the desire to procreate (Gn. 2:8, 24, 25). While individuals may live fulfilled lives in the absence of one or more of these, they remain basic to human life as a whole.

Procreation itself appeared later in the creation account than did the other needs of man as a sexual being. This demonstrates that children are not an essential part of every marriage, nor are they the sole reason for sexual intercourse. This is a salutary point to bear in mind when confronted by couples who 'demand' a child, regardless of the means employed. There is no hint in the Bible that a marriage is meaningless in either God's sight or in human terms in the absence of children.

Nevertheless, the procreative urge is built into our biological, that is our created, make-up. The desire on the part of a woman to be pregnant and to give birth to a child is an essentially human desire. The strength of the urge in many women reflects what a woman is in the image of God. A fetus, and subsequently a child, is part of the woman in a profound way. It is perhaps impossible for a male to understand this, and it has biological, psychological and even spiritual implications for the woman herself. This underlines the gravity of induced abortion on the one hand, and of giving up a baby for adoption on the other.

By itself, of course, the desire to bear a child does not exempt one from making ethical decisions. It does not condemn abortion under all circumstances, any more than it condemns giving up a baby for adoption. Neither does it suggest that a single woman or a lesbian couple should bear children. What it does is direct our attention to what for many women is a very powerful and very understandable desire. This, in turn, stresses the gravity of the choices that are repeatedly being made in the reproductive area, and are accentuated by the ever-increasing choices being held out by modern reproductive technology and also by the influence of social pressures.

In the Old Testament procreation was emphasized by God: 'Be fruitful and multiply . . .' (Gn. 1:28). It is not a question of *having* to do this, but of co-operating with God in bringing new humans into existence. This is signified by the 'woman' (the companion) in the creation account who is named Eve, the 'mother of all' (Gn. 3:20). We are co-creators with God and, as Paul Simmons has expressed it in his book: *Birth and Death; Bioethical Decision Making*,[13] creation has become procreation. As we bring children into existence, we are working hand-in-hand with God and are experiencing something of the outworking of our biological destiny as human beings. Understandably therefore, children are viewed as a blessing and a gift from God.

Childlessness in Biblical Times

If this is so, what about the converse? What about infertility? Sarai and Hannah in the Old Testament illustrate the plight of those who considered themselves to be infertile. Hannah demonstrates the agony, despair and social ostracism of the infertile (1 Sa. 1:5–18). She pleaded with God to remove her barrenness, and when her prayer was answered she regarded the child as a special gift from God (verse 20) and she was overjoyed (2:1). In the Old Testament there are indications that sin and infertility were associated, although when we turn to the New Testament we find Christ's specific teaching against such inevitable associations in the case of blindness (Jn. 9:1–5).

What is fascinating for us is to consider the lengths to which some of those in Old Testament times went to circumvent childlessness. The cases of Abram and Jacob have been referred to in chapter 1. These are not examples of surrogacy, as is frequently contended, since the maidservants in both cases played a continuing role in the family circle and also in the rearing of the children borne by them. In theological circles it is termed the patriarchal pattern.

An alternative also found in the Old Testament is the institution of levirite marriage, which required that if a married man died before having children, a surviving brother should marry and impregnate the widow (Dt. 25:5–10). The child would be regarded as the child of the deceased. An illustration of this institution is provided by Onan and Tamar in Genesis 38.

The patriarchal pattern is a form of representational begetting – one woman bearing a child on behalf of another woman, while levirate marriage is concerned with carrying on the family name. Both indicate the importance attached to child bearing in Jewish society. The question we need to ask is whether this reflected, on the part of the people concerned, faithfulness to God, or was it an outcome of their own desires or of the pressures of their society.

Perhaps the most clear-cut instance of representational begetting is provided by Abram and Sarai. God had promised Abram that he would have a child, and that ultimately his offspring would be countless in number. Quite specifically, Abram had been told that a son would 'come from your own body' (Gn. 15:4); it was this child rather than a servant in his household who would be the heir (Gn. 15:3). Ten years later however, Sarai his wife had still not borne him a child (Gn. 16:1). She was despondent, and had already planned an alternative strategy – to provide her own maidservant as a substitute, enabling Abram to have a child through her.

Abram succumbed and accepted the remedy proposed by Sarai. Her desire to build a family through Hagar was soon to falter, as she had to contend with Hagar's pride and rivalry, her inability to deal with her own hatred and envy, and Abram's unwillingness to shoulder his share of the blame (Gn. 16:4–6).

The family tensions during Hagar's pregnancy and after the birth of Ishmael do not bode well for this means of producing a child. There are however, mitigating circumstances in this instance. While it is perfectly true that it bore witness to a wilting of Abram's faith, the promise of Genesis 15:4 could possibly have been fulfilled in this manner. After all, Abram was the father as promised on that previous occasion. This practice was known in that society and, with hindsight, it also has to be acknowledged that the sons born to Jacob in a similar way (Gn. 30:1–22) were to count as full members of his family and as heads of tribes.

Nevertheless, in acting like this, Abram was guided by a lack of faith and by the urgings of Sarai. This emerges very clearly in the New Testament where Hagar's son is described as being born in 'the ordinary way' and not 'as the result of a promise' (Gal. 4:23), Hagar and her son are used there as illustrations of self-effort in religion (Gal. 4:22–27), as opposed to the way of faith and promise. Even Ishmael, Hagar's son, would have a restless existence with no ultimate goal, and he would never be a light to the nations (Gn. 16:10–12). Abram however, would continue to be responsible for Ishmael (Gn. 16:15–16).

This case therefore, fails to provide us today with automatic justification for using a third party in reproduction. It has to be seen in its historical and spiritual context, and this provides some questions we would do well to ponder.

Whatever we make of these particular devices to circumvent infertility, they illustrate God's concern for the infertile. It may well be legitimate, therefore, to search for remedies to overcome it. What does come through in the Old Testament is that the goal of these procedures was to strengthen the family unit, even if some of the attempts were misguided. We have to decide whether these Old Testament devices have any relevance for our quite different form of society, and if so, whether they provide us with guidelines for practices of gamete donation.

There appears to be no suggestion that we should actually employ these Old Testament practices today, especially in view of the involvement of sexual intercourse by a third party and the possible involvement of polygamy. Can we learn anything, though, from the importance to one society of providing a family with an heir, when the demand in our society is to provide a husband and wife with a child? This raises the issue of the nature and extent of the family, to which I shall turn later in this chapter.

We are still left with the question of how far we should go in attempting to alleviate infertility. Regardless of how we end up answering this question in specific instances, a general principle within which we need to work is that the availability of a technological procedure is never sufficient reason for using it. Somehow or other we are going to have to put together biblical principles and directives, and the intertwined threads of infertility, technological expertise and the challenges of gamete donation and embryo research.

Adoption as a Biblical Pattern
While adoption is generally thought of solely in terms of a social and legal procedure by which a child becomes a member of another family, it has deep roots in Christian theology. In

order, therefore, to explore the dimensions of adoption, I shall commence with its theological roots.

James Packer[14] writes: 'Adoption is a *family* idea, conceived in terms of *love*, and viewing God as *father*. In adoption, God takes us into His family and fellowship, and establishes us as His children and heirs. Closeness, affection and generosity are at the heart of the relationship.' Adoption, in this sense, is referred to on three occasions in the New Testament (Rom. 8:14, 15; Gal. 4:5; Eph. 1:5), its emphasis being that all true Christians are the sons (children) of God.

The one aspect of adoption relevant for our discussion is the light it throws on the grace of God, in terms of which God adopts us out of free love – not *because* of what we are, but *in spite* of what we are. Adoption is the supreme expression of God's kindness, in that he welcomes into his family those who are not fit for a place in it. God adopts because he chooses to; he is under no obligation to do so, and we – by what we are – do not deserve to be taken into his family. Nevertheless, he showers us with his love and concern. To quote Packer again: 'God receives us as sons, and loves us with the same steadfast affection with which He eternally loves His beloved only-begotten [Son]. There are no distinctions of affection in the divine family. We are all loved just as fully as Jesus is loved.'

The emphasis of the New Testament is that we are taken into God's family not because of any virtues we may possess, but because of God's own love and grace. We are adopted children, not natural ones, and our adoption stems from God reaching out to us and bringing us into his family. As a consequence, we are no longer slaves and outcasts, but sons and heirs of our heavenly father (Gal. 4:4–7).

In more general terms, God is recognized as the father of the fatherless (Ps. 68:5, 6). This has had direct implications for social practice, since care of the fatherless (orphans) was commanded repeatedly in the Old Testament (*e.g.*: Ex. 22:22; Dt. 10:18; Ps. 82:3; Is. 1:17). Moreover, one of the sanctioned uses of the tithe was for the provision for orphaned children (Dt. 26:12). God's people were blessed only as they met the needs of orphans (among others), and judgment was pronounced on those who oppressed orphans (Mal. 3:5). In the New Testament James used, as one of the tests of true religion, a person's concern for orphans – alongside help for widows, and spiritual integrity and uprightness (Jas. 1:27).

It follows from this that caring for the needs of deprived children is both a moral responsibility and an ethical imperative demanded of us by the biblical evaluation of the worth of individuals. This has been a constant theme in Christian circles for many hundreds of years, epitomized by the establishment of orphanages. As early as the second century it was said in defence of the Christians that they loved one another, cared for the widows and rescued the orphans from those who would do them violence.[15]

Adoption is a natural extension of this concern for orphans; it is, in fact, an ultimate expression of caring for those who have no parents of their own to care for them. It is the willing provision of a family for those who lack one of their own. Expressed in this way, the adoption of a child has much in common with the biblical doctrine of our adoption into God's family, or conversely, the biblical teaching on adoption owes a great deal to the social practice of adoption.

Throughout this discussion there have been two prominent emphases – the openness of God in accepting into his family those who are undeserving, and the obligation placed on the followers of Christ to assist children and others in need. From here it is but a short step to the establishment of orphanages and acceptance of the practice of adoption.

The issue confronting us is whether adoption as we know it today is simply concerned with the welfare of the adopted child. If not, what else is involved?

Adoption in Contemporary Society

Most adoptive parents have traditionally been infertile couples, or alternatively, couples who for some medical reason have decided against having children (or further children) of their own. For as long as there was an ample supply of babies awaiting adoption within the community concerned, the desire of couples for a child (or children) and the needs of the babies available for adoption converged. Although the desire to avert childlessness would probably have been uppermost in the motives of the couples concerned, this fitted in very well with the welfare of the adoptive children who were accepted into families rather than left to face a future of institutional life. There were of course difficulties, since certain children – notably those with mental or physical handicaps, and those with a different cultural or ethnic background – were not readily accepted for adoption. In this regard, the social practice of adoption has generally fallen short of adoption in biblical terms.

These problems with adoption have been markedly accentuated over recent years, as the number of 'acceptable' babies available for adoption has dropped dramatically in countries with liberal abortion practices, and where single parents are accepted. The result has been an increasing emphasis on one particular motive for adoption, namely, the overcoming of childlessness. There is no longer any problem in finding suitable adoptive families for 'acceptable' babies; the social problem of meeting the needs of these children has therefore, all but disappeared. With this trend, the face of adoption has changed: its role in overcoming childlessness has come to the fore, as has the plight of the 'unacceptable' babies.[16]

Not infrequently, it is argued that pregnant single women (very often teenagers) seeking an abortion, should be counselled to continue with the pregnancy, and make the child available for adoption. In this way the fetus's life will be saved, and a childless couple will be provided with a child. While I accept that there is considerable merit in both these consequences, we need to be aware that this view of adoption is quite different from the traditional one. Instead of the needs of an existing child being met by being made part of a family, a child is now being brought into the world in order to meet the needs of a childless couple.

I am well aware that this is only part of the issue, since a fetus's life is also being saved; nevertheless the way in which the argument is expressed is putting the spotlight on the couple longing for a child. In general social terms, this may be quite acceptable. We need to realize, however, what it is that we are doing; we are providing a couple with a child which is not genetically theirs, and we are doing this for the reason that they desire a child. In moving in this direction we are accepting the notion that the nuclear family need not be a genetically homogeneous unit. This is being done with only limited regard for humanitarian reasons arising from the welfare of the child.

Not all adoptions today fall into this category. Those of children with medical problems, or with generally unacceptable ethnic origins, may be notable in their humanitarian concern. So too may some adoptions of children from non-

Western countries, although a multitude of considerations frequently needs to be taken into account in these instances.

It is my contention that contemporary adoption enshrines a range of awkward ethical dilemmas, many of which are also encountered (sometimes in more extreme forms) in the new reproductive technologies. For the couple seeking a child for adoption, various choices confront them: between a healthy child and one with some form of handicap; between a child with their own racial characteristics as against one with different racial characteristics; between a child unrelated to them genetically (the adopted child) as opposed to one completely or partially their own in genetic terms but conceived using some artificial means. The couple also needs to consider the motives behind whatever choice they make.

Adoption also involves another party, and this is the woman whose child it is – the biological mother. While it is easy to advocate that a woman (frequently single and frequently a teenager) with an 'unwanted' baby gives up the baby to a couple longing for one, the biological and psychological bonds between the biological mother and the child are still broken. We should be aware that the arguments used to justify this will have relevance for arguments used in favour of surrogate motherhood. While there are immense differences between the two situations, there are also areas of overlap that we would be foolish to ignore.

Adoption is a multi-faceted procedure, with implications for the biological mother, the child, and the adoptive parents. All are persons deserving of our concern and consideration. Somehow the welfare of all involved should be protected, and their good should be assured. This is not easy when there are conflicting hopes. Within a Christian perspective the overriding concern should be with the weak and defenceless. These are the baby and, very often, the biological mother. This is the other side of the infertility coin, and it is one we need to take seriously. If we fail to do so in the sphere of natural conception, we shall find it difficult to cope with the pressures of artificial conception.

Nature of the Family

Biblical Perspectives
In the Old Testament the term 'family' is a broad one, encompassing three types of units.[17] The largest of these was the tribe,

next came the clan, and the three or four generation site-resident family was the smallest. In broader terms, God regarded the nation of Israel as a family, which was derived from a single ancestor, Jacob, or from his grandfather, Abraham (1 Ki. 12:24).

Israel had twelve tribes, which appear to have varied in size from a few thousand (Dan) to 100,000 (Judah). They were territorial units, and they probably played an important political role in the country. The tribes themselves were subdivided into clans, of which there were about 60. Each clan probably numbered 3,000–10,000, and it again was a territorial unit. On reaching the promised land after the forty years in the wilderness, land was given out on a clan by clan basis (Jos. 13–19), the size of the land allocations being directly proportional to the size of the tribe and clan (Nu. 33:54–56). So important were the clans to the society, that they remained intact until the late monarchy period. As might be expected from this, the clans served a range of important functions, with economic, industrial and legal roles, and also with roles in caring for the poor and needy.

The smallest unit, the family, was a three or four generational group living in several households on the same plot of land. This is what Michael Schluter and Roy Clements refer to as the '3G-family'. The members of a 3G-family were not all related to each other, since adoption appears to have been a common practice as a means of drawing the poor, the needy and foreigners into the kinship system. It has been estimated that a 3G-family would normally consist of 10–30 people. Each family had an adult male at its head. It is in this context that the purpose of levirite marriage (Dt. 25:9–10) can be appreciated. According to this, the deceased man's brother was to marry the widow in order to retain the family name and the identity of that particular 3G-family.

The Old Testament knew nothing of the conjugal or nuclear family. Each married couple may have lived in a separate house, although the man's parents would have lived in a neighbouring house as part of the same 3G-family. Its nucleus was what we know as the 'conjugal family', with its emphasis on the man-wife relationship (Gn. 2:24); its head was the 'grandfather/elder' who occupied a prominent position on local political and judicial councils.

What emerges from this Old Testament model is the place of

the extended family within it. As we move to the New Testament we again find that the extended family, with its wider kinship bonds, plays a prominent role in the life and ministry of Jesus. The genealogies of Matthew 1 and Luke 3 place Jesus himself in the context of the family-centred traditions of Israel. Jesus was of the tribe of Judah and of the clan-city of Bethlehem (Mi. 5:2; Mt. 2:6), and he grew up within an extended family (Mk. 6:3–5). In his teaching Jesus evoked responsibilities within the extended family framework, as when he denounced the Pharisees for finding ways by which adults could avoid financial responsibility for their parents (Mk. 7:8–13), or when he instructed the rich young ruler to honour his father and mother (Lk. 18:20).

Many of Paul's instructions and comments can be interpreted in the context of the extended family. His repeated references to 'brethren', and to fellow Christians as children, son, sister and mother all bear out this point. God's relations with his people are compared to those between 'adult' children and their father (Gal. 4:1ff; Eph. 4:13ff), while the church is described as 'the household of faith' (Gal. 6:10). The mistreatment or neglect of parents (by adults) (Rom. 1:30; 1 Tim. 1:9; 2 Tim. 3:2) was again indicted as godless and faithless.

Implicit in all this teaching is the importance of relationships within the extended family. Indeed, in the Old Testament, this family pattern was a means of institutionalizing love within society. The conjugal family must be seen as an integral part of this wider network, which helped to provide stability and protection for conjugal family relationships. The extended family also provided direction in economic and political matters.[18]

This discussion may seem to have taken us a very long way from the new reproductive technologies. In a way, it has; and yet, one of the greatest challenges posed by the new reproductive technologies is to the 'family'. The control which can now be exerted over reproduction means that the production of children can be divorced more and more readily from the context of the 'family' and from the marriage relationship. A major difficulty however, is that discussions rarely get beyond the conjugal or nuclear family, with the result that unrealistic expectations are placed on the nuclear family. This is particularly evident when infertility and childlessness are threatening the stability of this family unit. A general principle to emerge from the biblical teaching is that there is a mutuality of relationships within the 'family', whether this be the nuclear family, the extended family or the church family. When such supportive relationships are absent, the pattern of life is a sub-biblical one. To expect a husband and wife to cope *in isolation* with the trauma of infertility, or with bringing up a handicapped child (or incidentally with many other social pressures ranging from unemployment through marital difficulties to chronic illness), is to place upon them a burden totally alien to Hebraic and Christian precepts. Unfortunately, in modern societies with their high level of social mobility, it is frequently very difficult to attain anything approaching this ideal. The corollary of this is that there may be instances where we have to accept that couples living *in isolation* simply cannot cope with some of these intense social pressures. A less-than-ideal social situation may make way for a less-than-ideal ethical answer to very hard social problems.

Before leaving these general issues concerning the family, a number of other topics require discussion. The practice of concubinage in the Old Testament stemmed from the desire for offspring, especially since this was seen as a heritage and reward from the Lord (Ps. 127:3). Concubines sometimes enjoyed the affection of their partners (Jdg. 19:1–3) and generally had the house privileges of a wife. The resulting child could share in the inheritance (Gn. 21:10), although this was not always the case and difficulties could ensue (Gn. 21:14).[19]

Polygamy was allowed in ancient Israel (Dt. 21:15ff.), although it is doubtful whether it was ever common. Post-exile Jewish teaching was basically monogamous, while in the New Testament monogamy is generally presupposed.[20] New Testament teaching is based on the creation pattern (Gn. 2:18 ff.), which is explicitly monogamous (Mt. 19:3–9; Mk. 10:1–12; 1 Cor. 6:16; 7:1,2; Eph. 5:22–33; 1 Tim. 3:2). In these terms, it appears that polygamous marriages in the Old Testament were concessions to the hardness and faithlessness of Israel (Gn. 16:4, 6; 1 Sa. 1:6; 2 Sa. 9:13; 1 Ki 9:1–8). They were never reflections of God's will, the progressive unfolding of which in the Bible reveals a move towards the original monogamous ideal, with its exclusivity of the relationship between one man and one woman in sexual love. It is in this union that the human needs of mutuality can be met, by providing the security of belonging to each other and the exclusive intimacy which such a relationship needs in order to flourish and mature.

Although the focus of the present discussion is the family, we have been brought inevitably to the question of marriage. In biblical terms this is regarded as an exclusive lifelong union of faithfulness between husband and wife, sealed in physical intercourse (Gn. 2:24). Although a marriage is enriched by the birth of children, it is not a legal institution with procreation as its goal.[21] Its essence is faithfulness to each other, reflected as this is by becoming 'one body' in a variety of ways, ranging from physical union to oneness of outlook in social, family, economic, religious and cultural matters.

Sociological Perspectives

The concepts of family and marriage crop up repeatedly within society, and so they have to be tackled from this perspective as well as from the Hebraic-Christian one. Unfortunately, there are no ready definitions, especially of the family. It may refer to a married couple alone, a married couple with children, three generations of related people, an unmarried couple with children, a married couple with adopted or foster children, a married (or unmarried) couple whose children have grown up and are living away from home, a solo (divorced, widowed or single) parent with children, and so on. From this range of possibilities it is clear that, while marriage frequently has a great deal to do with the family, this is not always the case.

Robert Snowden and collaborators at the University of Exeter recognize two essential ingredients in family life.[22] These are: an exclusive sexual relationship; and, the birth, nurturing and upbringing of children. For them, family and marriage are concerned primarily with issues surrounding procreation. Taking this further, they argue that familial relationships normally imply a shared genetic background. The genetic link is a direct one in the case of children and their parents, and an indirect one where the birth of children unite previously unrelated sets of kin. In this way direct and indirect genetic links are important in establishing 'family' relationships, although such relationships are possible in the case of childless couples and their respective in-law kin.

Within 'normal' family situations, there are a number of assumptions. These include the identity of the mother and father, their respective roles in being the biological (genetic) parents of the children as well as their social parents, and the exclusivity of their sexual relationship. These assumptions are shattered by artificial interventions into the reproductive process, although as I pointed out in chapter 1, they are also shattered by adultery and adoption. Doubts arise over the identity of the parents, when the genetic link between the two parents and their children are broken, or when all stages in the reproductive process are not carried out in the same woman.

Under normal circumstances the genetic and nurturing functions of parents are difficult to separate. Once a division is created between these functions, difficulties in identity may well ensue. This is because a division has been created between the child's *past* in terms of family history and its *present* in terms of current family relationships. The crucial role of nurturing the child after its birth (the obvious face of parenting) may be carried out by those who have had no involvement in the child's past. This is when doubts are expressed about the child's *real* parentage or about the father's status as the real father (as in AID).

Whatever the child's genetic status, and whatever genetic links there may or may not be with the (social) parents, a successful family environment is one in which the relationships are based on respect and trust. Relationships of this calibre are crucial to the well-being and healthy development of children. Without them family life disintegrates and is rapidly undermined. In general, important support is provided by society's recognition of marriage and the family (including non-genetic relationships such as in adoption). If society were to conclude that family relationships were no longer worth supporting, the implications for family life could be far-reaching.

Implications for Contemporary Society
From the prior discussion a number of points have emerged to direct us in our discussion of specific issues in the coming chapters.

First, *monogamy is the ideal pattern in marriage.* If this is so, it follows that the ideal family pattern is one in which there is genetic continuity between the parents and children.

Second, *the extended family has a great deal to recommend it.* In our contemporary societies it may encompass not simply different generations of the one genetic family, but a nuclear (genetic) family together with one or more unrelated individuals such as single people, infertile couples, foster-children and young people. Although extended families may take many different forms, a central feature of them should be a welcoming atmosphere with trusting relationships. It is this mutuality of support and care that is important. In this way, the loneliness and isolation of the single person or the childless couple may – to some degree – be overcome, while the excessive demands made by children on the parents of a large family or on a solo-parent may be alleviated.

The quality of the relationships existing within the nuclear or extended family is the critical element in the nurturing of children. It is this that provides an appropriate context within which a child may begin to realize its potential. Once this is established, it can be seen how less-than-the-ideal genetic patterns can be accommodated. While genetic continuity within a family (in its narrow context) may be the simplest situation to deal with, the lack of such continuity can be handled in the context of loving, accepting relationships. It is within this framework that the adopted or fostered child can flourish, as can the child born out of wedlock, or reared by a step-parent, or conceived and born with the aid of a diverse range of reproductive technologies. The fundamental questions from a Christian perspective can then be seen to centre not so much on the technology *per se*, but on the context in which it is used and the family environment in which the offspring will be reared.

4

The Fetus,
my Fellow Traveller

All the issues raised by the new reproductive technologies involve, in one way or another, the status of the embryo and fetus. There is no escape from this perplexing and demanding topic, and I shall devote both this chapter and the next to a consideration of it. In the present chapter I shall describe some of the major features in the development of the embryo and fetus, with especial emphasis being placed on the development of the nervous system. Throughout this chapter I shall confine my attention to biological considerations.

Development of the Embryo and Fetus

The term 'embryo' refers to the human conceptus from fertilization until eight weeks gestation (the usual biological definition) or, as in some recent literature on ethical issues, until implantation at two weeks gestation. I shall adopt the biological definition, with the result that the term 'fetus' refers to the human conceptus from eight weeks of gestation until separation from the mother at birth (figure 1).

An additional term which has recently crept into discussions of research on the embryo is 'preembryo', referring generally to the embryo during the first two weeks of gestation (preimplantation embryo). The danger of this usage is that it gives the impression that there is a fundamental *biological* difference between the embryo before and after implantation. This does nothing to clarify the very difficult issues surrounding the early embryo, especially when research on early embryos is

Figure 1   Diagram to show the major stages in the development of the human embryo and fetus.

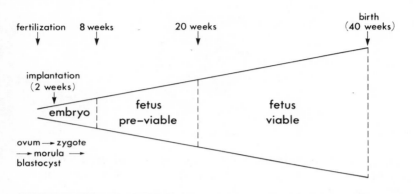

contemplated. To describe a preimplantation embryo as a 'pre-embryo' is just as misleading as to describe it as an 'unborn child'.

The fetal period is further subdivided into previable and viable periods. The term 'previable' refers to a fetus showing signs of life but not having the capacity to survive after separation from the mother. A fetus is generally considered to be previable when under 20 weeks gestation and weighing less than 400 grams (although these figures are relative and vary from one country to another). An embryo between two and eight weeks gestation may be regarded as a previable fetus. The term 'viable' is used of a fetus having the capacity to survive and sustain independent existence.[1]

These definitions provide no more than a framework for the overall development of the prenatal individual. In order to provide some of the major developmental landmarks, we shall have to look a little closer at the timing and sequence of development.

Fertilization is the fusion of a sperm and an ovum. This is achieved by penetration of the outer layers of the ovum (corona radiata and zona pellucida) by the sperm, so that the sperm is engulfed within the cytoplasm of the ovum. These processes induce the ovum to complete its maturation, one facet of which is the joining of the male and female pronuclei (figure 2). When this is completed, the fertilized ovum is known as a

Figure 2   Fertilized ovum showing two pronuclei.

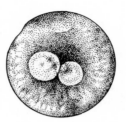

zygote. Fertilization occurs 24 hours or less after the ovum is released from the ovary, and it usually takes place in the uterine tube.

The zygote divides into two daughter cells (blastomeres) within 30 hours of fertilization (figure 3). Continued division occurs until at three days a ball (morula) of 16 or so cells is formed. The morula enters the uterus shortly after this. It lies free in the uterine lumen for one or two days, by which time it consists of 50–60 cells. During this time a fluid-filled cavity gradually develops within the morula; when this is established the whole structure is known as a blastocyst. Some of the cells form a structure that, later on, will form part of the placenta.

At about six days the blastocyst adheres to the wall of the uterus, following which some of the outer cells of the blastocyst begin to invade the uterine wall. This is the beginning of implantation. Two or three days later the amniotic cavity

Figure 3   The fertilized ovum (zygote) has divided into two cells (blastomeres).

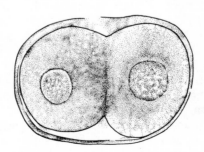

makes its first appearance. These events continue, so that by 12–14 days implantation is complete, and a primitive placental circulation has developed.

By 14 days after fertilization the embryo is still a flat two-layered disc, although the first indication of the future head end of the embryo appears at about this time. A structure known as the primitive streak develops as a midline thickening at 15–16 days. Important early features of the nervous system make their appearance just after this; these will be described under 'Development of the Brain'.

From this point onwards, a welter of events begins to take place. Since these are far too numerous and complex to describe in detail, I shall concentrate on various major events rather than attempt an exhaustive description.[2] By day 28, the embryo is 4–5 millimetres long (crown-rump measurement), and is 'C' shaped. The head, tail and arm-bud can be distinguished, four pharyngeal arches are present, and the heart bulges prominently (figure 4). By days 40–42 the embryo is 20–22 millimetres long and external features are becoming recognizable (figure 5). By day 46, the arms and legs are

Figure 4   Embryo at day 28. Crown-rump length 4–5 millimetres.

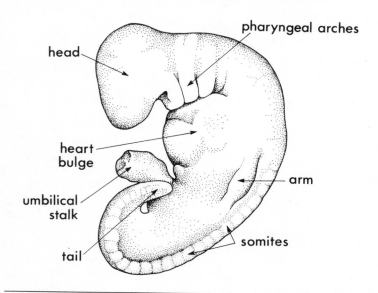

Figure 5   Embryo at days 40–42. Crown-rump length 20 millimetres.

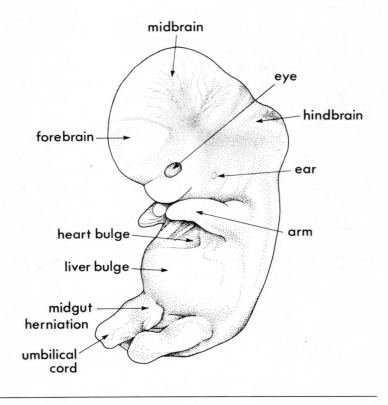

clearly seen, the fingers and toes have formed, eyelids have almost covered the eyes, and the external ear is advanced in form. Internally, there has been considerable development in organs such as the heart, lungs, gastrointestinal tract, and kidneys. Using ultrasound, the first movements can be detected at seven weeks.

The fetal period commences in week eight, and is characterized by rapid growth of the fetus (especially over weeks 9–20) and also by further differentiation of the organs and tissues formed in the embryonic period. Over weeks 9–12 there is a doubling of body length, fingernails appear, and the midgut which was herniated into the umbilical cord (figure 5) returns to the enlarged abdominal cavity. Distinguishing features of the external genitalia appear in week nine, and are distinctly male or female by week 12. Also by week 12, the ear has moved from the neck onto the head, and the eyes have moved to the front of the face (figure 6). The crown-rump length of the fetus is of the order of 80–85 millimetres.

At week 13 the fetus may suck its thumb, while by 16 weeks the skeleton can be clearly seen on X-rays. Over weeks 17–20 fetal movements can be felt by the mother ('quickening'), while the relative proportions of the parts of the lower limb are reached. Over weeks 21–25 the face and body generally assume the appearance of the infant at birth (figure 7); fetuses born prematurely towards the end of this period are usually viable. At this age fetuses are between 200–250 millimetres long (crown-rump measurement).

Figure 6   Fetus at week 12. Crown-rump length 82 millimetres.

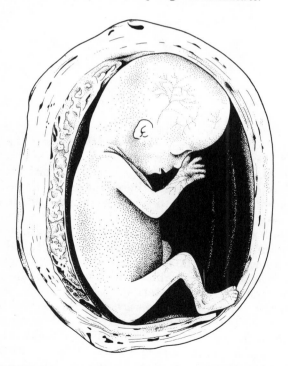

Figure 7   Fetus at week 24. Crown-rump length 228 millimetres.

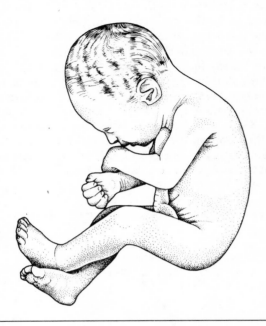

One further aspect of fetal development which may be of some consequence in analysing the status of the fetus is the development of the primary sexual characteristics. Although the genetic sex of an embryo is determined at fertilization by the kind of sperm that fertilizes the ovum, there is no morphological indication of sex until the seventh week, when the gonads begin to acquire sexual characteristics. The early genital system is similar in both sexes and initially all normal human embryos are potentially bisexual. This period of early genital development is referred to as the indifferent stage of the reproductive organs. The external genitalia are not distinctly male or female until the twelfth week of gestation.

Interesting as these landmarks are, they still provide relatively little information on essential aspects of embryonic and fetal development. This is because they are confined to external characteristics. In order to make progress with this investigation, we shall have to turn to the nervous system and how it develops.

Development of the Brain

Some of the major features of brain development are illustrated in figure 8. In chronological order of appearance the following landmarks are worth noting.[3]

Figure 8   Major features in the development of the brain up to 30 weeks of gestation.

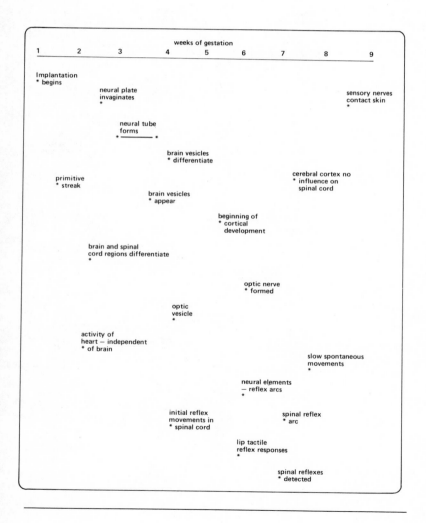

weeks gestation

| 10 | 11 | 12 | 13 | 14 | 15 | 16 | 17 | 18 | 19 |

thalamus
* enlarged

cerebral hemispheres
override * diencephalon

cerebellum
* established

optic chiasma
well-developed
*

cerebral cortex
* not functional

palms of hands
respond to
* stroking

EEG-limited
cortical areas
*

movements depend on
* spinal cord

face sensitive to
* touch

first cortical
sulci * appear

neurons multiply
* _____ *

most of body
surface sensitive
* to pain

most reflexes
* present

primitive respiratory
movements on electrical
stimulation
*

weeks gestation

| 20 | 21 | 22 | 23 | 24 | 25 | 26 | 27 | 28 | 29 | 30 |

stimulation of brainstem
induces body movements
*

some synapses
* present

cerebral cortex
inactive; controls
movements at
* birth

pupillary reaction
to light
*

migration of neurons
into cerebral cortex
* complete

hearing
mechanisms
complete
*

increase in secondary
sulci and gyri
* ──── ─ ─ ─ ➤

further sulci
appear
*

some mature synapses
in neocortex *

respiratory movements
begin
*

beginning of growth spurt
* ──── ─ ─ ─ ─ ─ ─ ➤

(glia, myelin, synapses)

skin reflexes
* appear

reflexes more
intense *

newborn
reflexes
present *

Three weeks. Two distinct regions appear in the developing nervous system, and these are destined to form the brain and spinal cord; the neural tube begins to form (figure 9); the earliest fetal movement occurs, in the form of activity of the heart (independent of brain function at this stage).

Four weeks. The open ends of the neural tube close; three primary brain vesicles (rudimentary regions of the brain) appear.

Five weeks. The optic vesicle (early forerunner of the eye) appears; further division of brain vesicles; the future cerebral hemispheres are visible, and the development of the cerebral cortex begins; the first neurally mediated reflex movements in the spinal cord occur.

Figure 9   Embryo at days 22–23. The neural tube (future nervous system) is fusing. At this stage the two ends of the neural tube are still open (anterior and posterior neuropores). The cephalic (anterior) end of the neural tube will give rise to the brain; the caudal (posterior) end of the tube will form the spinal cord.

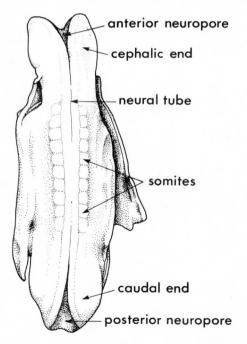

anterior neuropore

cephalic end

neural tube

somites

caudal end

posterior neuropore

Six weeks. There is enlargement of the cerebral hemispheres which can be recognized as distinct entities (figure 10); the principal neural elements for reflex arcs are present; the optic nerve is formed.

Seven weeks. There is still no influence of the higher centres (cerebral cortex) on lower centres (spinal cord); reflex responses of the lips to touch appear.

Eight weeks. The cerebral cortex begins to acquire its typical cells; spinal reflexes can be detected, and there are reflex responses (*e.g.* arm movements) in response to mechanical stimuli; spinal reflex arcs can be recognized for the first time as distinct structures; there may be slow spontaneous movements of the arms, legs and trunk, that are not dependent on sensory stimulation for their initiation.

Nine weeks. Sensory nerves make contact with the skin.

Figure 10   A transilluminated embryo at week 6, to demonstrate main brain regions at this stage.

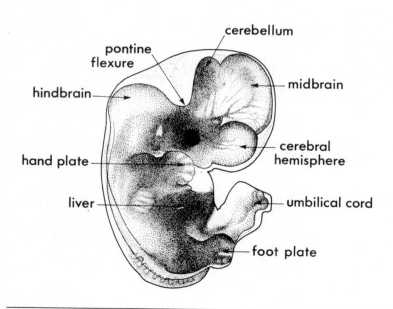

Ten weeks. The spinal cord attains its definitive internal structure; the palms of the hands are responsive to light stroking.

Eleven weeks. The face and extremities are sensitive to touch; the enlarging cerebral hemispheres override deeper structures such as the thalamus (figure 11).

Three months. The brain has its major structural features, and the spinal cord has cervical and lumbar enlargements; the neuroglial cells (supporting cells of the nervous system) begin to differentiate; the thalamus enlarges and the optic chiasma is well-developed.

The multiplication of neurons (nerve cells) occurs between 12 and 18 weeks; the entire body surface (except for the back, and top of the head) is said to be sensitive to pain by 14 weeks; primitive respiratory movements can be elicited by electrical stimulation of the brain stem (medulla); there are breathing movements; very immature electroencephalographic (EEG) activity can be obtained over limited areas of the cerebral hemispheres.

If there is sensitivity to pain at 14 weeks, this is a long time prior to the development of the cerebral cortex. At this early stage pain is poorly localized, and probably reaches the level of consciousness within the thalamus (a structure deep within the cerebral hemispheres). It is not known what the nature or extent of any painful sensations at this age may amount to.

Figure 11   The brain at 11 weeks gestation. The surface of the cerebral hemispheres is smooth.

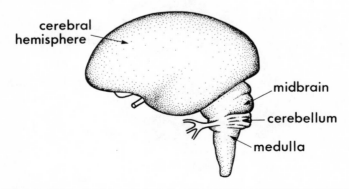

cerebral
hemisphere

midbrain

cerebellum

medulla

Four months. Myelination (laying down of insulating material around nerves) begins in the spinal cord; all reflexes, except for functional respiration and vocal responses, are present; movements of the fetus depend exclusively on spinal cord activity, since the cerebral cortex is not yet functional; the commissures (nerve connections between the two sides of the brain) are completed; the main regions of the cerebellum are established.

Five months. The migration of neurons into the cerebral cortex is well under way, so that it assumes its typical layered organization; the first two sulci (fissures) appear on the surface of the cerebral hemispheres; skin reflexes, such as the grasp reflex, appear.

Six months. Some synaptic connections (between neurons) are present and may be functional; the EEG still has an immature pattern and shows considerable periods of inactivity; respiratory movements begin; tendon reflexes are localized; a sucking reflex is present; all parts of the ear necessary for hearing are present.

Seven months. Reflexes are more intense, and there may be crying; all newborn reflexes are present; stimulation of the brainstem can induce bodily movements; the cerebral cortex is still inactive, and it does not control movements until birth; there is a rapid increase in the development of convolutions (irregularities due to the appearance of sulci) on the surface of the cerebral hemispheres (figure 12); beginning of the growth spurt of the brain, with the multiplication of neuroglia, the formation of myelin (in the brain), and the production of synaptic connections between neurons.

Eight months. Although there is rapid development in all areas, the EEG is still relatively immature at 32–36 weeks.

From this cursory description of brain development, the overwhelming impression is of its gradualness – and also of the staggered manner in which it comes into being. The nervous system of the three-month-old fetus is quite different from that of the seven- or eight-month-old fetus, let alone of the two-year-old child. It is quite mistaken to look on the nervous system of the three-month-old fetus as though it is simply a miniature version of the young child's brain. It is very incomplete, and its

*Figure 12   The brain at birth. The cerebral hemispheres are well-developed
and many sulci (fissures) are present on their surface.*

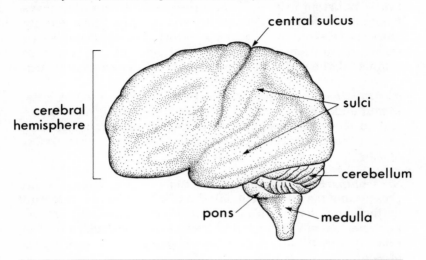

functioning is at a totally different level from that of the late
fetus or young child.

What follows from this is that, at present at least, it is
impossible to recognize a distinct point of transition from a
'non-brain' to a 'brain', or from a non-functioning nervous
system to a functioning one. This does not mean that there is
no such transition point theoretically, only that it is not possible to talk meaningfully about one in practical terms.
Whether or not this will ever be possible is a matter for debate.

What is possible are some generalizations. Among these are
the following: reflex activity appears long before 'conscious'
activity; the spinal cord develops much earlier than the cerebral hemispheres, which are only capable of controlling movement at about the time of birth; each function first appears in
an immature form; neurons appear fairly early, although they
mature and make contacts with each other much later on (in
the latter three months of gestation). The immaturity of the
cerebral hemispheres even at eight to nine months gestation is
demonstrated by the relative immaturity of the EEG tracings
at this late stage of fetal life.

In assessing brain development, particular emphasis should

be placed on certain features, such as myelination (development of myelin around nerve cell processes), synaptogenesis (development of synapses, that is, connections between neurons and the development of networks between neurons. This is because these developments are essential constituents of an adequate physical basis for higher mental functions.

Myelin consists of fatty layers surrounding the processes (axons) of many neurons, and it is responsible for speeding up the passage of nerve impulses, thereby increasing the efficiency of axons in their signalling function. The development of myelin is essential for the normal development of the brain and spinal cord, and it may even be that an individual's acquisition of behavioural and psychological capacities is dependent on the extent of myelination of appropriate brain regions.

The timing of myelination varies in different parts of the human central nervous system. It is first seen in the spinal cord during the fourth month of gestation, although even here it may not be completed until a few months after birth. In the brain the laying down of myelin commences at different times in different systems from seven months of gestation until a few months postnatal. For instance, myelination in the commissural fibre systems connecting the two sides of the brain commences in the fourth postnatal month, while in the association areas of the cerebral hemispheres (the regions that provide the physical basis for higher mental functions such as thought and the use of language) it begins towards the end of the third postnatal month.

Synapses are the points of connection between neurons and serve as the sites where information is passed from one neuron to another and where information may be modified (figure 13). The number of synaptic contacts in the human nervous system is unimaginably large, and is thought to be of the order of 10^{14} (one thousand million million). These connections are crucial for the functioning of the nervous system.

The first synapses to be described in the human nervous system have been at eight weeks gestation, although these are very few and far between and they are unlikely to be functional. A more characteristic description is of a few synapses at 23 weeks gestation in the cerebral cortex. In general however, the major production of synapses commences during the

*Figure 13   Diagram **a** is a surface view of the side of an adult brain, showing motor, sensory and visual areas. Diagram **b** is a view of the layers of the cerebral cortex of the motor area. The neurons (nerve cells) are arranged in various layers, and a large number of their processes (dendrites) are depicted. Diagram **c** is a higher-power view of a dendrite and one of its spines, where a synaptic connection is made with another neuron; diagram **d** shows the ultrastructural appearance of this synapse, with the spine of the dendrite on the left and the enlarged termination of the axonal process of the other neuron on the right.*

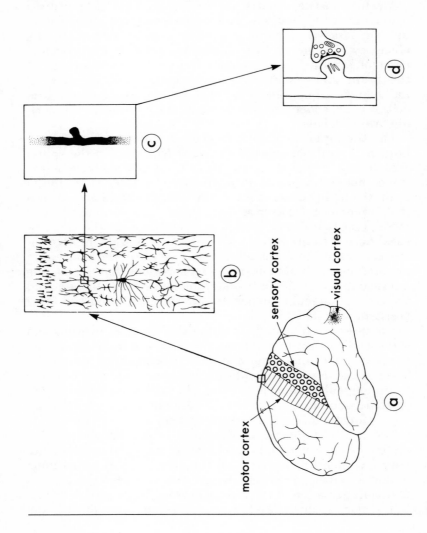

seventh month of gestation, and continues until about 18 months postnatal.

Before synaptic connections can be formed, neurons must put out their processes, known as dendrites (figure 13b). This is because most synaptic connections are established on dendrites. Generally, dendrites branch repeatedly, giving to the neuron a tree-like appearance. Since most of the synaptic connections between neurons occur along dendritic branches, the way in which dendrites develop is a good indication of how synapses are forming.

When a new-born human's cerebral cortex is examined, the region with the most mature neurons is the motor cortex; this is followed by the main sensory region, after which comes the visual cortex (figure 13). In a study of the brains of infants born prematurely, with a gestation age of 33 weeks, it was found that certain types of neurons (large pyramidal and giant stellate cells) in the visual cortex had relatively well differentiated dendrites, with prominent spines (where synaptic connections are made).

Also of importance for the functioning of the nervous system is the nature of the networks made by large numbers of neurons – within any one brain region and also between brain regions. It is the complexity and extent of these networks in the human brain which are probably its most distinctive characteristic. In the motor cortex, which is the most developed area of the human's cerebral cortex at birth, there are three major types of network. Of these, just one of them – the system linking the cerebral cortex with deeper regions of the brain and the spinal cord – develops prenatally. The remaining two systems link up groups of neurons at different levels within the cerebral cortex, and are fundamental to the development of higher mental functions. They, however, develop principally during the first two years after birth.

These findings have been corroborated by others dealing with the sequence of development of neurons in different layers of the human motor cortex (figure 13). In general, it appears that neurons within the deeper layers of the cortex appear first (5 months gestation), with those of the more superficial layers appearing by 7 months gestation. The motor cortex however, is not fully mature even at 8 months postnatal. These data fit in very well with the overall developmental pattern shown by the neuronal networks. The complexity of neuronal circuitry, so essential for the manifestation of human attributes, only emerges as a feature of the human brain during the first two years after birth. This is especially true of the circuitry within any given cortical layer, and it is this circuitry that is critical to human development.

Specific Issues Raised in Fetal Development

Fertilization
To most people it seems obvious that fertilization occurs when a sperm and ovum come together and that this takes place at some specified and, in theory at least, identifiable point in time. From that point onwards, human life exists. But is this as unequivocal in biological terms, as we frequently like to think?

About one thing we can be sure: each new human life represents a continuation of human life in general. It is not the creation of life. Rather, it is the bringing into existence of a new and unique embodiment of human life. To recognize this is not to denigrate the meaning or the value of each human life, but it does place it in perspective. We do not create life, either naturally or artificially; we have nothing like that sort of power. We simply act as agents, bringing a new generation of human beings into existence.

In this sense, human life does not begin at any specific stage of development, whether this be with the ovum, sperm, blastocyst, embryo, fetus or at birth. Neither does it begin with the first heartbeat, the first appearance of brain function, or at the time of viability. Human life is potentially, or actually, present at all these stages. Of course, for a new individual to appear, an ovum and sperm must come together and fertilize. Once fertilization has taken place, the nascent embryo represents the first expression of what may emerge much later on as a recognizable individual. But from what stage can the embryo be meaningfully referred to as an individual member of the human species?

The significance of *fertilization* is that, once it has occurred, the ovum becomes active and the genetic individuality of the embryo is established by the combination of genes from each of the parents. The resulting one-celled embryo, or zygote, is still capable of splitting to form two individuals. This twinning potential remains for as long as two weeks after fertilization.

The first cell divisions of the fertilized ovum produce a cluster of equivalent cells (blastomeres), which are not at this stage integrated into a multicellular organism. This non-integrated state persists for a few days after fertilization. During this period it has been demonstrated in mouse embryos that one or more cells can be removed from an early embryo without affecting the outcome of development – a complete mouse is born (see Epilogue). A few more days of development pass before the cells which will give rise to the embryo proper can be distinguished from the cells which will form the placenta.

Fertilization signifies the commencement of a new individual human life. From a practical standpoint, however, it is not possible to know when this has occurred (except in IVF). As a result, many obstetricians regard implantation, which is completed two weeks after fertilization, as signifying the point at which a new human life can be detected. This is because, prior to implantation, a woman is physiologically unaware of her pregnancy, the first signs of which occur towards the final phases of implantation.[4]

In other words, in clinical terms, fertilization marks the theoretical commencement of a new life, whereas implantation is much closer to its commencement in recognizable terms. And so, if the term *conception* is used, it can be equated either with fertilization (the usual situation) or with implantation.

Both definitions I have considered are biologically plausible, although the equating of conception with implantation is a more useful one from a biological standpoint. Whatever position we may adopt on this matter, neither conception nor fertilization is such a straightforward concept as frequently imagined by non-biologists.

Genetic Uniqueness
In spite of these uncertainties, it is tempting to argue that the data of genetics prove, without any shadow of a doubt, that once the ovum and sperm have united, a new individual human being exists. Many Christians, in asserting the personhood of the embryo, place considerable reliance on the genetic uniqueness of the newly fertilized ovum from day one of development. This is taken by some as basic data (scientific, embryological or genetic), from which there can be no rational escape.[5]

We can certainly agree that, in the vast majority of instances, the genetic constitution of the embryo is different from that of all other human beings. In this sense, each embryo is an individual. An embryo's genes constitute the building-blocks upon which that new individual human being will be built.[6]

But this is not the whole story. We, as adults, are far more than our genes. We are what we are as a result of a myriad of factors, including our genetic inheritance, the environment of the uterus in which we developed, the family and culture in which we grew up, the influence of our friends, the education we received, and the direction and moulding of God. To emphasize an individual's genetic constitution as being the hallmark of what that human being is and represents, is a step in the direction of genetic fatalism. We do align ourselves very closely with the quality of our genetic endowment, and our sense of self to some extent derives from this, but it is not everything.

This is poignantly demonstrated by identical twins who, while having identical genetic constitutions, are still individual human beings. Not only this, but division of the embryo to form identical twins can occur as late as 14 days into gestation. The argument that genetic individuation marks the unmistakable beginning of human life at fertilization will not therefore, suffice in some instances. Against this, it is argued by some that individuation is a long drawn-out process, and that it is imperfect in some cases.[7] Unfortunately, this is irrelevant when discussing whether the genetic constitution of the embryo is the complete basis of every individual's uniqueness.

The difficulties posed by identical twins for the notion of genetic uniqueness go further than this. Their lack of genetic uniqueness presents two additional problems.

First, the embryo which comes into existence at fertilization has no future existence as an embryo-fetus-adult. The individuals we recognize as identical twins started their existence as offshoots of that original embryo, some time after fertilization, and it is these two resulting embryos that have futures as embryo-fetus-adult.

The second problem is that identical twins lack genetic uniqueness. Do they, by the same token, lack value as human persons? Should we treat them as less than full human persons because they lack something most of us possess? The answer given by all civilized people is 'no'. They possess as much value as any other human persons, simply because they are persons made in the image of God. This, however, demonstrates that their status stems not from their genetic status, but from what they *are* as persons and from the dignity bestowed upon them by God. But if this is the case with identical twins, is it not also the case with everyone else?

Besides identical twins, the view that genetic uniqueness throws light on the moral status of the embryo has to contend with yet further considerations. The genotypes of an unknown number of embryos appear to be established some time after fertilization. These include mosaics, and chimaeras. For instance, mosaic trisomic embryos (with three pronuclei) may revert partially to diploid (with two pronuclei) long after fertilization. Also, androgenetic embryos (those with two male pronuclei) are originally triploid at fertilization. In other words, the genotypes of some embryos change within the first few days of embryonic life.

Some products of fertilization with a unique human genotype have no value as human beings. An example is the hydatidiform mole.[8] In this instance, fertilization is either dispermic (involving two sperms) or involves a diploid spermatozoon. The pronucleate ovum is, therefore, triploid (three pronuclei). At syngamy the female pronucleus is excluded, so that the embryo develops with a diploid set of paternal chromosomes. The result is a hydatidiform mole, which has no potential as a human person, and which probably never had any potential because of the aberrant nature of its fertilization. A growth of this nature is not treated as valuable simply because of its unique genotype. Rather, its lethal consequences to the mother are taken into account and it is removed. Once we have accepted this course of action however, we have conceded that, in some instances, the uniqueness of genotype is not everything.

Pregnancy Wastage
This is defined as the loss of an embryo or fetus during the period of gestation. In other words, it is the failure of a fertilized ovum to result in the birth of a living newborn.

Estimates of the frequency of pregnancy wastage vary enormously. In a large number of studies carried out over the past few years, frequencies reported have varied from 5% to 78%.[9] This variation in estimates is due to a variety of factors, including biases associated with the type of data collected, incomplete data, and extrapolation in order to make data complete. One of the main factors is the difficulty in detecting a pregnancy in the early weeks of development, especially prior to implantation. One of the most rigorous studies undertaken[10] used different life table methods to compute and analyse a common set of data (the records from New York City in 1963 and 1967). This yielded a pregnancy wastage estimate of between 25% and 75%, with the most likely figure being a higher one rather than a lower one. The most commonly accepted range would now be in the vicinity of 50% to 75%.

The significance of the rates of spontaneous fetal death is that, for a 25% mortality, 1.3 pregnancies are required per live birth. For a 50% mortality two pregnancies are required for one live birth, while for a 75% mortality four pregnancies are required.

In an attempt to put many of the available data together, James Schlesselman in 1979[11] suggested that 16 per 100 ova fail to be fertilized. Of the 84 ova which are fertilized, 15 fail to implant, leaving 69 implantations per 100 ova. Of these embryos 42 are alive one week later, 37 at the sixth week of gestation, and 31 at birth. The loss therefore, is 69% when the ovum is taken as the reference point. If fertilization is used as the reference the loss is 63%, whereas the loss is only 55% in terms of implantations. Working from the 42 embryos viable at two weeks after fertilization, the loss is 26%.

Spontaneous abortion, fetal death, trophoblastic disease, ectopic pregnancy, and prematurity are all forms of pregnancy wastage. Of these, spontaneous abortion is the predominant form, with 90% of pregnancy wastage occurring during the first trimester of gestation.

In order to illustrate what these figures mean in real terms, we can use, as an example, the American figures for live births.[12] In 1983 there were 3,614,000 live births in the USA. If a 50% prenatal mortality rate is assumed, this means there would have been 7,228,000 pregnancies in order to achieve 3,614,000 live births (two pregnancies for each live birth). By the same token, there would also have been 3,614,000 spontaneous abortions. If a 75% prenatal mortality rate is used, the number of pregnancies rises to 14,456,000 for the same 3,614,000 live births (four pregnancies for each live birth). In this case, the number of spontaneous abortions is of the order of 10,842,000.

In using figures such as these, I am not attempting to give to rough estimates a facade of accuracy they most certainly do not possess. I am also aware that, in some respects, these figures are simplistic. They do not take induced abortions into account, although if this was done the figures for spontaneous abortions may actually increase. On the other hand, there are factors besides spontaneous abortion responsible for some pregnancy wastage – as I have previously mentioned – and these would reduce the figures a little.

In round figures, and using a fairly conservative estimate, it is not unreasonable to think that, in 1983, there may have been about five million spontaneous abortions in the USA. For the sake of comparison, and without making any comments in this section, it might be noted that the present annual rate of induced abortions in the USA is of the order of 1.5 million. I shall return to this matter in chapter 5.

The question which needs to be asked in the present context is why there is this astronomically high rate of pregnancy wastage. The crux of the answer is to be found in *chromosomal abnormalities*. The frequency of these in spontaneous abortions has been reported to vary from 8 to 64%, the most frequently quoted overall figures being 40 to 50%. This variation stems largely from the ages of the abortuses examined. For example, in a study by Boué and Boué in the mid-1970s[13] 66% of abortuses between two and seven weeks of age had an abnormal karyotype, this figure dropping to 23% between 8 and 12 weeks. A review of seven studies carried out between 1970 and 1975[14] estimated that the frequency of chromosomal abnormalities in spontaneous abortions decreased from over 60% in the earliest recognized states of pregnancy to less than 5% by the end of the second trimester.

It has also been found that both the rate of spontaneous abortions and the frequency of chromosomal anomalies among abortuses increase with maternal age. For instance, it has been estimated that among recognized pregnancies spontaneous abortions rose from 16 per 100 pregnancies among 20–24 year old women to 37 per 100 pregnancies among 35–39 year olds.[15] In a similar manner, the frequencies of chromosomal anomalies per 100 spontaneous abortions rose from 59 to 74 in the same age groups.

What emerges from studies of chromosomal anomalies is that the mechanisms for eliminating them during pregnancy are extremely efficient. For instance, it appears that over 99% of chromosomal abnormalities are eliminated through spontaneous abortion or fetal death. This figure is arrived at by comparing the number of chromosomal abnormalities at birth (six per 1,000 live births) with the number at implantation (estimated at 890–1,113 per 2,226 implantations required for 1,000 live births). On a percentage basis, 99.3–99.5% have been eliminated.[16]

Over 90% of chromosomal anomalies fall into three categories.[17] Trisomy (the presence of one extra chromosome) accounts for 40–45% of chromosomally abnormal specimens in humans, the most common occurrence being trisomy 16. The absence of a sex chromosome (45,X anomaly) is found in 20–25% of spontaneous abortions. This has a prenatal mortality of about 98%. Polyploidy refers to the presence of complete extra sets of chromosomes. Of these, triploidy occurs in 15–20% of chromosomally abnormal abortuses, and tetraploidy in another five percent. Only about one percent of triploid conceptuses reach term.

Concept of Brain Birth
The concept of 'brain birth' or of 'brain life' has been elaborated in an attempt to find some point during brain development that will mark the commencement of brain functioning and, therefore, of the fetus as a human person. In this section it is not my purpose to assess the usefulness or otherwise of this concept as an indicator of the beginning of human personhood – that is dealt with in chapter 5. Rather, I shall confine my attention to a consideration of whether the notion of brain birth is a meaningful one from a biological point of view.

The idea that there is some point during development when the brain begins to function is modelled on the converse situation, namely, that at some point the brain ceases to function. Over recent years criteria have had to be formulated to determine 'brain death', because of modern medicine's ability to maintain a patient's cardiopulmonary functions almost indefinitely. Inevitably, the problem which has had to be faced is to decide when an unconscious patient who is still breathing (with the aid of artificial ventilation), is dead. In order to do this, doctors have resorted to the brain and to the question of when it is 'dead', that is, when it shows no signs of any function. When the brain is dead, so, it is argued, is the person; the human life of that particular individual has come to an end.

If it can be determined when the brain ceases to function, can it also be determined when the brain commences its functioning? The analogy is a powerful one, and we would be unwise to overlook its attractions. It is not unreasonable to argue that, at some particular stage during development, numerous discrete functions come together so that the rudimentary nervous system begins to function *as a nervous system*. It may still be very immature, and yet its overall functioning is recognizable as the functioning of a nervous system. A picture sometimes used is that of a few rocks tumbling down a mountain-side. A few rocks do not constitute an avalanche. And yet when the momentum is sufficient and enough rocks are involved, an avalanche is underway. The small isolated phenomena have become something quite different. In much the same way, the individual neural phenomena become integrated into a brain-like phenomenon at some point during development – a brain has been born. One writer[18] has expressed it this way: 'Once a human fetus has developed a brain capable of consciousness its biography ... has begun.'

The question confronting us is not whether this makes sense theoretically, but whether there is any way in which it might be recognized in practice. I believe it is essential that we address the issue in this particular way, since a consequence of the approach adopted by some is that the embryo/fetus is a non-person prior to brain birth, and a person thereafter.[19] We shall also have to decide, not simply whether it is or is not possible to recognize brain birth at the present time (with current knowledge and understanding), but whether it will ever be possible to recognize it; is it a recognizable phenomenon?

I have dealt with landmarks in the development of the brain in a previous section, and I shall not repeat them here. What I need to do however, is to outline the criteria currently employed to recognize brain death.[20] This is the essence of the brain birth analogy, and it needs to be followed as far as possible. Of the various definitions of brain death in current usage, the following criteria are helpful:

An individual who has sustained irreversible cessation of all functions of the entire brain, including the brain stem, is dead:
(i) In the absence of artificial means of cardio-pulmonary

support, death (the irreversible cessation of all brain functions) may be determined by the prolonged absence of spontaneous circulatory and respiratory functions:

(ii) In the presence of artificial means of cardio-pulmonary support, death (the irreversible cessation of all brain functions) must be determined by tests of brain function.

Cessation of brain function is tested by monitoring for electrocerebral silence. The electroencephalogram (EEG) criteria must be observed for a minimum recording period of 30 minutes at a time, when the clinical criteria have persisted for at least six hours. These criteria should be reexamined and confirmed on a second occasion at least six hours later. These criteria however, may be inapplicable for children under five years of age, since there are indications that the immature nervous system can survive significant periods of electrocerebral silence.

It is at this point that the limitations of using EEGs to identify brain birth become apparent. When the EEG is used to determine the loss of brain function, it is dealing with an essentially all-or-none phenomenon, whereas the EEG when used to determine the beginning of function is concerned with a progressive function. During development it has to tell us when an *acceptable* level of functioning is present, not when *some* functioning is present.

The difficulties are compounded when the characteristics of the EEGs of premature babies are analyzed. Such studies have been carried out since the late 1950s, and data are now available on premature babies from 24 weeks of gestation onwards. Most of the data however, come from infants 28 or even 33 weeks of gestation and older.[21]

Premature infants with gestational ages less than eight months have long periods during which the EEG reveals no activity (figure 14). During the rest of the time, brief periods of slow waves alternate with shorter periods of electrical silence or low-amplitude activity. The slow waves appear independently over the two hemispheres, and are irregular and variable in form in the youngest babies. Spindle-like patterns with frequencies of 12–20 cycles per second, and shifting spiky waves are prominent in the youngest premature infants, but have more or less disappeared by term. Prior to eight months gestation, stages of wakefulness and sleep cannot be differentiated, whereas in older infants cerebral activity is generally continuous. Gradual changes in EEG characteristics occur over the first few years of postnatal life, until adult patterns are seen in most wave patterns by seven to eight years of age. Cerebral rhythms, however, tend to be more labile in children than adults, often being suppressed or augmented locally for varying periods of time.

Figure 14   Electroencephalographic (EEG) patterns of premature infants.

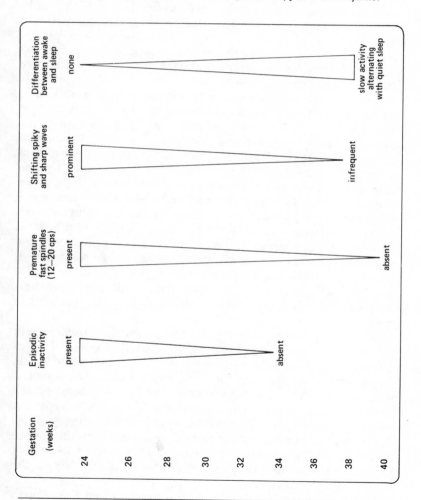

EEGs from premature infants of varying developmental ages, therefore, provide much the same picture as that provided by a study of the developing brain, and this is that the acquisition of an adult state of affairs is a long drawn-out process. The EEG appears to be particularly unhelpful, since the electrical inactivity of brain death is a normal feature of the developing brain, albeit for periods of time lasting from a matter of seconds to a few minutes. This lasts until about 32 weeks gestation. If the EEG is to be taken as a guide to brain birth it is a highly conservative tool, placing the emergence of the semblance of an adult pattern at 32–36 weeks gestation. Since premature infants can survive, with assistance, from as early as 20 weeks gestation, the relevance of the premature EEG patterns has to be questioned.

How does the study of brain development help in this matter? As we saw in a previous section its dominant feature is that different systems are laid down at different times, and these are not coordinated until relatively late in development. This is illustrated in figure 15, from which it can be seen that some developmental sequences can only occur once the preceding sequence has been completed; for example, b follows a, c follows b, and e follows d. This diagram also shows that some sequences, such as g and h, occur late in development, while h is not completed until after birth. If brain birth is placed at time '1', only sequences a, d and f are present, and even these have not been completed. No other sequence has commenced. At time '2', all the sequences are present, except for g and h. By time '3', which is late in development, all developmental sequences are in place, even if further development is still to occur.

Quite a different matter is presented by anencephaly (absence of the cerebral hemispheres), which raises a host of intriguing issues. Although newborns with this condition do not live any length of time, fetuses survive until they are born due to the protection and nourishing environment of the uterus.[22] These fetuses can survive, therefore, *in utero* without any form of cerebral functioning. This suggests that cerebral function until birth is not necessary for the active maintenance of the bodily functions of the fetus. If this is so, it is only at birth that the brain can be said to assume responsibility for the control of our existence.

There is, therefore, no simple answer to when brain birth

Figure 15   Illustration of the sequential manner in which the brain develops. **a–h** *represent distinct sequences implicit in the development of the brain. For an explanation, see text.*

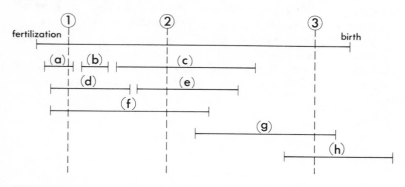

occurs, except to say that if it is placed very early, such as at '1' in figure 15, numerous phases of development will not even have appeared. If the concept of brain birth is a valid one, I consider it should be placed when most developmental sequences have at least started, for example, at '2' in figure 15. By reference to the specific data shown in figure 8, I would very tentatively place brain birth at approximately 24–28 weeks of development.

This is, of course, an arbitrary conclusion. It is at odds with those who have put the emergence of the brain at 12–30 days,[23] around 40 days[24] or eight weeks.[25] It is also at odds with those who consider that the brain of the new-born is incapable of a capacity for thought and rational deliberation, and therefore bestows upon the new-born a non-personal status.[26] Herein, lies our dilemma. The concept of brain birth is used to demarcate the transition from non-personhood to personhood, and this weighs heavily on the point at which it is placed. In this discussion I have attempted to ignore this consideration, although this does not mean that my placement of brain birth at 24 to 28 weeks gestation is correct.

We come back again then, to the value of the concept of brain birth. If we wish to use it as the demarcating point between non-personhood and personhood, we are left with what, to most people, is an embarrassingly late point. But to make this point much earlier than six months, and especially around six to eight weeks, is to utilize criteria quite unlike those employed for brain death.

My conclusion is that the notion of brain birth is a misleading one. We cannot get away from the major differences between a progressive phenomenon which is leading somewhere new, and a once-and-for-all phenomenon which is the final point of an existence that is now at an end. In biological and clinical terms we are dealing with quite separate worlds, and it is confusing to attempt to use the one as a model of the other.

5

The Fetus: Master or Servant?

Prenatal Human Life – Biblical Guidelines

In discussing the biblical data on fetal life, considerable emphasis is generally placed on a few biblical passages. These are considered by some so crucial, and also so self-evident in their interpretation, that the mere act of quoting them demonstrates in unequivocal terms that 'human life commences at conception'. It is my intention to take matters rather slower than this, and to attempt to discover what general principles we can glean from the biblical writers before applying these principles to contemporary issues. The principles which emerge about prenatal human life should also be viewed within the context of the biblical guidelines on human life in general (see chapter 3).

While I shall not limit my attention to just a few biblical passages, it is worth quoting at length some of those frequently considered to be crucial.

'Your hands shaped me and made me. Will you now turn and destroy me? Remember that you moulded me like clay. Will you now turn me to dust again? Did you not pour me out like milk and curdle me like cheese, clothe me with skin and flesh and knit me together with bones and sinews? You gave me life and showed me kindness, and in your providence watched over my spirit' (Jb. 10:8–12).

'For you created my inmost being; you knit me together in my mother's womb. I praise you because I am fearfully and wonderfully made; your works are wonderful, I know that full well. My frame was not hidden from you when I was made in the secret place. When I was woven together in the depths of the earth, your eyes saw my unformed body. All the days ordained for me were written in your book before one of them came to be' (Ps. 139:13–16).

'Before I was born the Lord called me; from my birth he has made mention of my name' (Is. 49:1).

'Before I formed you in the womb I knew [chose] you, before you were born I set you apart; I appointed you as a prophet to the nations' (Je. 1:5).

'When Elizabeth heard Mary's greeting, the baby leaped in her womb, and Elizabeth was filled with the Holy Spirit. In a loud voice she exclaimed: "Blessed are you among women, and blessed is the child you will bear! But why am I so favoured that the mother of my Lord should come to me? As soon as the sound of your greeting reached my ears, the baby in my womb leaped for joy"' (Lk. 1:41–44).

In the light of these passages, as well as others to which I shall refer, it is possible to make a number of general statements.

1. *The biblical writers include the fetus within the human community.* The unborn are expressions of the promises of God, and play an essential part in many of the purposes of God. The beginnings of adult human life are to be found in the unborn, and there is a continuity of life before and after birth. There is even a hint that our creation as individuals 'in the womb' is a reminder of the importance of justice within society (Jb. 31:13–15).

2. *Conception (fertilization) is repeatedly recognized as a gift of God* (Gn. 4:1; 16:2; 29:31,32; 30:22,23; Ru. 4:13). It is an act of creation, in which both humans and God have their essential parts to play. In the Old Testament, God is frequently seen as opening or closing the womb (uterus), within the context of faith and of his own purposes (see Chapter 3).

3. *The knowledge and care of God extend to the fetus.* This is brought out as God's servants look back at his concern for them throughout their own fetal life, exemplified by David's awareness of God's care of him prior to his birth (Ps. 22:9, 10; 139:13), and also by the way in which God's sovereign purposes for Jeremiah were enacted before his birth (Je. 1:5). David also confesses that his sinful nature was present

before birth: 'Surely I have been a sinner from birth, sinful from the time my mother conceived me' (Ps. 51:5). An additional feature of the biblical evidence is that the experiences of God's servants point to an awareness of being the same person both before and after birth. In a more general sense, the picture of human development and aging is used to refer to the nation of Israel being upheld since before birth (Is. 46:3).

4. *God's purposes did not commence at fertilization; they commenced in eternity.* God 'saw' David long before he was formed in the womb (Ps. 139:15,16); God chose Jeremiah and consecrated him as a prophet long before Jeremiah's body took on the form of a human being (Je. 1:5). In similar vein, Paul argues that the followers of Christ were chosen by God, not at the beginning of their earthly existence, but before the creation of the world (Eph. 1:4; 2 Tim. 1:9).

5. *The fetus is recognized as an essential part in the continuum which makes up the prenatal and postnatal facets of a human life.* For instance, as Gordon Wenham[1] has pointed out, the struggles of Esau and Jacob in the womb of Rebekah prefigured their struggles in later life (Gn. 25:23). Samson's mother was told to abstain from alcoholic drinks during her pregnancy (Jdg. 13:7). This was relevant to his life as an adult, since he was to be a Nazirite and therefore would be forbidden to drink wine.

6. *The importance of the fetus in the unfolding of the life of an individual is supremely brought out by the incarnation of Jesus, who commenced his human existence as an embryo.*[2] The angel of the Lord told Joseph: 'Do not be afraid to take Mary as your wife, because what is conceived in her is from the Holy Spirit' (Mt. 1:20). Even the life of the Son of God was, for nine months, enshrined in the life of a fetus.

These principles provide insights into God's purposes in the lives of those who emerged as, and were ordained to be, significant in God's kingdom. God protected them in the mother's uterus as well as in postnatal life, and this is set forth in a spirit of praise and worship. The context in which we read about God's concern for the unborn is always one in which there is a living relationship between God and one of his people. Job, in perplexity, confessed that God had made him in the uterus, and yet he failed to understand God's purposes for him (Jb. 10:8–12). He even wished that he had been stillborn

(Jb. 10:18,19). There is nothing neutral about Job's approach to
God's oversight of him before birth, and this is typical of all
other biblical references to God's actions in the history of the
individual.

These biblical passages touching on fetal life are confessions
about God and his purposes. They do not impart information
about the precise status of fetal life, although by implication
they provide helpful pointers to the attitudes we should adopt
towards fetal life. In Ecclesiastes we even get an admission of
agnosticism about embryological events: 'As you do not know
the path of the wind, or how the body is formed in a mother's
womb, so you cannot understand the work of God, the Maker of
all things' (Ec. 11:5).

The question facing us is whether the biblical teaching
enshrined in these passages provides us with a complete guide
to God's providential dealings with prenatal humanity. To
some, it appears that it does. For instance, Gordon Wenham[3]
writes that 'the child in the womb is a human being enjoying a
personal relationship with God'. John Stott[4] contends that the
fetus is 'already a human life who, though not yet mature, has
the potentiality of growing into the fullness of the individual
humanity he *already* possesses'. The significance of both these
conclusions is that they are based on the passages I have
quoted (although in both instances the principal passage referred to is Psalm 139), and these are interpreted as applying to
every single fetus ever conceived. The personal history of God's
servants, and the unique events surrounding the incarnation
of the Son of God, have been transmuted into a general principle relating to the status of all fetuses.

And yet, numerous questions remain. There is much that the
biblical statements leave unsaid. They tell us nothing
explicitly about those numerous embryos and fetuses
spontaneously lost during the early stages of prenatal development (chapter 4). They fail to tell us the significance of determining precisely when human life begins, and they do not
address the question of whether a very early embryo is a
person with the rights of a person. They provide no data about
the individuality of the unborn as a whole, nor about the
significance of the unborn human relative to that of the adult
human. They do not provide specific guidance in assessing the
relative merits of a five-day-old embryo, a five-month-old fetus
or a five-year-old child. Care also has to be taken with claims

about the nature of biblical teaching on the unborn, since these claims themselves may raise yet additional difficulties. For instance, what does it mean for a five-day-old embryo to 'enjoy a personal relationship with God'? Similarly, what does it mean to claim that a five-day-old embryo 'already possesses individual humanity'?

There appear to be major silences in the Bible on the status of the unborn, and we would do well to ponder these silences before proceeding any further.[5] We have to ask ourselves very seriously whether specific references such as the ones I have quoted lead to concepts like 'the sanctity of human life' or 'the inviolability of fetal life'. Do they, by themselves, inevitably lead to the view that all fetuses from their earliest existence have an unqualified right to protection under all possible circumstances?

As I have already indicated, this is where difficulties arise, since many argue that the biblical passages quoted above demonstrate unequivocally that 'human life begins at conception'. At face value this straightforward statement is unexceptional, perhaps even self-evident. However, it is emphasized in the context of the abortion debate where it is regarded as synonymous with the statement that 'fetal life is inviolable'. The end result is the contention that abortion is homicide, for no other reason than that it terminates a genuine human life.

It is evident from this progression of reasoning that the conclusion being drawn from these biblical passages is that fetal and adult life are synonymous under all circumstances, and regardless of the stage of development of the fetus. It is frequently claimed that no moral distinction can be made between them; they are always of equal value, and both – one imagines – are inviolable. If this is the case, it follows that to destroy a five-day-old embryo is precisely the same in ethical terms as killing a twenty-year-old adult in cold blood – both constitute murder. Moreover, whoever carries out the destruction is a murderer.

Once again therefore, we have to ask whether any biblical passages are this explicit. Do they categorically teach the equivalent status of fetus and adult? Four pieces of biblical data are repeatedly quoted in support of the belief that they are equivalent.

1. Exodus 21:22–25 is freely used to teach the parity of mother and fetus, and yet it has lent itself to a variety of opposing

interpretations by biblical scholars.[6] A pregnant woman becomes involved in a fight between two men; she is hit and the result is a miscarriage. The critical issue concerns the nature of the penalties to be exacted by the husband for injury to the woman and the death of the fetus. According to one group of scholars a distinction is made between the death of the fetus and the death of the woman, on the ground that fetal life is not equivalent to an adult human life. If a fetus died a fine was exacted, the level of the fine being determined by the husband and the judges. On the other hand, if the woman was injured or died, the law of punishment in kind (*lex talionis*) was applied. According to Exodus 21:12, anyone killing a baby, child or adult was considered a murderer, for whom the death penalty was exacted.

An alternative interpretation is that, where injury or death occurs, *lex talionis* applies to both the fetus and the mother. And so, in the case of Exodus 21:22, there was to be a demand for damages for causing the woman to go into premature labour. The following verses exacted further compensation if either mother or fetus suffered physically. The resulting principle is that mother and fetus were considered of equal value.

Whatever interpretation is the more appropriate, (and this depends a great deal on the translation consulted), this seems a slender basis on which to build a whole theology of the fetus. Moreover, the biblical writer was dealing with the regulations within a covenant community, and his primary concern at this juncture was with the nature of the punishment to be inflicted for injury incurred following accidents or fighting. He was not dealing with the status of the fetus as such, nor with its relative importance compared with that of postnatal human life. This passage, then, is dealing with unintentional abortion brought about by personal conflict, and not with deliberate abortion carried out for a whole array of motives. Whatever principles may be extracted from this passage, therefore, cannot be applied as they stand to the extensive array of grounds for induced abortion in contemporary society. Neither should it be concluded that intentional abortion is far worse than unintentional abortion, and is therefore automatically condemned in this passage without the need for further discussion.

The difficulties encountered in moving from this Exodus passage directly to abortion in contemporary society are considerable. There are even greater difficulties in applying it to the status of the embryo and early fetus (and to questions relating to the disposal of embryos). The miscarriage at the heart of Exodus 21:22–25 must have been of a relatively well-developed fetus, perhaps six-months or older. Had the miscarriage been of an embryo of just a few days or a few weeks gestation, the woman may not have been aware of her pregnancy, let alone of a miscarriage. To extrapolate from the miscarriage of an older fetus to the status of an embryo a few days old involves a major leap, which has to be justified on the grounds of legitimate biblical interpretation.

2. A second illustration of biblical evidence adduced in favour of the equivalent status of prenatal and postnatal human life is the incarnation. Thomas Torrance[7] writes:

> In the Apostles' Creed the Christian Church confesses faith in Jesus Christ God's only Son our Lord, 'Who was conceived by the Holy Spirit, born of the Virgin Mary. . . .' It acknowledges as one of the central truths of the Christian faith that in his Incarnation in which the Lord Jesus assumed our human nature, gathering up all its stages and healing them in his own human life, including conception, he thereby gave the human embryo a sacred inviolable status from the very beginning of his or her creaturely existence.

I have already argued that I believe the incarnation to be important in the stress it places on the integral part played by fetal life in the life of a human being as a whole. Our lives as individuals commenced at fertilization, just as the life of Jesus as a human being commenced at fertilization. Nevertheless, it is difficult to see in what way even the incarnation, in isolation from other biblical teaching, provides us with the significance of a few days of embryonic life in the absence of any ongoing individual human life.

I imagine that the incarnation bestows an inviolable status not only upon the fetus, but also upon life-after-birth. After all, Jesus was a man as well as a fetus. If this is so, it has to be asked what the concept of inviolability signifies. A straightforward definition of the term includes ideas such as 'to be kept sacred from being profaned and treated irreverently, or from being disregarded, or treated with disrespect'. A strong interpretation of this term leads to the belief that both fetal and adult human life should never be taken and that human beings (both prenatal and postnatal) have a right never to be deliberately killed. A weaker definition of the term states that all human life deserves our utmost respect, and that, under all normal circumstances, human life is to be protected and cared for.

What then is the practical outcome of the concept? The stronger interpretation seems to suggest that there are no circumstances whatsoever in which human life is to be taken, even in self-defence at an individual level, or in response to aggression at a national level. It also seems to imply that fetal life is never to be taken, even when the fetuses belong to women of an opposing faction in warfare. It also means that abortion is never justified, even when the mother's life is in danger. In practical terms, however, exceptions to this general rule crop up in all these circumstances, from which it appears that our actions are being governed by the weaker (and not the stronger) interpretation of inviolability.

And what about self-sacrifice; where does it fit in? Jesus did not regard his own life as inviolable, in the sense that he was prepared to sacrifice it for a greater good. Such self-sacrifice does not treat human life as sacred, since it is seen within the broader framework of the good of mankind. Does this help medical decision-makers when confronted by choices between saving or sacrificing one life rather than another? If human life is never to be deliberately taken, choices such as these could appear to pose impossible burdens in some situations. Nevertheless, they become possible when inviolability is regarded as giving to human beings the utmost respect possible, even though this is sometimes not total protection.

Undue emphasis on the conception of Jesus as undergirding the inviolability of fetal life also comes up against the knotty biological problem that the conception of Jesus was quite different from the conception of all other human beings. If the conception of Jesus did not involve the fertilization of an ovum by a sperm, why should his conception as a *biological* phenomenon become the basis of a *theologi-*

cal statement about the status of all normally-conceived fetuses?

3. Further biblical data used to justify the significance of the fetal existence of Jesus is the account in Luke's Gospel, in which John the Baptist as a six-month-old fetus in his mother's womb 'leaped for joy' (Lk. 1:41–44). One interpretation of this is that it was a special movement inspired by the Holy Spirit, and that the six-month-old fetus was Spirit-endowed. Gordon Wenham[8] takes this further and argues that the fetus's joy was prompted by the two-week-old embryo of Jesus, although the response could equally well have been to the coming of Mary. Wenham's conclusion is that 'Mary is *already* mother of Christ'.

There can be no doubt that this passage indicates that God was at work in John the Baptist's life, even prior to his birth. This is consonant with much other biblical teaching. It is however, a major leap from this passage, which describes a unique event, to the contention that all fetuses ever conceived have precisely the same status as that accorded postnatal life. If we are searching for a direct application of this passage, it would appear to teach that all fetuses are filled with the Holy Spirit, rather than with their universal rights and privileges. Such an interpretation would appear to be quite unwarranted, and detracts from the theological significance of the six-month-old fetus of John the Baptist as being Spirit-endowed.

4. One further point from Luke's account is that the word *brephos* used to describe the unborn John the Baptist is also used to describe the newborn Jesus and the infants brought to Jesus for blessing (Lk. 1:41,44; 2:12,16; 18:15). Again, this is used to argue for the humanity of the fetus, and for the view that personal identity begins at conception. This conclusion does not appear to follow from the use of this particular word, since it refers to just one instance of older fetal life and then to infants and children. It certainly underscores the significance of older fetuses, but again, can this legitimately be used as the basis of a vast generalization about fetal life as a whole and about the inviolability of all fetal life? To argue in this way is to make the same sort of leap as involved in using Exodus 21:22–25 in the same way (see point 1 above).

Fetuses as Persons

Clearing the Ground

Up to this stage in the discussion I have resolutely adhered to biblical concepts and specific biblical principles. I have deliberately steered clear of biological data. I have attempted to draw out of the biblical record major clues about the nature of human life in general and, in the light of these, some specific teaching on prenatal life. My concern has been to explore how far the biblical writers take us, and to follow them this far but no further. For this reason I have been reluctant to accept the position adopted by many evangelicals that human life, by which they mean full human personhood, commences at fertilization. I am not convinced that this is a viewpoint necessarily endorsed by the biblical writers.

The point at which I have arrived is that the principles provided by the biblical writers provide us with many important hints about how we should view embryonic and fetal life. They do not however, provide us with guidance on many of the minutiae; neither do they tell us how to act in borderline cases. Nevertheless, they are critical to our ethical stance on the unborn.

The biblical principles also need to be augmented with scientific ones. It is impossible to discuss specific issues in bioethics without being adequately informed on the scientific data. However, when speaking as Christians, this needs to be acknowledged. It is all too easy to give the impression that our viewpoint is solely derived from the Bible when, in fact, it is heavily dependent on a particular interpretation of biological observations.

Analysis of the scientific data has led to the emergence of three schools of thought: the genetic school, the developmental (or gradualist) school, and the social consequences school. The *genetic school* emphasizes the genetic uniqueness (or, as some would phrase it, the genetic particularity) of each embryo; it is this alone that constitutes the humanity and personhood of an embryo or fetus. The *developmental (gradualist) school* recognizes that genetic capacity alone is insufficient to speak meaningfully about the fetus as a person; a requisite degree of development is also required, together with an appropriate environment. The *social consequences school* contends that society decides what value should be placed upon fetal life, since humanness is in part determined by the degree to which a person is accepted and recognized by others.

Of these three schools of thought, the first two have strong biological components and so can be analyzed, at least in part, by considering biological parameters. Some of these have been touched on in chapter 4. Biological considerations alone however, will not provide a definitive guide to one's view of the embryo or to the manner in which the embryo is to be treated. This brings in philosophical perspectives, especially concerning the priorities to be espoused within the human community, and the respective emphases to be laid on prenatal and postnatal human life.

And so, while it is helpful to divide views on the unborn into genetic, developmental, and social consequences schools of thought, it would be misleading to suggest that each of these is based on just one predominant idea. The genetic school could equally well be referred to as the *conception school*, since the emphasis in this case is on conception as the beginning of human personhood. Considerable weight is placed on genetic uniqueness by those holding this position, although comparable weight is given to a view of personhood that sees it as indivisible from its initiation in the newly formed embryo.

In the case of the developmental school, some proponents of this position lay great stress on the development of the brain, as they search for the first manifestation of consciousness or thought. For them the emergence of such a point during development marks the beginning of human personhood and therefore of human value and human rights. By contrast, others who may be classed as belonging to the developmental school recognize within the developing fetus a gradual increase in its potential for full personhood. For them, there is no point at which a fetus *becomes* a person, and hence there is no stage at which it was ever a non-person. Although both positions are developmental ones, there is considerable difference between them in practical terms. Once again therefore, it is misleading if this important distinction is overlooked.

Although the social consequences school stands in its own right, it contributes to the other schools of thought. For instance, considerable impetus for the genetic school stems from the belief that any other standpoint will devalue the fetus (and perhaps human life in general) in the eyes of society. This is a social consideration, and not a biological one. The developmental school also relies on social considerations when it is contended that an older fetus is worth more in society's terms than is a younger fetus or an embryo. Although important biological landmarks may underlie this judgment, the value placed on consciousness, thought or sentience is, in part, a socially-determined one.

Personhood of the Fetus – Evangelical Contributions
While it is tempting to launch directly into a discussion on 'personhood', the complexity of the topic and my own inability to deal adequately with it make this impossible. In addition, the specific area of concern in this book – the personhood of the fetus – is even more difficult to unravel, and the state of the debate on this topic is at an even more rudimentary level. Whatever is written at present must, therefore, be viewed as tentative. This is the beginning of what will undoubtedly be a long-drawn-out debate.

While evangelicals are agreed on the biblical data underlying this debate, as set out in 'Prenatal human life – biblical guidelines', their views on the personhood of the fetus are diverse. This is amply illustrated by the conflicting views of Oliver O'Donovan, Regius Professor of Moral and Pastoral Theology in the University of Oxford, and of Donald MacKay, Emeritus Professor of Communication and Neuroscience at the University of Keele. Although I shall deal with the views of a variety of evangelical scholars, O'Donovan and MacKay are good examples of the two ends of the spectrum.

(a) *Fetuses are persons.* O'Donovan[9] appears to claim that the fetus has personhood from the moment of conception, with the result that we must commit ourselves to its care in spite of the fact that its personhood will only be revealed later in personal relationships. In contrast, MacKay[10] considers that the fetus becomes a person possessing rights and demanding care when nervous system development has reached a point at which 'brain birth' can be said to have taken place.

O'Donovan sees a radical dichotomy between what he describes as the Christian view of the human person with its emphasis on continuity and historicity, and the modern view based on the importance of a qualitative assessment of human beings. O'Donovan argues that 'we discern persons only by love, by discovering through interaction and commitment that this human being is irreplacable'.[11] In this way we commit ourselves to children in the womb and to the severely handicapped, unlike 'the modern thinker' who makes distinctions between human appearances, human qualities, and between persons and pre-persons.

More specifically, O'Donovan[12] argues: 'we can recognise someone as a person only from a stance of prior moral commitment to treat him or her as a person, since the question of what constitutes a person can never be answered speculatively'; he further comments that 'we know someone as a person as that person is disclosed in his or her personal relations to us'. What is critical to O'Donovan is the element of personal engagement, since no observational criteria (such as brain activity, respiration or heartbeat) can, according to him, provide any information about personhood. The word 'person' therefore cannot be reduced to any one dimension; to do so is, in O'Donovan's view, a category mistake. Neither does personhood develop, since it is not a qualitative phenomenon; it is 'substance'.

In considering fetuses, O'Donovan utilizes the concept of commitment, according to which parents treat the fetus as a baby and in this way know their child as a baby. In this commitment we recognize fetuses as persons, and this, for O'Donovan, is appropriate; since we are responding to what he describes as the 'human face' – the immediate self-presentation of humanity. In responding to how we recognize the fetus as having a 'human face', O'Donovan resorts to embryology and to what he views as a major discontinuity at conception 'when the parental genotypes borne by the two gametes re-form into a new genotype, the distinct endowment of the new conceptus'. In the light of this knowledge he concludes that we can recognize the human face in the blastocyst and zygote.

O'Donovan's stance, therefore, is an amalgam of the genetic and social consequences schools. He concedes that no scientific evidence proves that the fetus is a person; this, he contends, cannot in principle be proved. Personhood cannot be equated with brain activity, genotype or implantation, although what is provided apparently is information about the beginning of individual human existence. It is this which provides the point when commitment to caring for the fetus is to begin.

In this way O'Donovan maps out his view of prenatal humanity, with its emphasis on commitment and its antipathy to observation and experimentation. All embryos and fetuses are, according to this view, to be treated as persons from conception onwards, regardless of any qualitative considerations. A crucial element in his argument is that the fetus has a human 'appearance'; it is *obviously* a person, just as the comatose individual is obviously a person, whereas the anencephalic infant is less obviously a person (since he allows for the abortion of such an infant). However, in shunning all scientific means of investigating brain activity or respiration, he is unable to provide any clues as to how this 'appearance' is to be recognized in borderline cases. Commitment to an individual as a person must have limits, such as when the comatose patient dies. One wonders what is the virtue of pronouncing that an individual is a non-person only when death is obvious to the layman. His refusal to utilize the concept of brain death questions the practical relevance of his view of personhood.

It seems that O'Donovan's aversion to scientific observation drives him in this direction. When it is applied to the embryo or fetus, no distinctions can ever be drawn between them – all are persons, because we are to be committed to all of them. What, however, are the consequences of our commitment? Does commitment *always* amount to maintaining a dubious pregnancy? Does it *always* lead to preserving the life of the fetus, regardless of severe handicap or maternal illness? Commitment to decide that a fetus is a person is one thing; commitment to determine how to treat that fetus is another, since our commitment to persons (prenatal or postnatal) does not inevitably lead to preservation of the person's life, under all conceivable circumstances. O'Donovan would agree with this, on the basis of a policy of 'equal protection'. This allows him to approve of abortion in the case of immediate or remote threat to the mother's life, and where there is 'total deformity' in the fetus such that no life outside the uterus could be achieved. These conclusions, however, are based on qualitative considerations (*e.g.* the self-conscious humanity of the mother demands more attention than the yet unconscious humanity of the infant [fetus]), in which judgment is being made between the respective demands of two persons deserving of equal protection. O'Donovan's reliance on commitment therefore, proves inadequate at certain points, although it leads him to reject all forms of research on human embryos on the ground that this makes them ambiguously human. This is a questionable conclusion, especially when the results of artificial procreation, IVF children (and adults), have to be related to as persons. This is also a relatively unconvincing way of demonstrating the need to treat embryos with dignity. It is difficult to see how we are to be totally committed to early embryos, even before their existence is evident and their chances of developing further are limited. Although O'Donovan rejects the force of the argument based on pregnancy wastage – on the ground that a statistical argument is irrelevant to discontinuity in individual identity – he has the problem of dealing with commitment to individuals, the existence of whom is uncertain.

O'Donovan's unwillingness to place any reliance on scientific approaches is curiously negated by his reliance on genetic data for determining the beginning of a new personal history at conception. For him, these are suggestive data, which are relevant to a discussion of personhood (since they indicate a major discontinuity at conception). By contrast, all other biological data serve to fragment the person and are consequently dismissed. Again however, he remains at the level of generalities, and does not consider whether *all* conceptuses are actually persons regardless of their karyotype (see chapter 4). I imagine he would invoke the concept of the human face. What this does however, is to place a question mark beside the personhood of each individual embryo, leaving the question of 'appearance' and therefore of 'commitment' to O'Donovan himself (and to each individual who has to make decisions about the fate of embryos and fetuses). One has to ask what general criteria can be gleaned from this approach, and whether it is of as much value as he suggests.

John Stott,[13] in picking up some of O'Donovan's theses, places them in a theological context. Stott's emphasis is on what he sees as the vital relationship between God and the fetus. This relationship, which confers personhood on the fetus, is nothing less than God's conscious loving commitment to it. This is God's grace, and it 'confers on the unborn child, from the moment of its conception, both the unique status which it already enjoys and the unique destiny which it will later inherit'. Stott continues: 'It is grace which holds together this duality of the actual and the potential, the already and the not yet.'

Stott, like O'Donovan, appears to accept that this position is based on faith. It is a position which protects the fetus and errs on the side of the fetus. Nevertheless, they concede that there is no way of categorically proving that the fetus is a person. In this vein Stott asserts that 'All Christians should be able to agree that the human foetus is *in principle* inviolable' (my italics). In this, they do not go as far as some who, on the basis of the genetic uniqueness of each individual fetus and/or of biblical teaching, see the foetus unequivocally as a person.[14]

One of the tantalizing features of most discussions on the personhood of the fetus is the lack of definition of what is meant by the term 'person'. While definitions are frequently not attempted or even alluded to, one gains the impression that personhood is regarded by some as equivalent to being a member of the species *Homo sapiens*, whereas for others it denotes quite specific intellectual abilities. These two approaches to personhood represent the two extremes in the debate, the former placing full personhood at fertilization, and the latter placing it at about one year after birth (figure 16a and b[iii]). From this it emerges that so many of the controversies about the new reproductive technologies and also about abortion stem from a lack of agreement on the status of the fetus as a person. This, in turn, may reflect radical differences in the value we ascribe to human life in general, although it remains to be demonstrated that the value society places on prenatal life has direct implications for the value society places on postnatal life.

For most people, personal life appears to signify more than biological life. At its simplest, this is expressed by placing greater value on human life than on non-human life. Conflict emerges when the distinction is drawn between personal human life and non-personal human life, although decisions about this have to be made routinely by doctors when dealing with what they consider to be irreversibly comatose patients, or when confronted by infants with major brain regions absent or with very severe handicaps.

It is at this point that some distinction has to be made. As we have seen, O'Donovan stresses the 'human face', the appearance of being a person. Lewis Smedes,[15] in an attempt to clarify this issue, does not define personhood but refers to our response to humans. He writes:

> I mean only to appeal to the intuition that an individual human being is more than the biological support system that provides the conditions of life for him or her. It is the person,

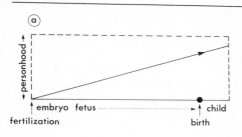

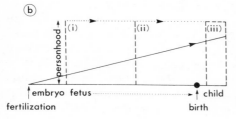

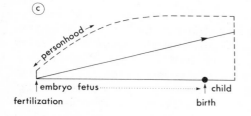

Figure 16   Diagrams to illustrate the major viewpoints on the personhood of the embryo and fetus. In all three diagrams the unbroken diagonal line represents biological development, with increasing maturity of the individual up to (and beyond) birth. The broken lines represent the personhood of the individual. In **a** the individual is regarded as having full personhood from fertilization onwards; no increase in personhood occurs at any stage throughout prenatal or postnatal life. In **b** personhood is acquired at some point during development; of the three possibilities depicted in **b**, (i) is some time during the embryonic period, (ii) is during the fetal period (around viability), (iii) is some time after birth; in each case, the embryo/fetus/child is considered to be a non-person prior to the onset of personhood. In **c** the embryo/fetus is regarded as an individual with the potential for full personhood from fertilization onwards; this potential increases during development so that by about the time of viability the fetus is considered to have value equivalent to that of a person; at no stage in **c** is the individual a non-person.

not the biological organism, that makes a claim on society for protection of its existence. We may not kill the biological organism as long as it is the base of individual personal life. The law protects the person. Jesus Christ died for the person. No matter how we finally describe the essential ingredients which lift a life into personhood, we must distinguish living person from bodily life.

(b) *Fetuses become persons.* Such approaches are, inevitably, subjective, although they are of considerable value in many situations. Nevertheless, the desire for greater specificity and objectivity is considerable. Donald MacKay,[16] for example, is not satisfied with the claims that the fetus is human, alive, and a divine work, or that it demonstrates continuity with post-natal human life. He accepts these claims, but is still not convinced that the early embryo 'is already a *person*, with the rights of a person'. Not only this, but he argues that there is no biblical evidence in favour of the personhood of *every* ovum that has ever been fertilized.

Against the background of Psalm 139, MacKay divides fertilized human ova into the X's and the N's. The X's are those that are spontaneously aborted 'at too early a stage for any of the minimal structures necessary for recognisably *personal* life .... to have developed'. The N's, on the other hand, are those embryos that develop into normal infants and adults. MacKay argues that it is only the N's that can eventually look back at their life-history and recognize the hand of God in all that has gone on previously (just as the psalmist did in Psalm 139). For MacKay, Psalm 139 has nothing to say about the X's of this world, from which he concludes that we have no biblical authority to claim that God views every fertilized ovum as a person. In the case of the X's, he asks, 'on what grounds could it be claimed that there *ever* was a person with personal identity?'

But if this is true, there must be some point during development when those fetuses which are going to 'make it' acquire the status of persons. MacKay recognizes a decisive moment in the maturation of the nervous system 'before which there is *nobody there*, but after which there is someone who is 'he' or 'she' as a personal cognitive agent, however limited in capacities'. In arguing like this he is not equating personhood with brain activity, since he regards the 'person' as belonging to a different category from neurons or neuronal networks.

MacKay concedes that there is no way of proving that an embryo or fetus aborted after a few days or weeks was never a person (any more than that there is evidence that such an embryo or fetus *was* a person). He believes, however, that no evidence from Scripture, science or experience requires us to make this type of commitment. What matters ultimately for MacKay is to ask what obligation God has placed on us with

regard to fetuses. He does not believe it is our duty to preserve
the life of every fertilized ovum, and he considers that in some
instances God may actually require us as his stewards to terminate the process by which a person would otherwise have
come into being.

This stance raises a number of considerations. The first is
that the specificity of the 'decisive moment' – the point when a
rudimentary brain comes into being – is not matched by ethical specificity. A decision has to be made not only on the
scientific question of when brain birth occurs (see chapter 4),
but also on the nature and extent of the obligations God has
placed on us in dealing with the pre-personal stage of fetal
development (figure 16b). The acknowledgement that there is
a stage when the embryo (and fetus as well, according to some
writers) has no personal characteristics of any description
places it outside the boundary of human protection. While this
does not inevitably allow us to do anything we like with the
embryo or early fetus (after all, research on experimental
animals is controlled by quite specific regulations in most
countries), it does alter the nature of our obligations towards
it.

The second consideration is that for MacKay, just as for
O'Donovan and Stott, the status of the fetus adopted by them is
one of belief, and also of commitment to this belief. While
MacKay emphasizes the lack of requirement to treat the
embryo and possibly early fetus as a person, O'Donovan and
Stott err on the side of the personhood of the fetus, even when
this is far from obvious in the early stages of development.[17]
Neither view by itself however, stands alone. Each has to be
offset by a commitment to human persons in general, whether
to fetuses in MacKay's case or to postnatal humans for O'Donovan and Stott.

MacKay's contribution to the debate on the personhood of
fetuses is a reminder that our own early history as embryos is
shrouded in mystery and uncertainty. We can reflect retrospectively on God's provisions for us as embryos, since each adult 'I'
has historical continuity with an embryonic 'I'. Nevertheless,
once we attempt to move prospectively from an embryonic 'I' to
a future adult 'I' we have to exercise great caution. While this
is theoretically possible, the ambiguity and uncertainty surrounding the futures of identified individual embryos are so
considerable as to render this a hazardous procedure. It is at

this point that MacKay's X's come into their own.

The question, which has to be asked concerning both the N's and X's in MacKay's description, is the nature of an embryonic 'I'. What does this mean? If the N's have an embryonic 'I' retrospectively, is this something that is bestowed only in retrospect? Or is there some meaningful way in which we can talk about an embryo as a person with a sense of its own destiny and future? Certainly, all embryos have a relationship to God; but what does this mean for those embryos which fail to develop beyond two or three weeks?

These are questions not just for MacKay but for all who would tread this treacherous path of discerning embryonic and fetal personhood. Whatever answers we emerge with will have to be able to meet the challenges of both the new reproductive technologies and abortion. They will also have to provide a balance between respect for the dignity of fetal life and for that of postnatal human life.

Lewis Smedes,[18] writing in the context of abortion and of respect for human life, skirts around some of these highly theoretical approaches to the fetus. He arrives at the conclusion that fetal life is person-becoming life. For him, 'the early stage of life's development is so remotely connected with the later stages that we cannot simply identify the early fetus as a person'. This leads Smedes to a gradualist position (figure 16c): 'The process of development not yet really begun leaves us with less than absolute certainty that we have a person as soon as we have conception. Growth into personhood is dynamic, gradual, complex; its beginning is obscure.'

Smedes is characterized, therefore, by a willingness to admit uncertainty about the embryo and early fetus. This prevents him from allowing this uncertainty to be converted into a presumption either in favour of the fetus or against it. In this way he is enabled to weigh up the demands of the fetus against the welfare of the mother, third parties, and the future child. In doing this, he is admitting that all these are integral participants in the moral deliberations that take place on human life. His concern is not so much with an abstract consideration of the precise status of the fetus as a person, but with the ways in which we treat both the fetus and mother. This does not lead to ready answers in conflict situations, but it takes seriously 'the ambiguity of not being something yet at the same time having the makings of what it will be'.

Personhood of the Fetus – the Wider Debate.
Although I devoted the previous section to contributions by
evangelical thinkers, it should not be concluded that these can
be readily distinguished from those of other persuasions. Evangelicals represent a broad spectrum of viewpoints spanning the
three major categories (a–c) outlined in figure 16. On the conservative side some evangelicals have much in common with
those speaking from a Roman Catholic perspective. However,
no evangelicals are as radical as someone like Joseph Fletcher
who would place the beginning of personhood at one year after
birth.[19] In the present section I want to widen the debate to
consider additional contributions to the question of the personhood of the fetus.

(a) *Fetuses are persons.* The official Roman Catholic position[20]
is that the embryo has human life potentially or incipiently
from the moment of fertilization, although tradition is not
unanimous on this matter. This position depends on biological,
philosophical and moral considerations. The biological evidence relates to data on the development of the embryo, the
philosophical reflection is on the nature of the human person,
while the rational moral reflection deals with the moral status
of the embryo.[21] An important argument is that, since it is
impossible to prove that personhood begins later than fertilization, moral prudence should err on the conservative side and
conclude that personhood probably begins at fertilization. Consequently, the embryo should be treated as a person, that is, in
the same way as we would treat a mature human being, from
the time of fertilization.[22]
    Some Roman Catholic theologians however, deviate in
minor ways from these principles. Charles Curran and Karl
Rahner,[23] for instance, consider that the embryo does not
become an individual until four to six days after fertilization.
Before this period, they consider that the embryo is 'only
potentially a human being'. It is worthy of respect, although
this is not as great as that to be accorded a mature human
being. A number of Roman Catholic theologians also consider
that hominization of nascent life should be related to the
development of the cerebral cortex. McCormick[24] has written
that, prior to this time, 'there exists merely a biological center
of life bereft yet of the substratum of a personal principle'.
    Also within some Roman Catholic thinking is the idea of the

embryo as a potential human person. Destruction of an embryo is the destruction of an organism with the potential to become an individual human person. While this concept is not confined to Roman Catholic thinking, as I shall discuss shortly, I shall consider here the way in which Teresa Iglesias[25] has approached it. She distinguishes between the process of development *into* a person, and the process of development *of* a person. In adhering to the latter concept, she contends that 'to be a human being is to be a person. There are no stages in our existence at which this identity does not hold . . . . It is in virtue of what human beings are right from the beginning of their existence that they must be accorded absolute respect and their lives treated as inviolable.' Underlying these conclusions is the idea of potentiality: whatever we now are, was present in potential form in the embryos from which we developed. Since we *now* have self-consciousness, the potential for self-consciousness must be present in all embryos. By this type of reasoning Iglesias arrives at the conclusion that 'the *kind* of life that the zygote has, because of the capacity it presently possesses, is *personal* life, that is, the life of a personal being or a personal subject'.

This argument, while not overtly borrowing from the genetic argument, has much in common with it. The impression is given that the embryo is a minute form of a mature human person. Everything is present in the embryo; all that is required is that it be provided with the opportunity to unfold. The embryo is the adult in miniature. A similar argument has been put forward by Robert E. Joyce in an essay: 'Personhood and the conception event'. The argument, in this case, is that every living, individual being with the natural potential for knowing, willing, desiring, and relating to others in a self-reflective way is a person. Since the human zygote is a living individual with the natural potential to act in these ways, it must be an actual person with great potential. For Joyce every potential is an actuality; as a result, the potential of a human conceptus to think and talk becomes an actuality. Similarly, he considers that no living body can *become* a person unless it already *is* a person.

We are once more back at a position whereby the personhood of the earliest embryo is indistinguishable from that of the adult. The question, however, is whether the capacity of *a* to develop into *A* makes *a* exactly the same as *A*. Quite obviously, the ability of an acorn to develop into an oak tree does not convert the acorn into an oak tree. Conversely, to destroy an acorn is not the same as destroying an oak tree. A three-day-old human embryo is not the same as a 30-year-old human adult; although the potential is undoubtedly there, the actual adult is far from realization.

To equate the potential with the actual is to flee in the face of the reality of biological and human development. In no other area of life do we do this. For instance, a student commencing a course of study has the potential to pass the final examinations, and this potential may ultimately be realized when the examinations are passed. In order to accomplish this however, a great deal of teaching and learning is required, and it is these alone that convert potential success into actual success. The student is changed in certain ways by the learning, so that the student who passes the examination is *different* from the student who turned up at the first class with a potential for passing the examination. While it would be unwise to push this analogy too far, it is important that we lay adequate stress on the learning environment as well as the enormous extent of biological transformation required to change an embryo into an adult. The person may be potentially present in the embryo, but its ultimate manifestation in the adult is of a dramatically different character.

Respect is due to the embryo because of what it is and, more strongly, because of what it may become (its potential). This follows, however, from its potential, and not because its potential has been converted into an actuality. Reliance on an embryo's potential does not convert it into a 'nothing', any more than the student in the above analogy is regarded as a 'failed' student or is excluded from further study on the grounds that he/she has not as yet passed the final examinations.

(b) *Fetuses are non-persons.* From these attempts at stressing the personal life of the embryo and fetus, I want now to consider the diametrically opposite position – that of regarding the fetus as a non-person. This is most clearly illustrated in utilitarian thought.

Peter Singer and Deane Wells,[26] in their assessment of the new reproductive technologies, consider the status of the embryo in the context of gamete and embryo wastage. As pointed out in chapter 2, they argue that there is no moral obligation to preserve the life of the embryo on the ground that it is not wrong to destroy either the ovum or sperm before they have united. This leads them to conclude that 'the newly created embryo is not entitled to a special moral status which makes it wrong to destroy it'. Even more provocatively, they suggest that the embryo be regarded as a thing, rather than as a person, until the point at which there is some brain function.

This drives them to a search for when brain function commences. What is significant from their angle are characteristics such as consciousness, autonomy and rationality. Of these, they consider consciousness to be the minimal feature. They write: 'As soon as a being becomes capable of feeling pleasure or pain, or of having experiences and preferring some kinds of experiences to others, that being has sufficient moral status to make it wrong to do certain things to it, for example, to inflict pain upon it unnecessarily.' What becomes important to determine is the degree of nervous system development which indicates consciousness. The complexity of this task has already been indicated in chapter 4, and it is surprising that Singer and Wells indicate that the brain function necessary for consciousness could not occur before the end of the sixth week after fertilization. This is an unrealistically early time, although they qualify this statement with the comment that 'it may eventually be shown that it does not occur until quite some time thereafter'.

In practice, therefore, these authors recognize the human embryo as a 'thing' for at least the first six weeks of development, and perhaps for very much longer. For them, the early embryo is not a bearer of rights, and as they remark in their discussion of ectogenesis, there is no difference in the moral status of the pre-sentient embryo and the embryo with its capacity for sentience removed.

While Singer and Wells do not discuss the embryo as a person, the result of their assessment is that the early embryo is a non-person. The only criterion they accept for bestowing personhood on an individual is the stage of development of the brain. It is this, and this alone, that guarantees any protection at all to individuals (both prenatal and postnatal). The ramifications of this position are considerable, and in the prenatal area they would allow extensive research to be conducted on embryos, and also procedures such as ectogenesis and cloning.

The underlying ethical principles espoused by Singer and Wells are expressed by them in these questions: 'What will lead to the kind of society in which the greatest possible number are able to satisfy their most important needs and desires? What will most reduce misery and suffering?'

Quite clearly therefore, when conflict arises something has to give way. Since embryos are provided with no protection at all, they do not feature in their own right in any calculations of misery and suffering. Their only contribution is to provide material for research endeavours aimed at reducing the misery and suffering of others. Singer and Wells therefore illustrate in a stark way the gulf between non-personhood and personhood and the transformation of the one into the other at some point during prenatal existence (figure 16b). For them, this is a move from no protection to some protection; what is not clear is the extent of the protection for embryos and fetuses even after brain birth has taken place.

Michael Tooley[27] has put forward a not dissimilar position on the embryo and fetus, although his major concern is to assess the acceptability of abortion and infanticide. Tooley draws a sharp distinction between *being a human being* in the biological sense and *being a person* in the moral sense; consequently, he concludes that not all human beings are persons. Instead, he enunciates the basic principle that it is wrong to kill innocent persons.

This, in turn, raises the inevitable question of whether or not the fetus (or, in terms of his concern with infanticide, the infant) is a person. Tooley's answer is that a person has the properties of being able to recall some of its past states, can envisage a future for itself and has desires about this, and has personality traits that do not alter in too drastic a manner over short periods of time. Tooley's application of this definition leads him to acknowledge that the adult members of some animal species, such as some primates and dolphins, possess these characteristics; whereas human fetuses and neonates lack them.

Tooley does concede, however, that human fetuses and neonates are potential persons. Having accepted this, he then argues that potential personhood only allows us to confer a right to life (for fetuses and infants), if we also accept the principle that it is wrong to refrain from producing additional persons. If one assumes that we are under no obligation to produce children (that is, contraception is acceptable), Tooley concludes that the killing of a fetus, a potential person, is no worse than using contraceptives. The following step in his argument is to claim that killing a neonate is no worse than killing a fetus; in this manner, he justifies infanticide. The details of the steps in this argument are beyond the scope of this book, and the conclusion itself is of only marginal interest in the present context. Nevertheless, it does illustrate one direction in which utilitarian thinking may lead.

Tooley also introduces a further category of beings; these are 'quasi-persons'. According to him, human infants become quasi-persons at about the age of three months. He is uncertain whether quasi-persons are morally any different from non-persons. If they are different and qualify for the right to life, we shall also have to recognize this right in both adult animals from a large range of species as well as in infants older than three months. Conversely, if quasi-persons do not qualify for such protection, infanticide may be permissible up to one year of age. One consequence of this conclusion is that, since in his terms, an adult baboon is a person or quasi-person, it is worse to kill a baboon in order to transplant its heart into a human infant than it would be to kill a normal two-month-old infant in order to use its body parts to save an adult baboon.[28]

It is not my intention to follow any further Tooley's arguments in favour of infanticide. What is important for my present purposes is that one of the grounds on which he builds his case is the non-personhood not only of fetuses but also of new-born children. While most of those who claim that early fetuses are non-persons would not accept Tooley's progression to infanticide, what is significant about Tooley is his insistence on the non-personhood of much older fetuses and even of new-born babies. He looks for a much larger and better-developed repertoire of behavioural patterns as a basis for personhood than do others. And so he can conclude that new-born humans are not persons since they lack a capacity for thought, self-consciousness and rational deliberation. At the neuro-anatomical level, the networks located in the upper layers of the cerebral cortex thought to underlie higher mental functions are not present at birth. In addition, bioelectrical patterns at birth are relatively unorganized.[29]

In arriving at his conclusions, Tooley overlooks what one commentator has described as 'the moral obligation to nurture'.[30] He fails to take account of the commitments humans have to the welfare and survival of infants and also, to varying extents, to fetuses as well. This is where the family and its obligations come in, since the newborn is totally dependent on the voluntary acts of responsible moral agents committed to its care. These interactions between the newborn and ourselves are essential for its survival and well-being. What they attest is that, even when the neurological and behavioural features of the newborn (or fetus) are inadequate on a biological scale of values, our commitment to love and care for one of our own is basic to what we are as humans living in community. In this we begin to see something of the Christian emphasis on our being made in the image of God.

This is the type of commitment envisaged by O'Donovan in his discussion of the embryo. My difficulty with O'Donovan is not with his emphasis on commitment, but with his insistence that this places upon us an obligation to treat all embryos and fetuses *as though* they are persons deserving of equal protection to postnatal humans under practically all circumstances. It was for this reason that I considered his position in the section: 'Fetuses are persons'. It should, however, also be evident by this stage that, in practical terms, I have far more in common with O'Donovan than I do with Tooley. The crucial factor is that of commitment, which I see as a fundamental theological one, even though there are undoubtedly differences between O'Donovan and myself in the degree of the commitment we advocate to prenatal humanity.

(c) *Fetuses are potential persons.* Crucial as the principle of commitment is, it does not answer all our questions about the personhood of the fetus, and this brings me to another perspective – the fetus as a potential person or, more strictly, the fetus as a being with the potential for full personhood. Although this has been alluded to in passing, it has not as yet been adequately explored.

According to the *potentiality principle*: 'If, in the normal course of its development, a being will acquire a person's claim to life, then by virtue of that fact it already has some claim to life.'[31] In terms of this principle, a potential person is an existing being which, while not yet a person, will become an actual person during the normal course of its development (figure 16c). A human fetus is a potential person, in contradistinction to an actual person (a normal adult human being), or a being with a capacity for personhood (a temporarily unconscious person), or a possible person (a human sperm or ovum), or a future person (a person in a future generation).

The potentiality principle asserts that potential persons, such as fetuses, have a claim to life, whereas possible persons cannot exercise such a claim. Furthermore, it accords full personhood to those with a capacity for personhood. On the other hand, the claim to life of a potential person may be weaker than that of an actual person.[32]

The potentiality principle takes seriously the continuum of biological development, and refuses to draw an arbitrary line to denote the acquisition of personhood. At all stages of development the fetus is on its way to full personhood and, if everything proceeds normally, it will one day attain in its own right full personhood. The fetus is regarded as part of a continuing process, the end result of which is the emergence of an individual human being characterized by human personhood.

Inherent in a potential person is a high probability of future personhood. With this goes a claim to life and respect, a claim that in very general terms may be proportional to its stage of fetal development. The claim is always present but, just as the probability of an older fetus becoming an actual person is much greater than that of a zygote becoming a person, it becomes stronger with development until at birth 'the potential person attains properties and relationships so close to those of actual persons that the consequences of killing at this point are practically the same as killing young persons'.[33]

The potentiality principle is nothing more than an attempt to find an approach to the fetus that takes serious account of the gradual nature of fetal development. In this, it stands in sharp contrast to other approaches which claim that the fetus becomes a person at some specific stage of development, whether this is at fertilization, implantation, quickening, or birth. In all these instances (except fertilization) the fetus is regarded as a non-person prior to this particular stage of development and a person deserving complete protection following it (figure 16b). Each of these views has major difficulties, and the potentiality principle was elaborated in an attempt to view the fetus in more realistic terms.

According to the potentiality principle there is no point in development, no matter how early on, when the fetus does not

display some elements of personhood – no matter how rudimentary (figure 16c). The potential is there, and it is because of
this that the fetus has a claim to life and profound respect. This
claim however, becomes stronger as fetal development proceeds, so that by the time of birth or earlier (viability) the
claim is so strong that the consequences of killing such a fetus
are the same as those of killing an actual person – whether
child or adult. Conversely, the fetus in the last trimester will,
when necessary, be treated as a 'patient'. Its potentiality in no
way makes this inappropriate.

Critics of the potentiality principle invariably want a hard-
and fast answer to 'when' the fetus becomes protectable. Such
an arbitrary line, however, is against the notion of this principle (figure 16c), according to which human life is *always* deserving of protection no matter how immature it may be. What
the principle does not do is allow the developing human to be
viewed in complete isolation from all the other humans
intimately involved with it, since *all* are to be treated – as far
as possible – as beings of dignity and as deserving of respect.

A fetus is never 'half a person' any more than a child is 'half
an adult'. Just as the child is on its way to adulthood, so the
fetus is on its way to actual personhood. In the same way as a
child is not of less significance than an adult, although it is
certainly different from an adult, so the fetus is not of less
significance than the young child (or adult). Nevertheless,
there are major biological differences between the early fetus
and child, and these differences are taken seriously by the
potentiality principle.

In ordinary life we recognize a difference between the accidental loss of an embryo or early fetus and the birth of a
stillborn child. Both entail the death of fetal life, and yet under
most circumstances the loss of a child which almost-made-it is
felt much more acutely than that of a child which had hardly-
begun-to-develop. The potentiality principle takes account of
the respective degrees of development lying behind these
responses. It never underestimates the significance of even the
earliest stages of fetal growth, but it does treat with seriousness the developmental continuum of which the fetus is an
integral part.

The potentiality principle *never* provides grounds for lightly
disposing of the fetus; this is not its intention. In terms of this
principle it is never legitimate to refer to a fetus as being '*only*

a potential human being (or person)'. Such condescension is foreign to the principle. However, when serious conflict arises between the welfare of the mother and that of the fetus she is carrying, it provides some guidance in assessing the weight given to the claims of the fetus, insofar as its degree of development is concerned. Nevertheless, this principle by itself never opens the door to abortion. The potentiality principle also confers respect on the early embryo. At no stage is the embryo a non-person (figure 16c). At no stage therefore is it of no value as an end in itself, neither can it ever be disposed of at will. This demonstrates that an interpretation of the potentiality principle within a Christian framework is a conservative principle; its aim is to conserve fetal life, and this is a feature of considerable importance when confronted by the new reproductive technologies.

Many Christians are suspicious of the potentiality principle mainly because they fear it will lead to a low view of the fetus. I have attempted to show that this is not the case.[34] Moreover, alternative views of the fetus require some serious analysis. For instance, if we ascribe actual personhood to a 13-day-old embryo, with complete protection for this embryo under all circumstances, what may be the consequences? What will happen when there is conflict between this embryo and the welfare of postnatal lives? Should the good of existing persons be sacrificed for that of life hardly-yet-begun? If we answer in the affirmative, on what scriptural principles is our answer based, and is it possible, in practice, to afford the embryo or early fetus complete protection?

The potentiality principle may not have the simplistic facade of absolutist positions. But we may find that in everyday existence we live according to it even when claiming to espouse a 'higher' view of fetal status.

Moral Significance of Developmental Issues

The many arguments and counter-arguments to which we have been introduced in the preceding pages have left us with a great variety of options. Some of these are of theoretical interest only, and may, or may not, have implications for the way in which we actually *treat* the embryo and fetus. Others however have very obvious practical implications, such as the justification of infanticide, abortion-on-demand, or ectogenesis. While none of these outcomes is of immediate relevance to the topics I am concerned with in this book, they are a very clear manifestation of a particular view of prenatal human life.

The status of the embryo and fetus appears such an insoluble problem to some people that they attempt to avoid it, and discuss the new reproductive technologies without taking it into account.[35] While I have sympathy with this response, it is an unsatisfactory one because discussions about what are allowable ways of treating embryos are based implicity, if not explicitly, on assumptions regarding the worth of embryos. Nevertheless, this response does pinpoint a commonly experienced despair, namely, that there is no way in which those with diametrically opposing views on the embryo and fetus will ever find any common meeting ground. The arid, and at times acrimonious, debate on abortion has been a cause of this despair, and there are signs that it is being repeated in the mushrooming debate on the new reproductive technologies (see chapter 2).

The question confronting us is whether there is any way out of this impasse. Even a brief glance at figure 16 is enough to pinpoint where the conflict lies. The contrast between a and b in this illustration is the contrast between complete protection of the embryo and fetus from fertilization onwards (a), and no protection at all for some period early in gestation or during the greater part of gestation (the period to the left of lines (i) to (iii) in b). As long as this stark contrast is maintained, and if complete protection or no protection at all mean what they appear to mean in practice, there can be no hope of reconciliation. We need to ask, however, whether in reality the contrast is as glaring as this. Is it possible to provide *total* protection for *all* embryos and fetuses from day 1 of gestation throughout the whole of the gestational period? Or are advocates of this position advocating something which is theoretically appealing but quite implausible in practice? For those who consider that the fetus acquires protectable status (or personhood) at some point during (or even after) gestation, the question has to be asked whether this allows others within society to do anything they wish to the embryo or fetus prior to this point? Is it true that for most people holding this position, the human embryo or fetus is of less value than an adult rat or adult baboon? Or is the prenatal human of considerable value, even if not of absolute value, prior to the development of a brain (at whatever stage that may be put)?

Unfortunately, both positions are all too frequently expressed in harsh simplistic terms, so that the unenviable 'either/or' choice is forced upon society. And this is where the third option – the fetus as a potential person – comes in (figure 16c). While this is not as clear-cut an option as the other two, and while it is expressed in different ways by different exponents and is also open to misunderstanding, it serves to emphasize that a middle way can be followed on the perplexing question of the status of the prenatal human. It emphasizes that, in practical terms, there is much we do not understand about both the biological development and the personhood of the embryo and fetus. The potentiality principle is not, of necessity, diametrically opposed to some expressions of the other two options, although it is not compatible with b(iii) and is probably not compatible with b(ii). Apart from these exceptions, it mellows the more strident expressions of *a* and *b*.

In Christian terms, our task is to determine which position (or even positions) can be utilized to express fundamental Christian aspirations regarding the embryo and fetus. I believe it is essential that the task is expressed in this manner, since the biblical data by themselves do not lead inescapably to just one of the positions. While they are frequently interpreted solely in terms of the view that the fetus is a person in the fullest sense of that term from day 1 of gestation, I do not believe that the biblical data take us so far. My reasons for this have been outlined earlier in the present chapter.

In practice the status we ascribe to fetal life reflects a mixture of theological, ethical and biological presuppositions. The duty of Christians is to be as loyal as possible to the diverse range of principles and teaching found in the Bible, allied to which are consistent ethical principles and reliable biological guidelines.

A Christian perspective must, it seems to me, start from the fundamental assertion that fetuses are human beings; they are genetically part of the species, *Homo sapiens*. Fetuses are one of us; or, perhaps more accurately, they are the earliest versions of ourselves.[36] Each one of us was once an embryo, and then a fetus. There is a continuity between the fetus and ourselves that we dare not deny.

Fetuses therefore, have a value in, and of, themselves, just as we have a value in, and of, ourselves. They achieve significance because they are one with us within the circle of humanity. The fetus throughout its development is important, and has both significance and dignity. There is a gap of profound dimensions between an unborn human and an appendix. An unborn human has the potential to become a fully-developed, mature human being, whereas an appendix has not. Once a fetus has been conceived, that fetus must be regarded with seriousness and concern. A new human life has commenced, and under all normal circumstances that life is to be nurtured and protected.

One aspect of our responsibility as human beings is to protect other humans, especially the weak and disadvantaged. Such protection should extend to the fetus which, in Paul Ramsey's words[37] is 'live enough not to be dead, not yet mature enough to be an infant, yet a human being enough to deserve protection'.

The question we are now left with is whether this protection should be absolute from day 1 of gestation onwards. Do the embryo and fetus, no matter what their stage of development, have exactly the same status as postnatal human life? Are there any differences between what we were as fetuses and what we are as adult humans?

Obviously there are differences between fetal human life and postnatal human life. Fetuses manifest few of the characteristics of human persons; their intellectual and rational abilities are limited or non-existent. They may be one of us, but they have yet to manifest the characteristics we expect of personhood and of beings made in the image and likeness of God.

If this argument is accepted, we can conclude that the embryo and early fetus are human beings, and have the full potentiality of growing into adult human persons. Useful as such a statement is though, it does not resolve the issue of whether the embryo and early fetus are persons, in the sense that we as adults are morally obligated to protect them under every conceivable circumstance.

What does the personhood of the embryo and early fetus amount to? In what ways do they, in their *present* state, demonstrate God-like attributes?[38] What value do they have in God's sight as embryos and early fetuses, especially when 50–70% of them (chapter 4) will never develop much further?

As we have already seen, Christians can be divided into three camps in terms of their position on the personhood of the fetus: all embryos and fetuses are persons, embryos and/or early fetuses are non-persons, or they are potential persons in that their significance is seen in terms of their potential for developing into mature persons (figure 16a-c). In these responses, there is of course very considerable overlap with the views of many others within society, although by and large, Christian thinking is biased towards fetal protection.

I believe that each of these positions is feasible for Christians, although each of them needs to be thoroughly worked out within a theological context. Before proceeding any further with this discussion, though, we need to clear a little more ground. And in order to do this, we shall have to consider again three topics dealt with in chapter 4; the moral significance of genetic uniqueness, pregnancy wastage, and the emergence of a functioning brain. In each of these cases, we need to ask what their implications are in ethical and theological terms.

Genetic Uniqueness
In chapter 4 I dealt in some detail with the limitations of the argument for personhood based on genetic uniqueness. My intention there was to demonstrate that this argument is not an infallible guide to what constitutes a person. While most individuals *are* genetically unique, some are not; moreover, of the conceptuses aborted spontaneously very early in development, some which are genetically unique could not under any circumstances develop into human persons. The argument from genetic uniqueness therefore, must not be made to say more than the biological evidence will allow it to say.

Quite apart from this, Christians need to beware of equating personhood with genetic uniqueness. Once this is done, the meaning of personhood has been radically altered. To reduce what we are as persons to what we are genetically is to involve ourselves in the most extreme form of reductionism. Granted that this is not what Christians intend, but if they are being consistent this is what they have ended up with. Human beings are more than their hereditary endowment, just as much as they are more than their brains.[39] While it may be quite correct to criticize those who equate the beginning of personhood with the emergence of a functioning brain, undue emphasis on the significance of genetic uniqueness demonstrates a similar uni-dimensional approach to the meaning of what we are as persons.

While our genetic endowment constitutes the biological foundation on which we are built, it is not more than this. The myriad facets of our experiences and learning that go to make us the actual persons we are cannot be overlooked in our desire to establish the personhood of early embryos. To do this is to lapse into genetic fatalism, by which we are predestined to be whatever is enshrined in our genes. It would be difficult to find any theological justification for this view, with its elevation of biological determinism and its downgrading of our actions and responses as the bearers of God's image.

It goes without saying that whoever is conceived by human persons is human, is a member of the species *Homo sapiens*, while most of such conceptions have the potential to develop into human persons. This, however, does not prove that all embryos and fetuses are persons in their present stage of development. In order to take this argument further it is essential to invoke the potentiality principle.

The genetic definition confuses potentialities with actualities.[40] Taken to its logical conclusion it equates the zygote with a person, since the zygote is bestowed with absolute value. But can the zygote bear this weight in practice? It is not a question of whether a zygote has the potential to *develop into* a human person, but whether it is *now* a person. But is this an example of claiming an absolute value for what has only relative moral worth?

Pregnancy Wastage

It is only in the recent ethical literature that any reference has been made to pregnancy wastage (often referred to as spontaneous abortion, one of its constituents), and then it has usually been in the context of induced abortion. The query raised by the enormously high levels of pregnancy wastage (see chapter 4) is whether this astronomically high natural loss justifies treating fetuses as inviolable. It is unfortunate, however, that it has proved all-too-easy to use this natural loss of fetuses as partial justification for deliberately destroying normal fetuses.[41] This I regard as a tragic misuse of the reality of pregnancy wastage. It is unacceptable to convert what is *natural* into a *moral* guideline. Simply because there are diseases 'in nature' does not mean that medicine should not attempt to cure them, let alone believe that it is obliged to induce them.[42]

Nevertheless, it would be short-sighted to overlook the significance of pregnancy wastage on this account. No matter how pregnancy wastage is viewed, it poses a major challenge to those with a high view of the fetus, and especially those who hold the view that a person in the fullest sense of that term comes into existence at fertilization. If this is the case, embryos or fetuses threatened with spontaneous abortion have just as much right to be protected as those threatened with induced abortion. Alternatively, if it is argued that fetuses are innocent and therefore should not be deliberately aborted, it would seem to be the case that fetuses about to be spontaneously aborted are equally innocent. On this basis arguments against the taking of fetal life by induced abortion should be matched by attempts to save fetal life that would otherwise be spontaneously aborted (attempts that go well beyond what is undertaken or even feasible by the medical profession at present). This is a necessary conclusion for all to whom fertilization endows innocent human lives with all the rights ascribed to persons, including a right not to be killed and a right to protection in life-threatening situations.[43]

From this it follows that those who ascribe to the inviolability of the fetus have a duty to do everything possible to prevent spontaneous abortions. Only in this way can innocent human life be saved. An adjunct of this is that medical research aimed at preventing spontaneous abortions should be given very high priority. Indeed, political pressure should be exerted towards encouraging research efforts to combat pregnancy wastage, as much as to opposing induced abortion. I am not advocating prolonging the dying process of irreversibly dying fetuses, but of giving serious consideration to ways in which research could transform condemned fetuses into healthy ones.

My intention in making these remarks is to underline the immense threat posed by pregnancy wastage to the fetus, particularly if the life of the fetus is thought to be inviolable. The question I am concerned with is whether the life of the fetus should, as a general principle, be given such an absolute status. Since, in the context of spontaneous abortion, the greatest loss of fetal life (approximately 60%) occurs within three weeks of fertilization, we are here considering the inviolable status granted to the early embryo.

Some dismiss this problem by comparing the prenatal loss of

human life to the high infant mortality rates in the Middle Ages or in developing countries in the 1980s. It is even suggested on occasions that these losses reflect the will of God; they are God's way of controlling overpopulation or of eliminating defects. However, if human life is precious, both categories of loss are tragic. To suggest that it is God's will that some humans should die (the prenatal ones) but that others should be treated and helped to survive (the postnatal ones) is to divide humans into two classes – one destined to die and the other to live. This is to do precisely what those who advocate abortion (however reluctantly) are accused of doing by strong anti-abortionists.

What we are left with is the loss of fetal life as a manifestation of a fallen world. There is however, a major problem with pregnancy wastage, and this is that the cause of the wastage in 50% of cases is chromosomal abnormality (chapter 4). To attempt to save every fetus about to be spontaneously aborted would mean allowing into life an astronomically large number (perhaps 2.5 million per year in the United States) of abnormal children. While this is not even feasible at present (even if anyone wished to do it), the question facing us is whether, theoretically and theologically, this would be justifiable. In this instance, to save life is to produce handicapped life. The 'protective mechanism' of spontaneous abortion would be overridden, thereby uncovering vast sources of developmental abnormalities. It is this element in the pregnancy wastage debate that makes it so different from efforts to decrease perinatal mortality rates, where to save life is (in most instances) to produce healthy, normal life.

This, I believe, is a strong argument against regarding every fetus as being inviolable. There remain many uncertainties in this whole area, and a great deal more attention needs to be devoted to it. Moreover, nothing I have written should be taken as an argument against devoting a great deal of money and effort to research on the nature and cause of chromosomal abnormalities. This, in turn, however will probably entail research on human embryos and it will certainly lead to genetic engineering. Whether those who espouse the inviolability of the embryo and fetus would wish to go in these directions is another matter.

We have reached the crux of the dilemma of pregnancy wastage. By its very nature it raises imponderable issues for the status of the embryo and fetus. For those with a high view of the fetus, but not an absolute one, it points to the urgent need for research aimed at reducing the incidence of spontaneous abortions and chromosomal abnormalities. For those advocating the inviolability of fetal life, it points in opposing directions – to the prevention of this wastage and the consequent birth of many defective individuals; and also to research aimed at combating chromosomal abnormalities, which by its very nature compromises the integrity of those embryos used in the research.

Emergence of a Functioning Brain

Use of the developing brain as the major criterion of when an embryo or fetus should be regarded as a person and therefore a protectable being is, as we have already seen, proving an increasingly attractive proposition for many schools of thought. However, at the biological level, the concept of brain birth has difficulties and it may not turn out to be nearly as helpful as is frequently imagined. It was on these grounds that I questioned the meaningfulness of the concept in chapter 4.

An ethical assessment of brain birth has to take seriously these scientific queries, and for this reason alone I have difficulties with it. There is, though, an additional factor to be taken into account. Once an embryo or fetus is designated as pre-brain-birth or pre-personal, it is removed from the sphere of human protection. The extent to which this occurs in practice will undoubtedly vary to a great extent, from those such as Donald MacKay who would probably afford it considerable protection, to those such as Michael Tooley who would appear to afford it little protection.

The difficulty lies in isolating the pre-brain-birth embryo or fetus entirely from the sphere of personal concern. This is something which does not occur when the fetus is regarded as a potential person, since in that case it always has some features of personhood. Once it is accepted, however, that it has none of the characteristics of personhood, it occupies a unique category. It has the possibilities of *becoming* a person; and yet this future perspective has no relevance at all for its *present* status.

It is this radical dichotomy between what a fetus (or embryo) *is* and what it *may become* that is intensely problematic. To class a living embryo as human material, in the sense in which an ovum or sperm is human material or a dead fetus is human material, is to miss completely the potential of the living embryo. It is for this reason that I cannot accept that a pre-brain-birth embryo is a non-person. This is a category mistake. Conversely, I cannot accept that the fetus is a person from fertilization onwards. As I have already indicated, this leads to major difficulties and is an anomalous designation that cannot be sustained in practice. This, too, is a category mistake.

What I am left with therefore, is a less-than-absolute stance on the personhood of the fetus. For me, this is summed up by the depiction in figure 16c. Although the potentiality of the fetus can be interpreted in a variety of ways, the conservative interpretation shown in this diagram accords with my own interpretation. This, I believe, is an expression of the biblical and theological views I have outlined in this chapter, and also of the biological data in chapter 4. I am not suggesting that this is the only way in which these data can be expressed, since any overall view of the status of the embryo and fetus is at best a tentative approximation of the complexities with which we are forced to grapple. What is essential is that any approach to prenatal human life should be a positive expression of essential biblical truths, should be consonant with our treatment of other human beings, and should be of practical value.

Fetuses in a Human Context
The diverse strands I have woven can now be drawn together and placed in the context of the real world in which we find ourselves. What are the implications of the principles I have been exploring? How do they help us sort out issues ranging from abortion-on-demand to research on the human embryo?

Fetuses under Threat
In an attempt to cope with attitudes towards the fetus, I shall put forward five propositions. The first is that *the taking of fetal life for reasons of social convenience is unacceptable*. Abortion-on-demand pays no regard to the value and dignity of the fetus, and is incompatible with any ethical system in which the fetus is seen as being one with us in the human endeavour. Our responsibility for such beings should lead under all normal circumstances to their protection. It is our duty to protect them from wanton and needless destruction. The recognition of

fetuses as 'the last of the unemancipated',[44] and some of the weakest and most defenceless members of the human community, leads inevitably to horror at the tragic slaughter of fetuses in which some societies are indulging.

Second, *fetal life is not of greater value than postnatal human life.* Opposition to abortion-on-demand need not be equated with absolute protection for the fetus under every possible circumstance. Human life in general does not receive absolute protection. It is true that the fetus is weak and defenceless, and therefore under all normal circumstances should be protected. But it is not only fetuses which are weak and defenceless. So are children brought up in impersonal institutions, beaten at home, malnourished in Ethiopia, enticed into smoking cigarettes or drinking alcohol by sophisticated advertising, or born with appalling physical deformities. The weak and defenceless are also young girls made pregnant by their fathers; and the men, women and children killed in modern wars, whether these be the many villagers killed in Vietnam or the far greater number who would be killed world-wide in a nuclear holocaust.

Any ethical system needs to pay serious attention to this endangered human life as well as that of fetuses. Although the wrongful taking of other human life is never an argument for the wrongful taking of fetal life, we must ensure that our standards pre- and postnatally have equivalent expectations.

My third proposition is that *the fetus is part of a human continuum extending from before fertilization and ending many years after birth.* The fetus, therefore, should never be made the sole object of ethical attention. In a fallen world there are often conflicting demands and interests, all of which need to be taken into account. All human life is precious, and as far as possible, our actions should bear testimony to the dignity and value of all individuals – fetal as well as adult; adult as well as fetal. Conflict will however, sometimes arise between the good of the fetus and the good of the mother and family, and perhaps even the good of society. Our ethical principles need to be such that they can cope with this conflict and still remain consistent with their underlying emphases.

In the fourth place, *embryos and fetuses are never just means to an end.* This principle assumes importance when research is contemplated on an embryo or fetus, and especially if an embryo is produced in the laboratory in order to be employed for research purposes. The respect due to the embryo and fetus suggests that we should be very careful before treating human embryos simply as a means to the end of the pursuit of scientific and medical information. The perspective I have developed leads to respect for an embryo for what it is now and prospectively. The early embryo is not nothing, even if it is not a mature human person. To isolate an embryo from its future dimension, and to treat it as though it was an end in itself *as an embryo* is to fragment the history of an individual human being.

From this it follows that *research on living embryos, with no therapeutic goal in view for the embryos concerned or even for embryos in general, can only be carried out by denying their possible viability and their potential significance as human beings.* Once this is done, however innocently by most researchers, no logically-consistent limits can be placed on manipulations of the unborn human. Of course, limits will be, and are now, placed on such manipulations, but of necessity some of them are highly arbitrary ones.

In the final analysis, we should be honest and admit that there is ambivalence, both ethically and scientifically, about the embryo and early fetus. We do not have a biblical warrant for undue dogmatism in this area; neither do we have sufficient scientific information for making categorical assertions. Faced with the mystery of our own beginnings, we begin to realize something of the mystery of human existence itself.

Innocence and Conflict

Fetuses are frequently referred to as being innocent, the implication sometimes being that there is a difference in kind between their moral condition and that of all other human beings. The difficulty with this concept is that it lends itself to viewing fetuses in a utopian context, thereby isolating them from the conflict inherent in the fallen world.[45] It is within this frame of reference that fetuses are regarded as inviolable. Within a world of conflict, however, this is impossible to attain. While the intention of those who maintain this position is laudable, and while we should not lightly discard this goal, fetuses are wasted in the natural course at a prodigious rate.

As I have repeatedly emphasized, this fact does not provide grounds for a low view of the fetus, and it certainly does not justify abortion-on-demand. Nevertheless, it is a reality with which we have to come to terms. Fetuses are no more inviolable than are postnatal humans. Both are part-and-parcel of a world in conflict; they are both destroyed and disfigured by disease, greed, envy, accidents, the unjust actions of individuals or societies, and selfishness.

Fetuses mirror what we *are* far more precisely than we frequently wish to admit; they, also, suffer from our greed and selfishness. They are one with us in the human endeavour; they benefit by our creativity and scientific expertise, and they are put at risk by our technological misadventures and short-term aspirations. As fetuses live with us, they experience the results of our faithfulness to God and our rebellion against him. In these terms they are no more innocent than we are. In a very real sense we can agree with the psalmist that they are conceived in iniquity (Ps. 51:5); the effects of mankind's rebellion against God affect them in their genetic make-up,[46] in the early divisions of the original cell, in their chromosomal patterns, in the uterine environment in which they spend the months of gestation, and in the ease or otherwise of labour and birth.

Fetuses are no more innocent than are infants and young children; both groups are weak and in need of protection. Moreover, both are owed the profoundest of respect because they are partakers with us of what it means to be human. In their weakness and defencelessness, we are called to place a wall of compassion and protection around them, and this we are to do to embryos, fetuses, neonates and young children. Similarly, we are to protect pregnant women, the handicapped and mentally retarded, the aging and the senile.

When viewed like this we begin to appreciate the appalling excesses of liberal abortion policies. At the same time however, we also begin to appreciate that fetuses are placed at peril by many other factors, and that fetuses themselves may place at peril other people within the human community (especially the mother). This is a manifestation of the human likeness that characterizes fetuses. If they were not so much like us, they would not constitute such a challenge to us.

If fetuses warrant our protection, which I believe they do, a host of ethical challenges emerges as a consequence. Some of these have already been touched upon. We are to strive to protect embryos and fetuses placed at risk by spontaneous abortion, although this will require a vast research effort and a major foray into genetic engineering. We are to do everything possible to bring about social changes that will lead to a reduction in induced abortion, in cigarette smoking and alcohol consumption during pregnancy, and also to a reduction in a vast array of environmental pollutants many of which threaten the health and welfare of embryos and fetuses. Yet another massive destroyer of fetuses and young children is malnutrition. And so one could continue, through the effects of teenage pregnancies, the consequences of atomic bombs and nuclear fall-out, and the insidious results of poor socio-economic conditions and inadequate housing.

To regard fetuses as innocent is to place them out of reach of the conflict inherent in the human condition. It is to make them something they are not. They are one with the remainder of us in the turmoil and grandeur of what being human is all about. They have the potential to be like us and to be what God would have us (and them) to be. They are not to be disposed of indiscriminately, even though as the earliest stages of what we are, they are in so many regards perplexing and ambiguous. It is no wonder, then, that the new reproductive technologies are themselves so perplexing and ambiguous.

6

Freedom to Bring Life into Existence?

Artificial Insemination by Donor (AID)

General Arguments
AID is a critical focal point within the debate on the new reproductive technologies. This may be surprising since it is not a new procedure and, compared with many of the other procedures in this area, it is technically very simple. Its significance stems from the acceptance it denotes of the use of a third party, that is, a donor. Hence, once AID is accepted as a legitimate procedure, there are no logically compelling reasons for denying ovum donations and possibly even embryo donations in IVF programmes.

Although AID is a widespread practice, it is very difficult to determine its extent. A few years ago it was estimated that well over 10,000 artificial inseminations (AIH and AID) a year were carried out in the United States. It has also been estimated that this technique has been successfully used in the United States about 300,000–350,000 times. In the United Kingdom in 1982, the Royal College of Obstetricians and Gynaecologists knew of over 1,000 pregnancies conceived and of 780 live births following AID in that year.[1] A recently published study for New Zealand[2] on the extent of AID between February 1982 and February 1983 revealed that 20 practitioners had received approximately 224 requests for AID, 159 women were inseminated with donor sperm, and 42 live births had resulted with a further 18 awaiting delivery.

Because of the response rate to the survey (68%), these figures are undoubtedly underestimates of the actual incidence of AID.

Arguments in favour of AID centre, as one would expect, on overcoming or at least bypassing the consequences of infertility. There is no doubt that AID enables a couple, where there is an infertility problem on the male side, to have a child they can bring up as their own and who is biologically the wife's child. Moreover, the wife has gone through all stages of the pregnancy, and so there has been bonding between mother and developing child. So, although the child is only 50% the couple's child in genetic terms, it is entirely the couple's child in environmental terms. This is also an important consideration where the husband does not wish to pass on a genetic defect to his children – where, for example, there is a history of Huntington's chorea on the male side of the family. AID may be contemplated by some couples in this situation, as an alternative to having no children of their own.[3]

When the trauma of infertility is coupled with the plethora of tests and clinical procedures the couple will have had to endure before the birth of the child, it is more than likely that the child will be loved and cared for. When viewed in these very straightforward and perhaps deceptively simple terms, AID should not be lightly dismissed as a serious approach to those desperately longing for a child. What makes AID even more attractive is that it is a relatively non-invasive procedure, requiring no anaesthesia or surgery. At this level of analysis nothing more could be asked of a technical intervention.

All the arguments are dependent on one basic premise, and this is that the source of the reproductive cell is of less importance than the love, care and nurture of children. In these terms, children constitute an essential element of marriage, so that the means by which they were conceived is of secondary importance.

Arguments against AID revolve around objections to the introduction of a third party into the marriage relationship. These objections are of two main types: one based on a particular view of marriage, and the other on psychological considerations.

For many, the introduction of a third party into the marriage relationship, even when limited to the sperm of an anonymous donor, means that a foreign element has intruded into what should be an exclusive relationship. The concern has frequently been expressed that this amounts to adultery, although the normal understanding of adultery is 'a breach of faith leading to the bodily sexual union of a married woman with someone other than her husband'. AID is not adultery in these terms. It has even been argued by proponents of AID that, since it is carried out with the consent of the husband, it is a mark of the stability of a marriage rather than the converse. Whatever arguments are employed, however, a third party is involved in the reproductive process, so that reproduction no longer depends solely on the generative capacity of the husband and wife alone. Whatever one's approach to this, there can be no escape from the fact that its acceptance entails nothing less than a complete revolution in society's attitude towards reproduction.

The second category of objection to AID centres on the reactions of the husband. He may reject the child on the grounds that the child may be a constant reminder to him of his own inadequacy and weakness. He may suffer from an acute sense of his own failure, and he may regard the child as belonging far more to his wife – the biological mother – than to him. He may also feel that he has failed his wife. These threats to the marriage relationship may outweigh any benefits stemming from the presence of the child. Such problems may arise, although equally well they may not. The issue is a purely pragmatic one. In practice it amounts not so much to an argument against AID, as to an argument for adequate counselling of the couple in preparation for AID and the birth of an AID child. It also has to be remembered that there are other family situations in which only one parent is genetically related to the child. An example is that of a step-parent, whose relationship to a child or children in a family may be perfectly successful (See chapter 1).

A very important consideration in looking at AID, as at all other reproductive technological procedures, is the position of the child. Perhaps the greatest danger here is a failure to cope with the secrecy surrounding the technique, and the deceit that is sometimes entered into by parents and family. Enormous care needs to be exercised at this point. The present difficulties stem in part from the legal position of AID, the question of the anonymity of the donor, the debate about what records should or should not be kept on AID births, and the nature of the information (identifying or non-identifying) which an AID child should or should not be able to obtain at the age of 18 or 20 years.

In general social terms, the issue raised repeatedly is the effect of AID on the couple and the child. Unfortunately, data are sparse principally because of the secrecy surrounding the procedure at all levels – from the anonymity of the donor to the desire of many couples to keep the AID a secret from their relatives and friends as well as from the AID child.[4]

An interesting investigation which throws some light on these matters is that of Snowden, Mitchell and Snowden from the Institute of Population Studies at the University of Exeter and published in their book, *Artificial Reproduction*.[5] In the early 1980s they undertook a study of 899 couples who had received AID between September 1940 and December 1980 in a service provided by one practitioner.

A total of 480 live children had been born through this AID service; 240 couples had one child, 101 couples had two children, 11 couples had three children, and one couple had five children. Although a considerable amount of data is available on the couples, including the number of inseminations, the rate of congenital abnormalities, reasons for discontinuing the AID, and the social class, age and marital status of the couples, these are of subsidiary importance for my purposes. Rather, I should like to concentrate on the effect of AID on the family.

For this part of the survey, the investigators succeeded in interviewing 57 couples who had given birth to an AID child between January 1977 and December 1980. The overall impression gained from the interviews was that the majority of the couples were extremely grateful for the AID child or children, and most had no regrets about their decision to employ AID. All the husbands and wives appeared to have accepted the children willingly and happily, and they found parenting particularly rewarding and satisfying.

When making the decision to have AID, most couples had also considered adoption. Most of the couples interviewed considered that AID was preferable to adoption, the main advantages in their view being that the child was more 'theirs' while in some instances the experience of pregnancy and childbirth was very important to the wife. Some emphasized that, while adoption was taking over responsibility for an existing child who had originated from outside their marriage, an AID child resulted directly from a decision made within their marriage. It was seen by some as being a social creation of their marriage, even if it was not a genetic product of the marriage. The child could also be passed off as their own child in a way in which an adopted child could not.

The major preoccupation of most couples was to ensure that people outside the medical profession did not discover they were having AID. This was because their overwhelming desire for children had driven them to meet this need by going outside the marriage relationship. Some of the fathers, in spite of their ready acceptance of the child, still experienced confusion over their paternity, while couples generally expressed concern that the donor's physical characteristics should match the husband's.

Of the 57 couples in this group only three had decided to tell the child of the AID conception when the child was older. Thirty three of the couples had told no-one outside the medical profession.

Another group of parents surveyed had AID children over the age of 18 years. Ten couples were interviewed, having 17 children between them the eldest of whom was 40 years of age. All these children were well loved and had brought considerable happiness to their parents. In seven of these families the AID had been kept a complete secret, but in the other three instances the children had been told. The reason for this was that the parents perceived that the children had a problem which could be alleviated by telling them the little they knew about the donor.

Seven young AID adults, who knew of their AID status from their late teens or twenties, were followed up in this study. The conclusion put forward by the authors is that these people were enjoying life and were happy to be alive in the realization that they owed their existence to AID. They were pleased to feel that their parents had wanted a child so badly that they had gone to the length of resorting to AID, and they were pleased that they were that child which had fulfilled their parents' wishes. The father/child relationship did not seem to have been damaged in these instances by the knowledge that AID had been utilized.

Ethical Analysis

The principal issues raised by AID centre around the introduction of a third party into the marital relationship. The third party, however, is represented by a product of a man's body rather than by the man himself as a person. Indeed, the donor has been carefully depersonalized in AID practice, so that there is no question of his entering the marital relationship as a recognizable person in his own right. In what way therefore, may a product of someone's body jeopardize the intimacy and mutual relationships of the marital bond? To take this further, it may be useful to compare gamete donation with blood donation or the donation of an organ. The donation of blood or an organ is a life-giving procedure, in which a person gives something of himself or herself in order to rectify a missing element in someone else. The donation of a gamete, especially sperm, is the giving of something of little significance to one's own life; in this sense, it means less to the donor than the giving of blood and much less than the giving of an organ. The effect of gamete donation however, may be much greater, since the end result is the production of new human life, rather than simply the repair of an existing life. Nevertheless, there are striking similarities between blood and gamete donation. The similarities between organ and gamete donation are less, since the giving of an organ, such as the kidney, is a self-sacrificial act, unlike gamete donation.

Another example of donation is adultery. In this case, a person enters the marital relationship as a person, and gives of himself to the wife. He not only donates his gametes, but also what he is and stands for as a complete person. A relationship is established, no matter how temporal and ephemeral. Adultery, therefore, is far removed from the clinical anonymity of AID or blood donation.

As we consider the spectrum extending from blood donation at one end to adultery at the other, AID appears to fit much closer to blood donation than to adultery. This does not mean that the two forms of donation can be equated, since we still have to face the significance of the donation of gametes. The element of new and future human life is implicit in gamete donation, and is this, in a sense, a giving of what one 'is' and 'represents'? It is certainly a giving of one's genetic uniqueness, or alternatively, a receiving of someone else's genetic uniqueness, into one's marriage. While this is not the same as the giving or receiving of gametes sexually and intimately in intercourse, the end result for the child is the same in genetic terms.

The donation of gametes in AID is made possible by the separation of the procreative and sexual sides of human existence. In more picturesque language it is the separation of baby-making and love-making. To a greater or lesser extent, all inroads into reproductive technology bring about this same separation. It is accentuated however, whenever a foreign gamete is introduced with the intention of producing an embryo. In this instance, the procreative aspect is no longer a product of marital love, since it would be non-existent without the foreign gametes.

Where, from a Christian angle, do we go from here? For some Christians, AID by mutual consent of married couples is not regarded as a moral evil. It may even be viewed as a great good in some instances, since it can be used to promote and preserve whole human personhood. Other Christians, emphasizing the third party element, recognize it as adultery in essence even if not adultery in fact.[6]

The conflicting opinions on AID within Christian circles have been well summarized by a Church of England Working Party[7]:

We differ . . . . on whether we see the genetic as the most basic manifestation of the personal and find the alienation of genetic parenthood from marriage a development which undermines the Christian understanding; or whether we judge that, although everyone is fundamentally influenced and limited by his or her genetic endowment, nevertheless the overriding factor is the social context which can assure proper love, respect and care. To this extent the question of genetic origin is not of fundamental moral importance, when compared with the question of how the child will be loved and cared for.

Enormous care must be exercised before approving AID. Its simplicity and innocuous appearance are deceptive. We should not accept the view that human beings can do anything they wish, and can solve all problems confronting them. Perhaps one of the supreme virtues is the ability, on occasions, to accept loss, inadequacy and suffering. This point has been developed by David Ison[8] in the context of marriage in the following way:

If the couple have promised to share all that they are and have, whatever that may mean, then they share together the infertility of one partner. The fertile partner in the marriage cannot procreate outside the relationship without refusing to share the whole life of the spouse, and is thereby refusing to accept the limitations their own marriage has placed upon them. AID breaks the exclusiveness of marriage in that it looks outside to find an alternative answer to the question of fertility when that already has an answer within the bond of marriage, unwelcome though that answer may be.

It is well known that marriages can be very successful even in the absence of children, although most would regard such marriages as deficient in a desirable element. The essential ingredients of a stable marriage, namely faithfulness between husband and wife and their love for each other, are nevertheless present.

AID introduces into the family unit only half an outsider, namely, a child carrying the wife's genes but not the husband's. In this regard, the child is more a part of the family than is the adopted child. However, in order to accomplish this, a biological bond between the husband and wife has been severed. AID involves therefore, a separation between the sexual and reproductive functions of the marriage relationship. This needs to be realized by all involved in AID procedures, whatever reactions it does or does not elicit in them.

The danger of this separation is that once human beings, and in particular procreation, are subdivided into a biological aspect that can be technologically manipulated, and a personal aspect that is above such manipulation, the integrity of human parenthood has been challenged.[9] This is not to argue that children produced by AID will not bring great happiness to a couple, nor that AID children will not develop and mature very successfully in the context of a loving and supportive family. The issue is principally one for society as a whole rather than for individual families. Widespread acceptance of gamete donations (including AID) could, in the long term, signify radical new directions for the family as we know it. This is a matter requiring urgent research, involving follow-up studies on AID children.

So far in this discussion, I have confined my attention to the third party element in AID. For many, this is the crucial one.

There are however, other factors to be considered as well. These revolve around the couple and their family, the donor, and the child.

In AID the husband and wife are participating in the social creation of a child – as opposed to the biological creation of a child. In this sense, they can legitimately refer to the child as 'our' child, since it is *their* decision that has resulted in the creation of a new human being. The child is, indeed, a creation of *their* marriage, as Snowden and Mitchell have clearly established in their book, *The Artificial Family*.[10] Novel as this is, it is the positive side of AID, and it is the element in AID that separates it so decisively from adoption. It is the stress placed on the husband's involvement in AID, even though he is no more than an onlooker biologically. When these two contradictory trends can be accepted by a couple, and especially by the husband, the creation of an AID child probably strengthens the marriage relationship. When this situation cannot be accepted at the personal level, the result may be disastrous for the marriage.

The effect of an AID child on a marriage appears to vary very considerably. It may provide the husband and wife with hope, even though the AID may not give them a child. On the other hand, the AID process or the AID child may be used as a weapon of attack and as a point of dissension in a failing marriage.

Perhaps the most contentious issue within the AID family (both the immediate and extended family) is the secrecy and deception of the AID. This is practically endemic within AID. Snowden and Mitchell[11] have written:

> It is this deception connected with paternity which is the source of all secrecy surrounding the practice of AID. It could be said that keeping the child in ignorance of its genetic origin, ensuring the donor remains anonymous, undertaking the AID process in a clandestine atmosphere and even keeping the fact of AID from friends, neighbours, and relatives stems from this fundamental issue of paternity.

The essence of the secrecy is that the husband of the AID mother wishes to be regarded as the *genitor* of the child as well as its *pater*, that is, the biological father as well as the social father. Whatever the reasons for this secrecy, it amounts to nothing less than deception.

It was pointed out in the previous section that the secret of the origins of the AID child are generally kept from all close relatives, and not just from neighbours, friends and the public at large. It has to be asked why this is the case, and what the repercussions may be for the child and family. While the legal situation concerning the donor and his responsibilities may be one reason for the secrecy, it is highly unlikely that this is the only reason. It may have to do with the feelings of the child in later years, the feelings of the husband, and the stress to the family associated with the stigma of conceiving a child in this way. The secrecy itself, however, may impose further stress on the family since the secret has to be maintained for an indefinite period of many years, and there is always the chance of a sudden disclosure of the secret.

Coping with stress of this order may be possible for a family in which the marriage is a strong one. Alternatively, many marriages may not be able to cope with it. There is also the far more general issue of the health of society. Although many individual families undoubtedly do handle AID children, and the secrecy surrounding them, very well, the issue of deception remains. These families are living with a 'lie', and this cuts to the heart of what normal family life in society is all about. This is deception on a grand scale, and it is being condoned by society. To quote Snowden and Mitchell again: 'The family depends for its existence on trust. Remove this basis for integrity and not only marriage and family life, but social stability is threatened at its very foundation.'

From a Christian perspective the institutionalization of deception must be seen as a very serious path along which society has embarked. This, just as much as the third-party element in the marriage relationship, strikes at the heart of Christian principles. The great difficulty with the deception is that it may be coped with perfectly adequately by some couples, whose marriages may be enhanced by one or more AID children. It is also true that AID could be practised more openly. Such a move, while in no way overcoming the objections of those who oppose it on account of the introduction of a third party into the marriage relationship, would remove one of the major difficulties posed by AID. This is because widespread deception threatens family life. The ready acceptance of the separation of biological and social parenthood, and the readiness with which deception is currently practised (even for the best of motives), means that the traditional family structure is being dispensed with.

This opens the way for lesbians and single women to have children by AID. In these instances, the aim of AID is to have a child in the absence of a husband. When used in this manner, AID becomes a means of dispensing with marriage, and – one imagines – the inconvenience of a husband and father.[12] It is not difficult to appreciate the ease with which AID can be used for a wide variety of social and philosophical purposes.

What emerges from this discussion is the complexity of the issues raised by AID. Far too little serious debate has been carried out with respect to this technique. Even the issue of the secrecy associated with AID has been trivialized. The desire to protect the anonymity of the donor is just one part of this question, and it needs to be distinguished from the confidentiality between the doctor ·and the AID couple, the secrecy within the AID family, and the secrecy between the family, their relations and society as a whole.

Relatively little attention has been paid to the *donor*, apart, that is, from the need to protect his anonymity. Excluding questions about the selection criteria of donors, and whether these have any implications for eugenic control, there are other serious ethical questions which have to be asked of the donor. Why is he willing to provide semen? Is he aware of the significance of this donation? Does he have no thoughts about the well-being of any resulting children? Does he have no moral responsibility for them? In the light of questions such as these, Dunstan has contended that, of all the people involved in an AID procedure, the donor is morally in the least defensible position.[13]

The donor is the biological father of the child, and yet he has no intention of ever acting as its social father. He deliberately removes himself from any such responsibility. The donor is viewing himself as providing a purely physical function, with no human or personal overtones for himself. Is this justified on the grounds that someone else is being provided with a service? Is it legitimate to allow the donor to be depersonalized in this way?

While it may be argued that donors come to no harm, little in the way of any data has been collected on donors. This also leaves unanswered the question of whether I, as a man, should care about what becomes of my genetic potential. Does it matter if it is used to provide a lesbian couple with a child? To approve the anonymity surrounding AID is to disclaim any responsibility for the ultimate fate of the semen or the resulting welfare of the child. Such a disclaimer must call in question any Christian view of human responsibility.

An offshoot of the donors' side of AID is the fee generally given to donors. Even if small, and ostensibly given as 'travelling expenses', it converts the donor into a vendor. Once again, this raises questions about the motives of such vendors, especially when the end-product is a new human life.

The AID child, as I have discussed previously, is a social creation. Not surprisingly, this child is a planned and a wanted child. So far, so good. By the nature of the situation however, the child is not the centre of concern – the couple who desperately want a child are. In many regards therefore, the AID child is not the object of attention, and it is for this reason that so little work has been undertaken in following-up AID families. It is also for this reason that the secrecy surrounding AID has been allowed to continue, with its overtones of keeping the child in ignorance concerning its origins.

We are back yet again at the question of secrecy. As long as this continues in its present form, there is no way in which adequate information can be obtained on the consequences of AID for the child (and later, adult). This is essential if society is to make an informed judgment on AID in terms of the resulting child. If we believe in the God-relatedness of all human beings, the AID child/adult should be of equal concern to society as the infertile couple contemplating AID. When the AID child's point of view is espoused, we must face the question of such a child's right to know something of its origins. At a time when adopted children are being guaranteed right of access to the names of their biological parents, on the grounds that their own interest demands it, is it legitimate to deny AID children the same right? As long as they are kept in ignorance of their status, there is no social problem. But there is a major ethical one, and this is accentuated by the fact that AID children have been *deliberately* created by society with an uncertain (and at present, unknowable) origin. This is virtually an unsolvable dilemma, and yet we ignore it at our peril.

The social and ethical complexities of AID are legion. It cannot be denied that the lives of some couples have been enriched by having children via AID; and yet the problems surrounding AID are almost unsurmountable. As a procedure, it appears to have been readily accepted by many within society, and while one may wish to condemn it outright, it is difficult to see justification for proposing that it be made a criminal offence. Even if it were, it would be impossible to police it. Its ethical and social ambivalence poses enormous problems, especially for Christians who need to be very careful that their condemnation of it does not also, by implication, amount to a condemnation of adoption, contraception, any form of reproductive technology, and even natural conception. Christians also need to beware that they do not judge the infertile much more harshly than they judge the fertile.

From what I have already written, it should have emerged that I am not convinced that there is unequivocal Christian teaching against AID. This is a reflection of the exceedingly complex nature of the AID debate. Although it is frequently narrowed down to an either-or choice, either the genetic argument or the social context argument, this is – I believe – an oversimplification. I believe it is unsatisfactory to condemn AID on ethical grounds in every conceivable instance in which it may be carried out within society; equally, I believe AID is not a viable option simply on the grounds that the resulting child will be loved and cared for. AID must be viewed within the context of both the family and society.

In the end, at a personal level, I come down against it. The reason for this is that I consider it is a superficial answer to childlessness, based as it is on the view that a couple's relationship is essentially a sexual and biological one, and that sexual intercourse is nothing more than a purely biological process. If this is all that sexual intercourse amounts to, the artificial, anonymous and impersonal aspects of AID are perfectly acceptable. It is a technological means of overcoming a problem rooted in a failure of biological or sexual functioning. Conversely, if sexual intercourse is regarded as more than a purely physical and psychological relationship, the artificial, anonymous and impersonal aspects of AID will amount to a threat to human relationships.

In these terms I hope it can be appreciated that AID may prove successful in individual families. Nevertheless, on a widespread scale, it has profound ramifications for society's view of the family. As a general principle, therefore, I am opposed to gamete donation as a routine response to certain forms of infertility.

In Vitro Fertilization – Simple Case

General Considerations
The IVF debate should not be viewed as an isolated pheno-menon in the biomedical arena. The ethical issues raised by this debate have much in common with issues being faced in many other areas concerned with the commencement of individual human life. They take us to the heart of the rela-tionship between much of modern biology and human society; they question the relationship between biotechnology and our perception of what it means to be human; and they bring us face to face with what, as individuals and as a society, we are prepared to trade in the pursuit of an improvement in various aspects of the quality of our lives.

Neither are all the issues raised by IVF new ones. Some, such as the moral status of the embryo and the twin issues of fetal harm and fetal consent, have been debated since the early 1970s.[14] Others, however, have emerged over the past few years or so, as the technical prospects in this area have moved rapidly into unexpected domains. Of particular interest in this context, is the multifaceted challenge presented by spare embryos.

The ethical context in which IVF should be discussed is not only that of the infertile couple, but also of the production of children by technological means. This may seem heartless, and possibly an irrelevant approach to those caught up in the despair and tragic helplessness of a couple longing for a child. I want to argue that the approach I am proposing is the only satisfactory one in the long-term. While it is true that the immediate context of the IVF debate is that of infertility, the power of the technology confronts us with questions about the nature, worthwhileness and usefulness of human embryonic material. This mixture of philosophical and pragmatic con-siderations cannot be evaded in the hope of short-term gains. The technological nature of IVF is inescapable.[15] It is a way around infertility rather than a cure for infertility. The tech-nological expertise solves the problem in a technological man-ner, so that each child produced by this technique – now and in the future – will have to be produced technologically. The solution to the human dilemma of infertility is being obtained by non-human technological means. This, by itself, is not a condemnation of the technique. Nevertheless, it is a movement in the direction of increased dependence upon technology. In the long run, this may have considerable repercussions for our view of our own humanness and of human relationships.

A specific consideration which needs to be raised at this juncture is the hormonal stimulation of women in IVF programmes, causing them to superovulate and produce a few ova in a single cycle.[16] The advantage of this in clinical terms is that a number of ova are available for fertilization. Once fertilization has been achieved, two or three embryos can be inserted in the woman's uterus in the current cycle, and – with the feasibility of freezing embryos – further embryos are available for insertion in one or more future cycles (if required). The attraction of the latter is that it saves the woman from having to undergo further hormonal stimulation, monitoring and a general anaesthetic in order to obtain further ova (although the development of ultrasound techniques for carrying out some of these procedures will dispense with the necessity of general anaesthesia in the future). The use of two or three embryos per cycle increases the likelihood of a pregnancy occurring, although the chances of multiple births (with all their disadvantages) are also increased.

An inevitable consequence of producing more embryos than may be required by the couple providing the gametes is the existence of 'spare' or 'surplus' embryos. If these are not required by the originating couple, they can be: (1) donated to another couple ('donated embryos'; 'prenatal adoption'); (2) used for research purposes; (3) dispensed with.

Since the present section is dealing only with what I have described as the simple case, that is, where the embryo inserted into the wife of the couple has been provided by the couple themselves, these possibilities are not of direct relevance. They cannot however, be ignored, since some decision has to be taken at some point about the fate of any spare embryos. What this illustrates is that the simple case of IVF in its true sense does not involve hormonal stimulation of the wife. It uses one ovum per cycle, and therefore one embryo per cycle.

The factor which has contributed to the production and use of excess embryos up to the present has been the lack of satisfactory techniques for freezing oocytes/ova. While early embryos (*e.g.* eight-cell embryos) have been successfully frozen and thawed for some time, the technique for freezing and thawing oocytes has just become feasible (chapter 1, footnote 2). When oocyte freezing becomes a viable option on a wide scale the clinical justification for fertilizing a number of oocytes at any one time will disappear. The simple case of IVF will then become far more attractive in clinical terms.[17]

Ethical Assessment
My discussion in this section is confined to the simple case of IVF.[18] The embryo is the couple's own embryo genetically, and no spare embryos have been produced. Reference to chapter 1 will confirm that, in genetic terms, this form of IVF is analogous to natural reproduction. No third party is involved; the child is the offspring of the husband and wife, who are its biological as well as social parents. The only difference between the two situations is that IVF is a technological procedure, enabling fertilization to take place away from the sexual domain of the human body. It is this which confers upon IVF its effectiveness in bypassing some forms of infertility, its power as a means of control, and its intrusion into the previously sheltered and protected world of human sexuality. Herein lies its hope for some and its repulsion for others.

The element of human control in IVF has elicited two quite different responses to the procedure. The amalgam of human intervention and a laboratory environment has led some to condemn IVF as dehumanizing, on the grounds that *baby-making* and *love-making* have been separated. Others however, have seen the planning as being supremely human, especially since an obstacle to marital and human fulfilment has been overcome.

It has been argued that the laboratory production of human beings is no longer human procreation, because the technological inroads have replaced the profoundly human characteristics of normal procreation. This movement away from the physical and sexual may deprive procreation of its human connotations, since it no longer involves the diversity of factors constituting human sexual love. This could well have implications for the family as a biological unit, because the wholesale transfer of procreation to the laboratory would undoubtedly undermine the justification and support which biological parenthood gives to the monogamous marriage. It has even been argued that once we start making human beings in this way, we stop loving them.[19] These are strong arguments against the indiscriminate and widespread use of IVF. However, those children who have been conceived by IVF have been the products of marital love. What has happened is that the meaning of marital love has been transformed. The failure of its physical side has deprived it of its full human connotations. Nevertheless, it is still love, and the birth of a baby via IVF gives it a physical side it could not otherwise have had. To argue that these desperately wanted children are little more than technologically-produced creatures bears no semblance of reality to the clinical situation.

IVF is a dramatic extension to the sort of interference found in delivery by Caesarean section, hormonal induction of labour, and AIH. It has to be admitted that there are major category differences between IVF and AIH on the one hand, and Caesarian section and the hormonal induction of labour on the other, since the former are concerned with bringing about conception, and the latter with making birth safer. Nevertheless, they are all illustrations of reproductive technology and, for most people, there are no objections to the other three as long as there are strong therapeutic grounds for their use. Each of them can also be used unwisely. IVF should never, therefore, be regarded as a routine procedure, even when it becomes far more widespread than at present.

An argument sometimes raised against IVF is that it is an artificial means of conception, as opposed to the natural means which is regarded as the only acceptable one. The concept of the 'natural' is, however, highly relative. If it is argued that it is not natural to have a baby by IVF, it is equally unnatural to use any technological form of contraception, to employ any medication during pregnancy to protect the developing fetus, or to vaccinate infants. Many facets of modern medicine are unnatural, and yet this by itself does not make modern medicine *per se* unethical.

It has to be accepted, of course, that, IVF is quite often a failure. Some couples who might be expected to benefit from it, fail to do so. The successes of IVF therefore, have to be balanced against the failures, those who are disappointed and frustrated at having their last hope of a child dashed. The human face of IVF is to be seen in this balance, not simply in the children born to happy and grateful parents.

I can see no inherent objection on these grounds to IVF, where conception by natural intercourse is impossible. This is because IVF enhances the procreative process as a whole. The potential of IVF lies in its ability to rectify a missing element in the union of husband and wife, so that it may be a legitimate means of healing in certain situations. Nevertheless, this does not justify its use as a way of bypassing the normal means of human procreation in the absence of a therapeutic rationale.

It can be argued, with some justification, that a technological form of reproduction is inferior to one involving the bodies and personalities of two individuals. If this is accepted, it should be resorted to only when 'natural' reproduction fails. There is no likelihood that either IVF or its technical off-shoots will become a panacea for human ills, because these technological innovations are as fraught with dilemmas as are other aspects of the human predicament.

There still remains a lingering doubt, and this revolves around the fate of the embryos utilized in IVF procedures. This doubt is a two-pronged one: the sacrifice of embryos during the development and continued improvement of the technique; and the dilemma about whether to implant an embryo observed to be abnormal in some way. The first problem has much in common with many clinical research programmes. In these, initial treatment using a new procedure in human patients is frequently relatively unsuccessful. The rate of success increases with experience as modifications are introduced in the light of the results obtained in earlier trials. This is ethically acceptable, as long as adequate animal trials have been undertaken before moving into the clinical realm, as long as the patient has been fully informed of the nature of the procedures and adequate informed consent has been given by the patient (or proxy), and on the clear understanding that there is potential benefit to the patient. While there are obvious differences between this general situation and that involving embryos in IVF programmes, there are also important similarities once a programme is well established, and on the understanding that the couple concerned are adequately informed about all aspects of the programme. It may still be argued that the very earliest attempts at IVF were unethical. The question then becomes whether that renders current (and, one imagines, all future) IVF procedures also unethical. This may well be a subject for ardent debate; if so, we need to ask what stipulations we apply in other areas. For instance, many have expressed concern at some of the circumstances surrounding the very first heart transplant operations; it is not often suggested, however, that present-day heart transplant operations are unethical on those grounds.

The associated dilemma is whether an embryo should be transferred to the woman if it is found to be abnormal. The concern here is that the disposal of such an embryo is the disposal (or, in the terminology of some, the killing) of a human person. Quite clearly, the issue revolves around the status of the embryo. However, even if one adopts the view that the early embryo is a human person in the fullest sense of that term, a number of points may be relevant. The first is that, at present, it is only possible to detect abnormality in an embryo if the embryo is not dividing; in other words, if it is dead. There must surely be no problem for anyone in that case. Of course, the time may come when it will prove possible to detect genetic abnormalities in an embryo. It would still be possible, I imagine, to allow the parents the final say, and allow them to opt for transfer of an abnormal embryo. In all probability, such an embryo would be aborted spontaneously relatively shortly after transfer (see chapter 4). The question must be asked, however, on what grounds would anyone make such a choice? By doing so, they would be sticking implicitly to the 'embryo equals person' dictum, and yet they would also be acting in the knowledge that this may bring a genetically disadvantaged child and adult into existence. In making this comment I am not prejudging the ethical acceptability or unacceptability of this choice; what should be realized, however, are its far-reaching consequences.

Putting together all the foregoing considerations, I conclude that IVF is legitimate in the simple case, that is, when the gametes are obtained from the husband and wife of a married couple. They should however, have already weighed up very seriously the pros and cons of possible childlessness and also of all the factors within IVF. A couple should not go unthinkingly in the direction of IVF, because it may be accompanied by far more tensions and difficulties than they had realized.

I view IVF as being ethically acceptable in the simple case because it allows a couple in a stable relationship, to have a child of their own; a child derived from their own bodies, an outcome of their commitment to each other. In this way, it serves a therapeutic purpose. This is an acceptable goal, but it must be seen within the context of family love and commitment. If it is used to allow everyone to have a child regardless of family ties and long-term obligations, it becomes a threat to family life.

These general conclusions are, I believe, equally applicable within the Christian context. The matter needs to be prayed about, and God's will needs to be sought for each *individual* couple. The goal for all Christian couples, regardless of their fertility or infertility, should be the service of their fellow human beings. We need to ask what God would have of us, and how we might best serve Christ who gave himself in the service of others. IVF in no way alters these fundamental equations.

And yet, some will still object. They will argue that it is the technological nature of IVF that constitutes the principal objection to IVF. What this amounts to is a rejection of traditional Christian attitudes towards the natural environment. According to these we are stewards of God's natural world, and as such are to develop and improve it for human purposes. We are to use the resources of nature responsibly, being constantly aware that these resources belong to God. We are involved with God in 'drawing out and developing the latent potentialities of nature ... controlling and humanising the natural forces that formerly oppressed humanity'.[20] In these terms it is not possible to rule out *a priori* alternative modes of human reproduction, provided that the intrinsic value of human life is recognized and preserved. This does not mean that all practical applications of this technology are necessarily good; they are however, possible and are subject to human control.

IVF brings us face to face with our freedom to bring life, by which I mean new individual human lives, into existence. IVF precipitates this issue because the new embodiment of human life stems from human ingenuity and the application of human intelligence and creativity. Human persons, who would not otherwise have existed, are brought into being as a result of a deliberate, rational set of procedures to bypass a pathological obstacle. Fertilization occurs as the direct result of an impersonal technique aimed solely at producing an embryo. The deliberate nature of the process and its scientific precision force us to ask whether we, as humans made in the image of God, are acting within our God-given mandate, or whether we are misusing our freedom and acting irresponsibly.

Before rushing to answer this, especially in the affirmative, we need to ask whether it is as major a departure as we might think from generally accepted ways of acting. To a greater or lesser extent, we exert control over the timing and frequency of conception. This reflects the freedom we exert over bringing new human lives into existence by entirely or predominantly natural means. Unfortunately, we often fail to realize the profundity of this freedom, or to appreciate its deeply religious dimensions.

In discussing IVF, it is easy to convey the impression that control over reproduction is exercised only when technological intervention is present. All too readily, the conclusion is reached that control equals technology, and both are against our best interests. It is sometimes suggested that any form of technological control over reproduction splits up the human person, so that we are made less than human.

These are damning indictments which are tacitly provided with a Christian veneer. Reproductive technology becomes an attempt by human beings to exert their autonomy and to proclaim their independence of the purposes of God. Reproductive technology comes to epitomize the endeavours of humanist man, in stark contrast to the Christian's emphasis on obeying the dictates of God.

But does reproductive technology, either in the form of IVF or contraception, inevitably lead to this end point? The fact that both IVF and contraception can be misused is not in question. This is true of all forms of technology; it is also true of all forms of human endeavour. But this is precisely what is to be expected of fallen human beings (see chapter 3). The difficulty with the anti-technology stance is that it isolates reproductive technology from other forms of technology; it also ignores all the non-technological ways in which we exert control over reproduction.

For those who reject technology *as a principle*, the rejection of all forms of technological inroads into reproduction is consistent. This, however, alters the argument completely, since IVF is neither worse nor better than microcomputers or nuclear power; contraception is condemned along with corneal grafts or pacemakers or artificial hip-joints. It appears though, that some regard reproductive technology as of a different character from automobiles or pacemakers or even microcomputers. Its human connotations have sinister overtones, although these are rarely spelled out in detail.

A related objection to IVF is that it may lead on to the other, even less acceptable procedures, and that we have no way of preventing this development. Such a contention is generally stated quite categorically, without any supporting data. If applied consistently this viewpoint amounts to a rejection of all technology, all forms of medical treatment, and even all scientific endeavours. Underlying this belief is a very pessimistic view of human beings, one that emphasizes their fallenness rather than their grandeur as creatures made in God's image. Such a view sees only the dangers of technology, and never its benefits.

How do we respond to the development of antibiotics? Do we focus our attention solely on their side-effects and the development of resistance by bacteria? Do we see the undue dependence of some on the 'wonders of modern medicine', perhaps at the expense of 'the hand of God'? Or do we recognize in them a revolutionary means of controlling a vast array of debilitating infections? Perhaps we may even say that they have proved a blessing – truly from God – as a way of improving the standard of health of whole societies, and the lot of millions of God's creatures.

It is not irrelevant to turn immediately from our response to antibiotics to our response to IVF. There are many similarities between the two, both positive and negative, and we would do well to ponder them. My point in making this comparison is to argue that we cannot accept antibiotics as a gift from God, and totally reject IVF as a gift from the same source. We would be unwise to use antibiotics for trivial reasons, and we would be unwise to consider employing IVF without very considerable thought and in extreme circumstances. And we may decide not to use either of them, just as we may decide to turn away from many other technological developments. Our decisions in these areas, as in all others, should be truly human ones – making use of all the information at our disposal, putting this decision in the context of our other responsibilities, and seeking always to serve others and to serve God.

IVF leads in directions we may not wish to go (see following sections), but these are not inevitable at the individual level. IVF also ushers in great benefits for some infertile couples, and in this regard it has much fewer ethical problems than AID. We should be grateful for IVF in its simple form, just as we should be grateful for surgical operations to combat cancer of the breast, stomach ulcers, or a ruptured appendix, and other procedures that provide limb prostheses or kidney transplants.

Neither is control over reproduction to be despised. An anti-technology fervour can lead to the advocacy of uncontrolled reproduction. The latter may not be a problem for the infertile, but it is a major one for the fertile. And it is also a major problem for Christians, with their high view of the individual, their emphasis on human responsibility, and the significance they place on the mutual care and concern that should exist between marriage partners. Procreation is just one outcome of the marriage relationship, and it needs to be seen within the framework of two people growing together, supporting one another, and serving others. It is within this broad context that contraception has to be placed, and it is within the same frame-work that any form of reproductive technology has to be viewed.

Control over reproduction is essential when marriage rela-tionships and responsibilities are approached in this manner, and when the neonatal mortality rate is low. This control may be technological, it may be 'natural'; the character of the con-trol is of secondary importance. What is important is that control is being exerted over the timing and number of child-ren a couple wishes to have. And such control is independent of the question of technology.

A final issue we should consider in this section is a couple's reasons for wanting or having children. When confronted by infertility, and a couple's very deep longing for a child, it is tempting to decry this and suggest non-technological means by which this longing might be satisfied. While this may be true (see chapter 8), we must beware of applying different stand-ards to the fertile and the infertile. The fertile may think little about their reasons for having a child (or another child), and the reasons – if verbalized – may be rather simplistic. The infertile, however, are forced to express themselves in poig-nant terms, and these may bring to the surface longings that give the impression of being self-centred.

Whatever we make of infertility, and whatever its cause in a specific couple, its effect is to curtail the freedom of the infertile in one very important part of their lives: they cannot bring new human life into existence. This brings us to the heart of what it means to be human, in that the control we normally exercise in one important aspect of human life is missing. Infertility is then, a religious issue, which raises questions of intense concern to each of us.

The desire for a child is not to be shunned, and attempts at overcoming or bypassing infertility are not to be dismissed as the whims of 'humanist man'. This does not mean they are to be satisfied regardless of marriage and family obligations, any more than other deep desires are to be automatically fulfilled. Nevertheless, the desires of the infertile for a child are to be treated with great seriousness.

It is at this point that an inconsistency frequently creeps into attitudes. For some, IVF and other reproductive technologies are suspect because they satisfy the longing for a child in a technological manner. Adoption, however, is not always suspect, although it too satisfies the longing for a child, albeit in a non-technological manner. I consider that the differences between these two situations are more illusory than real. As pointed out in chapter 3, the main goal of adoption in many of today's societies may well be to satisfy the desire for a child rather than to help a child who would otherwise be destitute or confined to an institution. To condemn the technological procedures while applauding adoption is to miss the crucial issue, namely, appropriate ways in which childlessness may be overcome.

The crux of the matter is therefore childlessness, the ramifications of which have medical, social, ethical, and theological implications. Some of these will be touched on in chapter 8. At this juncture, the point to note is that IVF can be just as legitimate a way of overcoming childlessness as is adoption. Each has its own set of ethical dilemmas, and neither should be embarked on lightly. Before either course of action is undertaken considerable attention should be given to alternatives, including the acceptance of childlessness, fostering, and the adoption of otherwise unwanted children.

In Vitro Fertilization – Spare Embryos and Donations

Spare Embryos

The question of spare embryos has become a crucial one in the debate on the ethics of IVF. It is no exaggeration to say that it has proved the catalyst to widespread opposition to these procedures.

The fertilization of two or more ova from a woman at any one time brings into head-on conflict pragmatic and ethical considerations. The pragmatic consideration that the simultaneous transfer of two embryos increases the possibility of successful implantation has to be balanced against the startlingly novel ethical question of our obligations regarding those embryos which are not transferred back to the woman from whom the ova were taken.

Clifford Grobstein[21] has summed up the ethical dilemma in this way: 'If it is moral to remove a human egg from a woman and fertilize it . . . . is it any less moral to do anything more to the subsequent early embryo other than to reinsert it into the uterus of its donor?'

A range of responses can be given to this seemingly straightforward question. We may contend that it is moral to carry out IVF, but that it is not moral to do anything with the resulting embryos other than reinsert them into the woman who provided the ovum. If we adopt this position, all ova removed from a woman and successfully fertilized will be reinserted.

On the other hand, it is argued by some that spare embryos do not warrant any particular protection and society is not obliged to bestow them with rights. Under these circumstances the spare embryos may be frozen and inserted in a later cycle into the donor, or they may be offered to another woman or to a surrogate mother, or they may be used as research tools.

Regardless of the use to which these embryos are put, the debate revolves around the issue of the status of pre-implantation embryos outside the maternal body. This, in turn, raises issues such as whether the pre-implantation embryo is a human being, a potential human being or potential person, an entity deserving limited protection since it manifests pre-individuality, or an entity deserving no protection at all.

These possibilities are a clear indication of the conflicting values of society in this area, a conflict that is far from a theoretical one. Whatever answers we give to these questions will determine what manipulations we are prepared to accept, and even encourage, on pre-implantation embryos. The dire urgency of these issues is highlighted by the use that is already being made of them for research purposes (see chapter 7).

The question of spare embryos cannot be separated, at the technical level, from the freezing (cryopreservation) of embryos.[22] There would be no spare embryos, if procedures were not available for freezing and subsequently thawing embryos. Cryopreservation of a pre-implantation eight-cell human embryo followed by thawing and transfer to the uterine cavity, with a resulting pregnancy, was first described in 1983. Techniques of embryo freezing are now able to preserve the embryo with a viability of 50–60%. The pregnancy rate following the transfer of a frozen thawed embryo is of the order of 7% per embryo transfer. Based on this data, each four- or eight-cell embryo which is frozen has a 7% chance of surviving freezing and of implanting after transfer. Some consider that the successful cryopreservation of human embryos helps overcome the wastage of spare embryos following hyperstimulation followed by fertilization of a number of oocytes. This is because a limitation in the number of embryos transferred per cycle is essential in order to minimize the risk of multiple pregnancy. It is also argued that the successful pregnancy rate following transfer of frozen thawed embryos increases the overall efficiency and success rate of IVF procedures.

Viewed in these terms, embryo freezing provides a means of increasing the clinical efficiency of IVF procedures in the simple case. Within this narrow confine, and excluding any consideration of the fate of spare embryos 'unwanted' by the originating couple, there appear to be no serious ethical objections to embryo freezing.

The dilemma from which we cannot escape, however, is whether it is possible to assess embryo freezing (and therefore spare embryos) within such a narrow compass. The couple who have provided the embryos will have to make a decision about the fate of any embryos they do not require. For them there is no escape from decision-making: about embryo donation, research using embryos they themselves have produced, or the discarding of such embryos. In the same way, the medical personnel responsible for the IVF programme, and any overriding ethics committees, will have to face a similar array of decisions. While these decisions may pose few problems for some people, this will not always be the case. Some on the medical side may welcome the possibility of having a ready supply of human embryos, on which research can be carried out. Indeed, it is more than likely that considerable pressure could be exerted on couples (if the final decision on the use of the embryos falls to them) to allow their embryos to be put to 'good use'. The discarding of spare embryos would probably be regarded as a waste of valuable human material.

This illustrates a danger that could well arise, namely, the overlapping of clinical practice (the use of IVF to achieve a pregnancy) and research (the use of IVF to increase understanding of certain developmental and reproductive processes). While this also occurs in other areas of clinical medicine, there are greater dangers in the overlap in this instance, due to the different nature of the consent required (consent regarding the disposal of an embryo versus consent regarding one's own future welfare or that of a child for whom one has continuing responsibility).

From this discussion it emerges that embryo freezing has repercussions not only for the couple's chances of having a child, but also for the embryo itself. It is for this reason that embryo freezing inevitably raises the question of one's view of the status of the embryo. The divergence of viewpoints on this matter within society cannot be ignored, since it will not be rapidly resolved.

Gamete Donations
AID has already been discussed in its own right. In general terms, it also serves as a paradigm of any other form of gamete donation. One's stance on AID will determine to a very considerable extent one's stance on the donation of ova and embryos. Nevertheless, there are some differences, and some account needs to be taken of them. Each of the two new forms of donation therefore, merits a brief discussion.

Unlike AID, both ovum and embryo donations are dependent on IVF. Each of them therefore, has to be viewed within the overall perspective of IVF. In most instances, the donors and recipients of the gametes will be, or will have been, in an IVF programme. When this is the case, the donors are themselves affected by infertility, and in this way are linked to the recipients (although in some instances ova may be obtained at operation when a woman's ovaries are being removed). At present, the donor's and recipient's cycles have to be closely matched for ovum donations, and so the strict anonymity of AID may not be possible.

1. *Ovum Donation.*

Ovum donation may be required for a number of reasons. The wife of an infertile couple may not have ova available or suitable (*e.g.* severe genetic disease) for fertilization. For example, there may be a congenital absence of ovaries, a congenital absence of ova or premature destruction of the ova within her ovaries, or her ovaries may have been surgically removed for a pathological condition thereby rendering her sterile. In ovum donation an ovum from another woman is fertilized with the husband's sperm and transferred to the wife's uterus. The wife will have been given hormonal medication to replace that which is normally derived from a natural ovarian source. The principle of this condition is analogous to the situation where the male partner is sterile because of his inability to produce sperm. In general terms, therefore, ovum donation is directly equivalent to sperm donation. In physiological terms, however, there is a difference in that the mother – in AID – has a direct physiological link throughout pregnancy with the offspring of her own genetic material; this is not the case in ovum donations.

2. *Embryo Donation.*

Embryo donation is relevant where the husband is azoospermic or where his sperm are incapable of fertilization; and where for her part, the wife has no ova of her own available for fertilization. The male and female gametes may be provided in the form of a spare embryo, or may be obtained from male and female donors and fertilized specifically for the purpose of providing an embryo for an infertile couple. Either way, we are dealing with the practice of 'prenatal adoption' (in contrast to 'postnatal' [conventional] adoption). Some argue that embryo donation has advantages over postnatal adoption, since it allows a closer relationship between the embryo and the couple through the wife and husband experiencing their own pregnancy. This is relevant because of the emotional bonding which is established prior to birth between the parents and infant.

Since ovum donation is directly equivalent to AID, there is little that can be added by way of new principles or insights. For those opposed to AID, there is no reason to believe that they will not be equally strongly opposed to ovum donation. Similarly, those in favour of AID will also favour it.

Although ovum donation will probably remain a relatively infrequent occurrence compared with AID, due to its dependence on IVF, it is neither more nor less forbidding than AID. Its dependence upon technology is greater than in the case of AID, but if IVF is accepted it is difficult to see why ovum donation should be rejected on these grounds. It will come far more into prominence when the freezing of ova becomes a widely available technique in many IVF programmes (see chapter 1). This will almost definitely transform the procedure into a feasible proposition, although it will remain limited due to its basis in IVF.

Embryo donation is tantalizing in its similarities to adoption as we generally conceive it. The most straightforward case is provided by a 'spare embryo' from a couple in an IVF programme. This embryo was originally a wanted embryo, since it was produced in an attempt to provide a couple with a child. It has, however, turned out to be superfluous to their requirements. What is to be done with it? Or, perhaps, the question should be rephrased, and we should ask, what is the most appropriate fate for this human material in terms of its potential for full personhood?

It is possible to escape from this dilemma by stating that surplus embryos should not be produced. I consider this to be the ideal situation. Nevertheless, if society determines that surplus embryos can be produced, at least under certain circumstances, there is no avoiding the predicament.

I shall deal with the research side of the issue in the next chapter. This still leaves two possibilities: embryo donation, or discarding the embryos. It is not my intention to pit the one against the other, since this would be a false choice. This is not to deny, however, that situations may arise where such a choice has to be made.

The similarities between embryo donation (prenatal adoption) and postnatal adoption (adoption in the conventional sense) stem from the 'wantedness' of a human organism (embryo or child). The adoption of an embryo enables the adoptive mother to experience the developing organism within her throughout gestation, an experience denied the adoptive mother in postnatal adoption. The mother is also able to give of herself to the developing fetus, since its environment is that of her own body. In many respects therefore, she provides for that fetus in the most profound of all ways. She is not the genetic mother, but she is the carrying and nurturing (social) mother. The adoptive father too is able to make a more direct contribution to the growing fetus than would ever be possible when adopting a child.

The principal motive for embryo donation (prenatal adoption) would undoubtedly be the longing for a child. There could, however, be a subsidiary humanitarian motive – the desire to give 'human life' to an already existing human embryo. In these regards, this form of adoption would have much in common with conventional adoption. However, the humanitarian side has an interesting twist – if an embryo is not provided with this particular opportunity for life (by this or another couple), its alternatives are non-existence (discarding) or use as a research tool. Neither alternative is in the individual embryo's best interests. With postnatal adoption, the alternatives for the child, apart from adoption by another couple, are either being fostered or spending much of his or her childhood in an institution. The alternatives may or may not be in the child's best interests, but they are not death. The anachronism about postnatal adoption in many Western societies today is that the child will not be as well provided for (from the point of view of life in a family) if it is already medically or culturally disadvantaged in some way.

For those who emphasize the fully personal status of pre-implantation embryos, it would seem that embryo donation should be the course to be preferred. Given the prior existence of these embryos, and the fact that they are no longer wanted by their biological 'parents', embryo donation appears to have much to recommend it. It may even be regarded as obligatory, if pre-implantation embryos are to be treated precisely as children and adults are to be treated. A corollary of this is that active steps should be taken to find adoptive couples for surplus embryos.

This pressure in favour of embryo donation (prenatal adoption) does not apply to those with a different view of the human embryo. If the pre-implantation embryo is regarded as of little intrinsic value, then clearly the fate of the embryo *for its own sake* is of no great concern, and can never justify prenatal adoption. If this form of adoption is advocated, it will always be from the point of view of the prospective adoptive parents, since it is a means of providing them with a child. This situation should be a salutary reminder that it is possible for adoption (pre- or postnatal) to be undertaken when the interests of only one of the interested parties is taken into account.

For those who, like myself, hold to a high view of the dignity and potential of the pre-implantation human embryo, but who do not equate it with full personhood, the question will be asked whether embryo donation is akin to sperm or ovum donation. Does it intrude into the marriage relationship, as they do? Would it be surrounded by the degree of secrecy and deception surrounding AID? How easy would it be to tell the child of his or her origins? What information would be kept about the couple donating the embryo, and would the child be in a position to make contact with the genetic parents? Would the genetic parents even contemplate this possibility at the time of allowing a surplus embryo of theirs to be used to assist another woman in an IVF programme?

Questions such as these begin to place embryo donation in a broader human context, into which the interests of the resulting child as well as of the genetic parents can be incorporated. Experience in tackling these issues is non-existent at present, and we would do well to hesitate before rushing in this direction.

While it is true that there is no intrusion of a third party into the marriage relationship in this case, there is certainly intrusion – of third *and fourth* parties. Embryo donation takes much further than any other procedure the separation of biological and social parenthood – a point which those who advocate embryo donation on the grounds of the inviolability of embryonic life would do well to note. For them, the conflict between two fundamental principles comes to a head with this procedure. Although it is true that the adoptive parents are on equal terms genetically with their child – neither has any genetic stake in him/her – they have allowed into the heart of their marriage an outsider. The question this raises is whether this particular intruder is a foreign element hostile to the exclusivity of the marriage relationship. It also raises the question of whether the wife is not, in essence, acting as a surrogate mother for the genetic parents – even though there is no intention of handing the child back (but will that ever happen?)

The good of the child, and of the genetic parents, dare not be overlooked by those searching for a Christian perspective on this matter. The dilemmas for the child have much in common with those experienced by the AID child, and they will not be repeated here. What is new however, is the position of the genetic parents. We need to ask in what ways they compare with a couple (or mother) giving up a child for adoption. On the face of it, the situation is totally different.

There is neither an unwanted child, nor one that cannot be adequately cared for; there is no lack of concern for an already existing child, nor for a fetus well on its way to postnatal existence. What there is, is an embryo with no potential for any further development unless it is placed in a woman's uterus; an embryo which was brought into existence in an attempt to give a couple a child of their own. This embryo is not an unfortunate end result of irresponsible sexual activity, but is an integral facet of the processes by which this couple may obtain a child. In this way it has far more in common with the natural means of conception, involving an enormous wastage of embryos (see Chapter 4), than it does with normal adoption.

Our response to this will inevitably depend on the status we ascribe to the human embryo. My intention in drawing out some of the issues is to emphasize the major differences between the situations of the genetic parents involved respectively in pre- and postnatal adoptions. Somehow these differences will need to be taken account of by those advocating embryo donation (prenatal adoption).

The discussion up to this point has dealt exclusively with embryos surplus to the requirements of a couple in an IVF programme. Embryo donation, using embryos specifically produced for this purpose from donated gametes, raises quite different considerations. I shall refer to this as *anonymous embryo donation*. In this instance, an embryo is being specifically *created* in the laboratory from the sperm and ovum of unrelated people, in order to be passed on to another couple. There is no personal interaction of any nature or at any level between the biological parents who, in turn, have no personal concern for the would-be social parents.

The process by which this embryo is brought into being has therefore been drained of all personal connotations, reducing it to an impersonal, technological transaction. Nothing truly human remains, all vestiges of human – let alone marital – relationships having disappeared. The transfer to a woman's uterus of an embryo produced in this manner can hardly be described as adoption, since the deliberate nature and reductionism of the procedure have drained it of all the range of meaning normally enshrined in the concept of adoption. There is no hint of humanitarian concern on the part of the prospective social parents, since their desire for a child has led to the deliberate manufacture of one in the absence of marital, social, or any normal human obligations.

A human embryo produced under these circumstances and for this purpose is an illustration of the excesses to which technology can be put. It highlights the way in which a human organism can be dehumanized, since it is being treated as an impersonal 'thing', and is serving the ends of someone else. Condemnation of anonymous embryo donation is not dependent on one's view of the status of the human embryo; it is an infringement of how human material (rather than just a human person) is to be treated.

Other concerns stemming from anonymous embryo donation centre on the welfare of the resulting children. This brings us once again to the dilemmas previously discussed in connection with AID, especially to the secrecy aspect and the question of whether there will be any provision for informing the children of their origins. The types of problems encountered with AID are intensified in this instance, and even if information were to be made available to the children the anarchic nature of their origins may have profound repercussions for their social and psychological development.

There are limits to the ways in which technological abilities are to be utilized, and these have to be determined by the human context in which the abilities are to be exercised. In this instance the *benefits* to the prospective parents (having a child) are to be weighed against the *losses* to the resulting child (conceived in the absence of any meaningful human relationships, and with an impersonal set of origins). Even if the prospective parents' motives are laudable, the means employed of achieving their desires are impersonal and clinically anonymous at almost every level. In this, there are similarities to

AID and ovum donation, but in the present instance the process of anonymity has been taken a step further. In those cases, an attempt is made to enhance the marriage relationship by using the gametes of one of the marriage partners. In this case, the gametes of neither marriage partner are involved. Neither has the embryo been conceived by (or for) another married couple (as in prenatal adoption). Anonymous embryo donation, therefore, even more than AID and ovum donation, demonstrates that there need to be limits to the lengths to which individuals and societies should go in overcoming childlessness.

Surrogate Motherhood

General Considerations

Surrogacy takes us further into the means that can be used to alleviate infertility. While it is not exactly the converse of AID, it is not unreasonable to look at it as such. The defect in this case is with the wife, who is unable or unwilling to conceive or is incapable of carrying a child to term. IVF can also be combined with surrogacy to overcome a fertility problem in the husband as well; this introduces a second form of surrogacy. In order to simplify terminology, it is most convenient to refer to the husband and wife of the infertile couple as the commissioning parents, and the third party, that is, the surrogate mother, as the carrying mother.

The classical form of surrogacy (partial surrogacy) is where the surrogate mother is also the genetic mother of the child; the husband of the commissioning parents provides the sperm, and so he is the biological father (see chapter 1). The classical form may or may not utilize artificial insemination.

As we saw in chapter 1, the combination of IVF and surrogacy (full surrogacy) means that an embryo from the couple wanting the child can be transferred to the surrogate mother, who then carries the embryo/fetus to term. Under these circumstances the surrogate mother is not genetically related to the fetus. I shall return to this distinction between the two forms of surrogacy in the next section.

Conditions from which the wife may suffer and for which surrogacy could provide a way forward include the lack of a uterus, severe pelvic disease, and a history of repeated miscarriages. It may also be contemplated where it is inadvisable for the woman to go through a pregnancy for medical reasons.

Surrogacy fills most people with alarm and horror. The overtones of purchasing a baby and of 'paying another woman to have my child' are grim and forebidding. The commercialization surrounding private agencies set up to provide this service, and the ever-present possibility of exploiting psychologically desperate infertile couples and financially destitute fertile women, have ensured that the whole topic of surrogate motherhood is clothed with mystery and intrigue. And yet I believe it has to be treated seriously, since it is one particular extension of the donation of genetic material. What happens in surrogacy is that it is not only genetic material that is donated (in partial surrogacy), but also a woman's body and whole person for the nine months of pregnancy.

Arguments adduced in favour of surrogacy stem from the hope it offers some couples of having a child genetically related to one of them (or, in full surrogacy, to both of them). It is a means by which the husband of an infertile woman can have a child, and is analogous to the means offered by AID for allowing the wife of an infertile man to have a child.[23] It can even be argued that if some infertile couples are given the chance of having children via technical procedures such as AID and IVF, it is discriminatory to deprive other couples of having a child at least partially their own via surrogacy.[24]

Although discussions of surrogacy are frequently conducted almost exclusively in terms of the financial gain of the surrogate mother, this need not be a predominant feature of the transaction. It is possible, therefore, to view the surrogate mother as a supreme example of self-sacrifice and altruism. The surrogate mother is prepared to accept the risks and constraints of pregnancy in order to help another woman.

While it would be generally conceded that the possibility of exploitation of the surrogate mother is a legitimate fear, it is also argued that this is not inherent in a surrogacy transaction. Where there is voluntary entry into such a transaction, surrogacy may not be as degrading as often suggested, especially if the payment covers costs rather than amounting to profit.

The arguments against surrogacy can be divided into those arguments also used against other procedures intruding into the marital relationship, and those specific to surrogacy. Opponents of any form of gamete donation will also oppose surrogacy on account of the introduction of a third party into the exclusive nature of the marriage bond, although in the case of full surrogacy this does not entail the intrusion of genetic material.

Opposition to surrogacy however, is much more widespread than this, since many who are prepared to accept the legitimacy of AID are unhappy with surrogate motherhood. The additional reasons for opposing surrogacy concern (1) the nature of the process itself, (2) the welfare of the surrogate mother, and (3) the welfare of the surrogate child.

1. *The Nature of the Process.*
    The distinction made between AID and surrogacy is the distinction between the impersonal donation of sperm – a product of one's body – and the highly personal giving of one's own body in pregnancy. It is this giving of oneself for another, in all probability for financial gain rather than in devotion to another, that is seen as demeaning and dehumanizing. The process itself is far more intimate and personal than any other form of donation, making surrogacy in the eyes of many of its opponents qualitatively different from the other reproductive techniques aimed at combatting infertility.

2. *The Welfare of the Surrogate Mother.*
    Closely allied with this objection to surrogacy is the objection concerned with the welfare of the surrogate mother. She is exposed to the risks of pregnancy for financial reasons, while she herself may also be affected by a deliberate misuse of pregnancy. The surrogate mother has voluntarily undertaken to bear a child, which she is contracted to give up at birth. In doing this she is allowing herself to be used as little more than a human incubator for someone else's child. Whatever the motives, it may be very difficult in practice to avoid such a relationship acquiring exploitive overtones. This is because financial interests are generally implicated in surrogacy arrangements.

3. *The Welfare of the Surrogate Child.*
    The welfare of the surrogate child is very much an unknown factor. The inevitable queries concern the consequences for a child of the knowledge that its genetic mother

deliberately produced it for its social parents, or equally, the knowledge that its social parents were prepared to have it brought into the world by another woman. An additional dimension is the knowledge that this transaction was a financial one; the child was bought by its social parents. Then there are difficult questions: Who is the child's mother? Why would the father go to these lengths to procure a child? Difficult as such questions are, they would be intensified if the surrogacy had been carried out to provide a single person or a homosexual couple with a child.

These considerations do not take into account the horrendous legal dilemmas of surrogacy, nor do they touch on the legal and psychological problems presented by a surrogate mother who refuses to hand over the child, or commissioning parents who reject a handicapped child. Basic to so many of these issues is the fundamental question of whether ultimately surrogacy is simply an illustration of one group of people – the commissioning parents – treating another group of people – the surrogate mother and the surrogate child – as a means to their own ends.

Ethical Assessment
Any analysis of surrogacy follows very closely on that of IVF and AID. Condemnation of both these leads inevitably to condemnation of surrogacy. Acceptance of IVF in no way warrants surrogacy. But what about acceptance of AID? Does this lead logically to an acceptance of surrogacy? As I have indicated, this is not the case since many regard surrogacy as having within it an exploitive or manipulative element from which it is virtually impossible to escape. An additional reason against surrogacy is that the relation of a child to the woman who carries it is extremely close, very much closer than is the relation of a child to its father. Hence the contrast between surrogate motherhood and AID.

However numerous our objections to surrogacy, a central one is the deliberate breaking of that intimate relationship between the biological or carrying mother and the child. Relationships are critical to what we are as human persons. Surrogacy therefore places the development of a crucial relationship in jeopardy, and it does this intentionally. Whatever the motives, surrogacy in the vast majority of instances is placing at stake one important aspect of human personhood. This is a very high price to pay for providing an infertile couple with a child.

Surrogacy arrangements generally stress that the surrogate mother cannot withdraw from the agreement. Once she has embarked on this course of action, for her there is no turning back. Understandable as this is from the perspective of the commissioning parents and the lawyers, it is an infringement of the woman's freedom. We should realize that she is not being asked to abide by a simple contract, but is being constrained to forego one of the most precious freedoms she possesses, that of expressing her humanity by rearing the child which she has nurtured throughout pregnancy and to which she has given life. This is of the essence of what a woman is as a human person created in God's image. To expect her to commit herself in advance to give up a child at birth, whatever the method of that child's conception or the reasons for it, is to demean her as a human being.

Such a restriction on a woman's reproductive functions is something we do not expect of a woman giving up a child for adoption. Freedom of choice has to be allowed, however awkward this may prove for those desperate for a child. This is simply a reflection of the Christian perspective that all involved in complex reproductive arrangements are human persons. This is true whatever we may think of some of these arrangements.

Contracts restricting the freedom of choice of the surrogate mother are therefore inimical to what she is as a being in God's image. This, it seems to me, is why any legal contract in surrogacy is unethical, and it applies regardless of the commercial nature of such contracts.

It may be asked whether surrogacy can occur within an extended family setting, undertaken perhaps between sisters or friends.[25] This is in contrast to surrogacy in the usual sense where the surrogate mother is unknown to the commissioning parents. The distinction is between surrogacy for compassion in the first case, and surrogacy for money in the second. Where relatives or friends are involved, the question of a rigid, legally enforceable contract does not arise. In this instance there may also be a meaningful relationship between the surrogate mother and the growing child, even though the child is no longer regarded as hers.

This is not an argument in favour of surrogacy, but this is a distinction that should be taken into account when generalizing about surrogacy. Surrogate arrangements, however informal and even when carried out within a 'family' context, are fraught with dangers and are never to be encouraged. Nevertheless, some cultural groups with close-knit communities may indulge in surrogate arrangements and yet would not approve of any of the new reproductive technologies. Such surrogacy is very far removed from the lucrative financial arrangements that make headlines and have all the makings of exploitation.

The welfare of the surrogate mother also needs to be considered from another angle, and this is her own reaction to the loss of 'her' baby. Far too little attention has been paid to this, or to the guilt and despair she may experience in later years. While the reactions of surrogates will undoubtedly vary, the loss of the child is as real for her as for the woman whose child has been adopted or the woman who has had a still-birth. In partial surrogacy, the surrogate is the biological mother. To dismiss her as anything less than this is to refuse to acknowlege her humanity, even if she voluntarily took on the role of surrogate with the most elevated of motives. This also highlights the difference between surrogacy within a family situation where the woman can change her mind, or where she will continue to have contact with the child, and commercial surrogacy where the break with the child is complete and final.

Full surrogacy, in contrast to partial surrogacy, introduces a complete divorce between the surrogate's carrying role and her genetic involvement. The child is no longer 'hers' in the genetic sense, although in order to accomplish this she has been depersonalized even further. She is now a human incubator.

One's response to this depends on one's response to the practice of surrogacy. If it is approved of, the elimination of the genetic component enhances the surrogacy element – the woman carries the child and nothing more. On the other hand, if surrogacy is disapproved of on the grounds of the depersonalization of the woman, full surrogacy is seen as accentuating the depersonalization process.

Full surrogacy therefore highlights one's view of the status of the woman as a human person. To approve of it is to assent to a procedure which allows one person to be put entirely at the disposal of another person or group of people. The fact that the woman is willing to act as a surrogate is beside the point; she is still being placed in a situation where her ability to fulfil a particular function is regarded as of greater importance than her status as a person. For society to approve such a situation (since this is within the framework of an IVF programme), is tantamount to accepting that some of its citizens are of less significance than others.

The technological imperative manifested by full surrogacy demonstrates the dangers of technology in the absence of an ethical imperative. Technological efficiency demands full surrogacy, but the cost in human terms is considerable. This is the case even without taking the child and its future into account. To move in the direction of full surrogacy is to be prepared to move in the direction of unfettered technology, with its threat to the meaning of human existence.

What this also shows very clearly is that there are limits to the lengths individuals and society should go to overcome childlessness. In the final analysis infertility and childlessness have to be seen as integral facets of human life as we know and experience it. We should not hesitate to assist infertile couples to have a child if it is at all possible, but there are limits to this endeavour, and the limits we set will reflect our priorities and will tell us a great deal about our presuppositions regarding human life. For me, these limits will demonstrate the importance of human relationships, the fact that marriage is worthwhile even in the absence of children, and the necessity for Christians to live in the light of God's promises and faithfulness rather than at the level of technical necessity. While it is undoubtedly desirable to enable a couple to have a child of their own, this is neither necessary nor essential for their lives as God's people.

7

Freedom to Manipulate Human Life?

Introduction

The realm of human prenatal research is a forbidding one, not only because of the innate complexity of the problems, but also because of the paucity of time over which these problems have been debated. However powerful and useful the traditions we have inherited in Western medicine, however precise the ethical principles devised by theologians and philosophers, we still find ourselves in a perplexing no-man's land between the traditional and the novel, between the accepted canons of our society and the unnerving technological wizardry of brash young biologists. The ethical literature in this area is sparse, with serious ethical analysis of human fetal research emanating from the early 1970s, and of human embryonic research from the late 1970s. Although current interest centres principally on research on the human embryo, it needs to be viewed against the background of discussions that have taken place concerning fetal research. This is important background information, since it provides helpful guidelines for principles and attitudes in the domain of the embryo.

I shall turn initially, therefore, to fetal research. My aim is not to analyse this issue exhaustively, or to come to any definitive conclusions. Rather, I wish to explore the nature of the questions and answers raised by the older fetus, as a prelude to a discussion of the questions raised by research on the embryo.

Definitions of the terms *embryo* and *fetus* and of *previable* and *viable* have previously been given in chapter 4. It should be noted that in the literature the term 'fetus' may be used to cover the period from implantation to birth, or even from fertilization to birth, rather than from eight weeks of gestation to birth. Definitions of viability vary, and all of them are arbitrary and subject to change. They may depend on age and weight, the viability line (in many discussions on the ethics of fetal research) being placed at 20 weeks gestation and a weight of 400 grams (300 grams in some definitions), and possibly on length (25 centimetres from crown to heel). Alternatively, it may be defined in functional terms, a 'viable fetus' being one capable of functioning as a self-sustaining whole, and being capable of independently maintaining its vital functions. Such a fetus will demonstrate a heartbeat, and its lungs will be capable of being inflated. These definitions of viability are a mixture of precision and imprecision, and yet they are among the best available at present. Once the notion of viability has been settled, at least for the time being, previability covers any fetus that fails to meet these criteria. Once research on the previable fetus is contemplated, however, it is essential that any definition of previability should err on the conservative side.

I am employing the term *research* to cover all aspects of the scientific study of embryos and fetuses, the object of the study being to discover new data and to formulate new ideas concerning how embryos and fetuses function. Research of this nature may simply involve observations of the growth and development of fetuses in different groups of pregnant women (*e.g.* in malnourished, compared with well-nourished, populations; or in one group of pregnant women receiving a particular treatment thought to aid the fetus in some way, against a similar group of pregnant women receiving a placebo), or by the use of ultrasound procedures may follow fetal growth in a large population of pregnant women. Another form of research is confined to a study of dead embryos or fetuses, in an attempt to learn more about the structure or functioning of tissues at various developmental ages and in different pathological states. This latter type of research is the domain of preclinicians and pathologists, and it may yield much useful information. In all these instances, it is possible to carry out a wide variety of research projects on fetuses, without in any way interfering with the normal development of individual fetuses.

Some research projects, however, also include deliberate

interference with the manner in which an embryo or fetus may develop. These usually involve the comparison of control and modified (experimental) groups. By the nature of this research, and because human material is being studied, the embryos and fetuses are not allowed to survive beyond the period of study.

Research of this latter type is better described as *experimentation*, in that the procedures are not directly beneficial to the embryo or fetus involved in the research. These experimental procedures, in turn, are not standard ones; their primary intention is to acquire scientific knowledge of benefit to persons other than the subject on whom the experimentation is carried out. This is sometimes designated *non-therapeutic research*.

An additional category of research is *therapeutic research* in which, although the treatment is not standard, the aim of the procedure is to benefit the subject on whom it is performed. For an embryo or fetus, this means that its goal is to improve the quality of the future life of that particular embryo or fetus, regardless of whether it does or does not prove successful. Therapeutic research, therefore, is a part of clinical practice, and has a great deal in common with therapeutic clinical research in many other branches of medicine.

In the remainder of this chapter it will be important to keep these different meanings of 'research' clearly in mind. It is difficult, however, to be completely consistent in their usage. Although I have mainly used the term 'research' in a general sense, I have allowed 'experimentation' to creep in where I know that non-therapeutic research is a major component of the research under discussion. It also has to be borne in mind that many other authors use 'research' and 'experimentation' interchangeably. I have limited use of the term 'therapeutic research' to the specific category of clinical research known by that term.

Fetal Research

Types of Research and Guidelines
In looking at the fetus as the subject of research procedures, we are confronted by a bewildering array of possibilities. These are outlined in figure 17. Such experiments may utilize fetal tissue, the fetus outside the uterus (separated whole fetus), or

Figure 17   This scheme illustrates the various stages at which research can be carried out on fetuses.

- **Types of tissue used**
  - -- fetal tissue
  - -- fetus outside uterus (separated whole fetus)
  - -- fetus inside uterus

- **Outside the uterus (following an abortion — spontaneous or induced)**
  - -- dead fetus
  - -- viable fetus
  - -- previable fetus

- **Inside the uterus**
  - -- viable fetus
  - -- previable fetus
  - -- no abortion planned
  - -- in anticipation of an abortion
  - -- during an abortion

the fetus inside the uterus. The latter two categories can be further subdivided: the fetus outside the uterus may be dead, viable or previable, while the fetus inside the uterus may be viable or previable. Experimentation on the fetus inside the uterus may be carried out when no abortion is planned, in anticipation of an abortion, or during an abortion.

In order to put fetal research into perspective, it is important to give a brief outline of the type of research that has been carried out over recent years. The literature is extensive, but three major types of experiments can be recognized[1]: those performed on the fetus in the uterus prior to abortion or normal delivery (type 1); those performed on the fetus in the uterus during an abortion (type 2); those carried out on the fetus outside the uterus following an abortion, and therefore following separation from the mother (type 3).

The first type of research may be performed at least one week prior to abortion or delivery, and includes an extensive range of non-invasive procedures. These would generally be regarded as therapeutic in character, the research being an offshoot of diagnostic or therapeutic procedures. Examples[2] are: the use of X-rays, amniocentesis and ultrasound in prenatal diagnosis; intrauterine blood transfusions for Rhesus incompatibility; studies of fetal behaviour including the fetal response to sound; retrospective studies on the effects of malnutrition on fetal development, and also of drugs (administered to the mother for therapeutic reasons) on the fetus.

One rather different type of study in this category were two prospective ones, reported in 1972, in which live rubella (German measles) vaccine was administered to the mothers more than a week prior to induced abortion. The aim of the studies was to ascertain whether accidental administration of this vaccine during pregnancy would have an effect on the fetus.

Another subset of type 1 research is that in which the research takes place just a few hours or days before an abortion or delivery. Some of the studies are therapeutic, and include prenatal diagnosis and studies for facilitating delivery. Other research however, is non-therapeutic and is allied closely to induced abortion. For instance, several studies have been designed to investigate the transfer of substances across the placenta. In these cases radio-isotopes, ethyl alcohol or steroids have been administered to the mother some hours before abortion. Subsequently, the aborted fetus was examined for traces of the substance in question. Among the compounds to be tested in this way were various antibiotics, ^{125}I-glucagon, and cortisol.

A minor extension of some of these studies makes them into a type 2 study, that is, a research procedure undertaken during an abortion. Placental transfer studies in this instance have consisted of injecting radioactive isotopes into the umbilical vein of the fetus during abortion by hysterotomy, and then examining the mother for the presence of radioactivity. The concern here is to discover whether compounds are transported across the placenta from the fetal to the maternal side. Other studies have examined blood flow within the fetal circulatory system, while yet others have concentrated on various aspects of fetal metabolism.

In the third type of study, abortuses are examined following separation from the mother. Since aborted fetuses may continue to live following abortion by hysterotomy or hysterectomy, some aspects of fetal physiology can be investigated. An example was the study of the circulatory system in the uterus and placenta using angiographic techniques (in which the blood vessels were outlined by the injection of a barium sulphate solution).

Another illustration of a type 3 investigation involved the removal of fetal organs and tissues from still-living fetuses immediately following abortion. The aim of studies such as these was to investigate the synthesis of certain substances in the liver and brain of the fetus. Yet a further example has been provided by studies aimed at prolonging fetal life employing a form of artificial placenta; the subjects were aborted fetuses.

In specifying these research endeavours, I have attempted to outline them in as objective a manner as possible. Most were carried out in the early 1970s, before guidelines were adopted in a number of countries on acceptable limits to fetal research (see next section). My use of them as illustrations must not be taken as in any way indicating my support for such experimentation. What they do is to stress the need for ethical assessments of fetal research, and the dire necessity of public debate and social regulation of this area. Having said this however, we should not jump to the conclusion that those carrying out research of this nature are grotesquely irresponsible. We may or may not agree with some of these procedures on human fetuses; nevertheless, the research is of a serious nature.

The types of fetal research just outlined raise a number of practical queries, quite apart from ethical ones. These include: the age of the fetus, and whether it is viable or previable; the therapeutic or non-therapeutic intention of the study; and the degree of risk to the fetus.

It was considerations such as these which led to the establishment of committees in various countries, and the subsequent publications of guidelines covering fetal research. These were issued in Britain in 1972,[3] in the United States in 1975,[4] and in Australia in 1983.[5] It is not my intention to look in detail at any of these. I simply want to extract from them some of the major proposals, as indicators of what society allows in this area. In particular I want to consider the use of the *live previable fetus*, since this is most relevant to a consideration of the embryo.

Both British and American policy documents permit experimentation on live previable fetuses, although limitations are imposed on such experimentation. The rationale for these experiments is, in the words of the American document: 'the development of important biomedical knowledge that cannot be obtained by alternative means'. Their justification therefore, stems from what is regarded as being the useful information they will provide. This is a 'good consequences' argument, the anticipated benefits of such research including knowledge concerning the transfer of substances across the placenta, the reaction of the fetus to drugs, enzymatic activity in the fetus, and therapies for preventing or offsetting congenital defects and for counteracting the disabilities associated with prematurity. Linked with this argument is an allied one, namely, that this knowledge cannot be achieved using animal models. The American document stipulates that 'investigation on pertinent animal models and nonpregnant humans has preceded such research', while the British report comments: 'The medical evidence we received showed that the whole previable fetus has offered an important opportunity that cannot be obtained in any other way for making observations of great value . . . .'

All guidelines build various safeguards into their provisions. These are of particular relevance to experiments carried out on the fetus *in anticipation of an abortion*. These provisions revolve around the stipulation that minimal, or no, risk be imposed on the fetus by the research. The British report argues: 'It is unethical to administer drugs or carry out procedures during pregnancy with the deliberate intent of ascertaining the harm that these might do to the fetus.' The major concerns underlying this limitation appear to be that the fetus may subsequently be born alive, or that the woman may change her mind regarding the abortion. The Australian guidelines come down against experimentation on the fetus destined to be aborted. The reason for this restriction is expressed as follows:

> There is little information available on the sensory awareness of immature fetuses and dissection of a previable but live fetus cannot be assumed to be without neurological impact on the fetus. Dissection of such a fetus could therefore be justifiably regarded as unethical and offensive. Ethical propriety requires that cessation of heart beat should have occurred before the commencement of any procedure on a previable fetus not aimed at its survival.

A different perspective is provided for experiments on the previable fetus *during the abortion procedure* or *following an abortion*. All three guidelines allow even potentially harmful research to be carried out under these circumstances. Again, there are stipulations, although these are of a different nature from those applying prior to an abortion. They include the stipulations that: the research should be justified, the method of abortion should destroy the fetus before its complete separation from the mother, the fetus should be less than 20 weeks gestational age, the research should not lead to any alterations in the abortion procedure, and the duration of life of the fetus should not be affected by the experimental manipulations.

While these guidelines also contain further stipulations (concerning parental consent for the procedures, the separation of the clinical and research teams, the role of therapeutic research and of research directed to fetal diagnosis in the uterus) the above points are the crucial ones for this discussion. What emerges is that these guidelines take a pragmatic stance, namely, that research on previable fetuses is justified under certain circumstances, within certain well-defined limits, and as a last resort.

Before taking these matters further, it has to be stressed that most discussion on fetal research revolves around research on the live previable fetus either inside or outside the uterus. Reference to figure 17 will show that, besides the live previable fetus, research is also feasible on the dead fetus outside the uterus and on the viable fetus either inside or outside the uterus. In general, most would agree that a dead fetus should be treated in the same manner as any dead human individual. Under these circumstances, research on dead fetuses (including dead aborted fetuses) is considered permissible under specified conditions, including the condition that consent has been given by the mother.[6] In the case of a viable fetus after delivery, even after an abortion, many would contend with the Peel Committee Report's statement that: 'the ethical obligation is to sustain its life so far as possible and it is both immoral and illegal to carry out any experiments on it which are inconsistent with treatment necessary to promote its life . . . .'

While it is not my intention to raise the abortion issue, it should be noted that the aborted fetus is in an anomalous position. There are two reasons for this. The first is that a normal healthy fetus in the uterus prior to the age of viability is deemed to be previable when an abortion is contemplated. As LeRoy Walters[7] comments: 'What renders the fetus non-viable is a human intervention which interrupts normal development'. The second reason is that the aim of an abortion is to terminate the life of the fetus. If such a fetus is born alive, the doctor's efforts are then to be directed towards saving its life. In other words, there is head-on conflict between the intentions of the mother and of the doctors. If the life of a viable fetus (infant) is to be saved, whatever the circumstances of its delivery, there is no room for any non-therapeutic research on such an infant.

Queries Raised by the Guidelines

A crucial facet of these guidelines is that, once the death of the fetus is inevitable – at the time of the abortion or subsequent to it – it can be exposed to risk. The argument appears to be that since the previable fetus is doomed, any harm resulting from the experimentation is of little consequence compared with the much greater harm caused by the abortion. Hence, if abortion is allowable, so is research on the fetus: the one follows inexorably from the other.

A utilitarian approach is also evident. According to this, the individual fetus is subordinate to the potential medical benefits resulting from experimentation. While none of the guidelines concludes that this legitimizes *all* experiments, it is the only reason given to justify *any* experimentation. The hundreds of thousands who may benefit from fetal research are seen as being of greater value than the relatively few fetuses that must be sacrificed in the process. The strength of this argument is accentuated by the inevitable demise of these particular fetuses, which are destined to be aborted.

In general, the various guidelines appear to adopt an intermediate position on the status of the fetus. They are not based on the view that the human fetus should be accorded the status of a person from the earliest stages of development, thereby debarring any experimentation on it. On the other hand, they appear to treat it as more than a non-personal organism, since they proscribe causing harm to the living previable fetus. Nevertheless, the reasons for this vary, and some of these are largely pragmatic and legal ones.

This intermediate position raises a number of general queries, which are of help in focusing attention on dilemmas inherent in fetal research. The first is this. The fact that the fetuses are doomed, that is, they are about to be aborted, plays a crucial role in all aspects of experimentation on live previable fetuses. The argument appears to be that, since these fetuses will never be able to realize their potential as fully-developed persons, it is legitimate to use them for the good of medical science, and therefore for the good of other fetuses that hopefully will realize that potential. But if this position is accepted, it has to be asked whether children and adults who are also doomed (for whatever reason) can be used for the good of medical science. Should experimentation on them be justified for equivalent reasons? Is the individual good always subordinate to the common good?

Some would argue that the answer to these questions is 'no' because they consider there are major differences in the status of prenatal and postnatal life. If that position is adopted however, difficulties still remain. And this brings me to my second query.

The fetuses which are doomed are doomed, in most instances, for reasons which originate outside the fetus. Except for those abortions carried out on account of suspected fetal abnormality, all others are undertaken when the fetus is – as far as is known – normal. The chances of a fetus becoming the subject of experimentation are unequal, depending as they do on a whole array of social circumstances. Does this make fetuses unequal, and how can we accommodate this inequality within our view of fetal status? Quite obviously, this inequality has nothing to do with the personhood or non-personhood of the fetus, or with the degree of its development. In experimenting on the fetus, then, are we simply using it for our own ends, however noble these may be; and does this inevitably have major implications for our view of children and adults? Can they, too, be used for the good of others when they are doomed, as a consequence of illness, starvation, accident or congenital defect?

This question highlights something which is emerging from these queries, namely, that the legitimacy or otherwise of fetal research is not dependent on the respective status of prenatal and postnatal life. Rather, it depends on the reasons for the termination of the life of the fetus, that is, in most instances on the legitimacy or otherwise of the abortion that brings the life of the fetus to an end.

Closely allied to this is yet another issue, and this is the nature of the parental consent to allow experimentation to be performed on the live previable fetus. This is generally based on the notion of the consent required to experiment on viable fetuses and children, that is, the consent of the mother or parents. Unfortunately, there is a difference between the nature of the consent in the two instances. With viable fetuses and children, the consent is for research on a being for which one expects to shoulder responsibility in the future. With the previable fetus however, the consent refers to a being for which the parents in all probability will not have to bear any responsibility in the future. In addition, since the parents have consented to abortion, the killing of the fetus, they hardly have the best interests of the *fetus* at heart (except perhaps when the abortion is on the grounds of severe fetal abnormality). It is unlikely, therefore, that any consent they give for non-therapeutic research on the fetus will have the same meaning as consent for similar research on a child whom they want to live and whom they hope to care for.

A premise underlying any non-therapeutic research on fetuses is that the consequences of such experimentation will be good; good, that is, in medical terms. This raises two problems. The first is how one decides that the prospective medical benefits will justify experimentation on live previable fetuses. The medical benefits that may follow from this type of research can only be surmised; they are not definitely known. In contrast, the destruction of the fetuses on whom the experimentation is carried out is inevitable, although most (if not all) of these would have been destroyed anyway because they are destined to be (or have been) aborted. The importance of this consideration, therefore, will depend on one's reservations regarding fetal research.

Another problem stems from whether the experimentation will have consequences additional to the narrowly medical ones; social consequences perhaps, especially long-term ones. Is there any possibility that experimentation of this nature will affect our view of human beings at other stages of development – from early embryonic stages through to old age? If such a possibility exists, how do we weigh this up against the *medical* benefits emanating from the experimentation? It may prove difficult for the medical profession and society to escape from the influence of the precedent-setting character of fetal experimentation. This is not an argument, in itself, against this type of experimentation, but it is a reminder of the importance of predicting as accurately as possible the probable long-term consequences of our actions as well as the obvious and direct short-term ones.

Ethical Assessment

Four major positions[8] have become evident on non-therapeutic research involving live previable fetuses before, during or after induced abortion. The view of each of the four on research of this nature is set out below:

1. It should not be carried out under any circumstances;
2. It should be allowed under exactly the same conditions, and to the same extent, as research permitted on children or on fetuses that will continue to term;
3. It should be permitted, and should not be as restrictive as that allowed on children and on fetuses that will continue to term; nevertheless, some restrictions should apply and some types of experimentation should be prohibited;
4. It should be allowed without any restrictions.

Paul Ramsey, a Protestant ethicist, epitomizes someone holding to the first position. He compares[9] the fetus to the *dying* (if the abortion is spontaneous) or to the *condemned* (if the abortion is induced), or to the *unconscious*. In his analysis Ramsey does not appear to keep these categories separate, his principal concern being with the analogy to the dying which covers not only spontaneously aborted fetuses, but also those dying as a consequence of induced abortion and unsalvageable prematurity. He contends that we should not inflict experimentation upon the dying, unless it is relevant to the death of *that* fetus itself. For Ramsey, fetal research is a violation of bodily identity and is a misuse of the dying. As such, it is considered by him to be irrelevant research, no matter how useful some of the information gained could be to an understanding of congenital defects or prematurity.

Ramsey's view of fetal experimentation stems from a more fundamental view, which is that of the status of the fetus. For him, it is a fellow human being which should be treated as one would treat a child. Hence, his opposition to experimentation on living fetuses is in line with his opposition to experimentation on children – even with parental consent.

Ramsey argues: 'It would be morally outrageous for future fetuses or children to be made to benefit from research on sacrificed fetuses. The research subjects are additionally misused if the experimentation is irrelevant to what caused their condemnation to be deemed just and necessary or electable.' The irrelevance of the research to the fetus concerned is brought out again when comparing the fetus to the dying: 'It is a kind of violation of bodily identity . . . . even to ask the terminally ill to consent to irrelevant research.' The fetus, as an unconscious subject, is considered to demand 'utter protection', since it is utterly helpless.

In equating the fetus with a child, Ramsey argues that we may not submit a child to procedures likely to involve any risk of harm, or even procedures that involve no harm but simply what he describes as 'offensive touching'. What Ramsey means by this is that a subject can be wronged without being harmed. This occurs whenever the subject (the child or fetus) is used as an object, and as a means to an end. It is for this reason that Ramsey denies the validity of proxy consent being given by parents to non-therapeutic research on a child or fetus. For Ramsey, to consent to a child being used as an experimental subject is to treat that child as 'not a child'. It is to treat the child as an adult person, and this is a violent presumption. Ramsey concludes therefore, that no parent is morally competent to consent that their child (or fetus) be submitted to any non-therapeutic research.

Richard McCormick, a Roman Catholic, contends that the issue of fetal experimentation can be separated – to some extent anyway – from the issue of abortion.[10] His position on the legitimacy of fetal experimentation is based on the concept of proxy consent. In terms of this concept, he argues that there are things we, and therefore children and fetuses, *ought* to do for others simply because we are all members of the human community. These include being subject to experimentation under certain rigidly-defined conditions. His position therefore, fits into the second category (allowing fetal research under exactly the same conditions as research on children).

McCormick argues for a position that allows experimentation on children where there is no discernible risk or undue discomfort. He writes: 'Experimentation may be legitimate if it left the fetus in no worse position during its dying than it is in as a result of the abortion.' McCormick however, will only allow this if the abortion itself is 'morally legitimate'.

The focal point of this position is provided by his acceptance of proxy consent in the therapeutic situation. Here, a parent may consent to an experiment on a child, if it is a reasonable presumption that that is what the child would wish if he or she was in a position to do so. This also applies, according to McCormick, to a fetus. He then extends this to experiments that are genuinely necessary for medical knowledge and that are calculated to be of notable benefit to fetuses or children in general. They may be legitimate, he argues, on one proviso.

This proviso is that the abortion is 'morally legitimate'. If it is, the fetus can be likened to a *justly condemned* individual. If the proposed experimentation involves no discernible risk to the fetus, proxy consent of the mother would be a defensible construction of the fetus's wishes. If there are discernible risks to the fetus, proxy consent is invalid. When, in McCormick's view, the abortion is not morally legitimate, the fetus can be compared to an *unjustly condemned* individual. Under these circumstances, experimentation is not valid. These arguments apply to experimentation prior to, during, or in the wake of, an abortion.

Both Ramsey and McCormick argue against a utilitarian position. Neither considers that the potential medical benefits of experimentation outweigh the concerns of the fetus. To do this would be to demean the fetus as a human being, regardless of the precise status we place upon it. It is to subordinate the good of the fetus as an individual human being to the presumed good of society; in this way non-therapeutic research erodes the protection of the individual. Both writers, in spite of their differences, refuse to allow the fetus to be put at risk.

A utilitarian position takes the form of a consequentialist argument, and can be expressed in terms of either the third or fourth positions on fetal research mentioned previously. If fetal research is allowed to proceed with few, if any, limitations, the justification lies in the good consequence that will follow from it – major advances in scientific knowledge and medical treatment that will be of benefit to all future fetuses and young children.

Against this have to be pitted the many unknowns or probable disadvantages of virtually unfettered non-therapeutic research on fetuses. It has to be demonstrated that unfettered research is required for these advances, when compared with what might be accomplished using stringently controlled research on human fetuses (as suggested above), allied with research on non-human experimental animals. The possible dehumanizing effects of highly invasive procedures on live previable human fetuses also require serious investigation, as does the possible precedent-setting nature of such work for equivalent procedures on postnatal humans.[11]

The close relationship between abortion and fetal research is interpreted by some as an argument in favour of research, even if it is of a limited variety. This is the position adopted by Marc Lappé and Willard Gaylin.[12] Once society has accepted the legitimacy of abortion, they consider that we acquire new moral duties, one of which is 'to rectify the costs of doing abortion by ethical behaviour, both in the manner in which abortions are done, and in the uses to which aborted fetuses are put'.[13] They consider that by using aborted fetuses to obtain important medical information of potential value to future fetuses, they are adding a moral good to a morally tragic situation (abortion). They make a case for very limited research on the living fetus, and emphasize the need for adequate research on laboratory animals, and that the human fetus should never be seen as a convenient or inexpensive laboratory animal.

Since the about-to-be-aborted fetus is doomed, Lappé wishes[14] to 'ennoble that death by utilizing it to serve its more fortunate fellows'. He continues: 'If the doomed fetus could be utilized to supply the information that could permit those same parents, or similar parents, a greater opportunity for a healthy, wanted child it would be a persuasive argument for experimentation.'

I have set out at length many of the arguments employed in this debate. In the light of these I would draw the following tentative conclusions.

1. *I do not object to research on dead fetuses, even if they are the result of abortions I would not consider ethically legitimate.* This in no way justifies or supports the reason for the abortion, and very considerable safeguards are needed to ensure that a research programme on fetuses is not used to justify any particular abortion or to give the appearance of respectability to society's attitudes towards easy abortion. To use tissues from dead fetuses for research aimed at benefiting

other fetuses and children is akin to using tissues from dead fetuses to provide much-needed hormones for presently-living children. It also has much in common with using tissues from dead adults for transplantation purposes or for research regardless of how those adults died (motor-cycle or car accidents, homicides, cerebrovascular accidents, or senile dementia).

There may well be differences of opinion among Christians on this matter. It needs to be stressed however, that different attitudes and practice do not stem from different views of the status of the fetus. Both research on tissues from dead fetuses, and the therapeutic use of such tissues, can be justified – in my opinion – by those holding a very high view of the dignity of human fetuses. As long as rigorous regulations apply to protect the interests of living fetuses, the use of tissue derived from already-dead fetuses (once appropriate consent has been given by the parents) is a means of using the tissue of dead fetuses to serve other fetuses whose lives can be saved or whose welfare can be improved in this way. This applies to already-living fetuses and future-fetuses.

2. *Viable fetuses, regardless of the circumstances under which they have been born, are human beings deserving of protection.* As has already been discussed, this raises major difficulties when the viable fetuses are the result of abortion for social reasons or on account of severe handicap. From a Christian angle, support and counselling of mothers confronted by this dilemma are urgently required. It may also involve being prepared to adopt children (handicapped as well as healthy) born in this way.

3. *Therapeutic research on live previable fetuses has as its aim the benefit of the fetuses in question.* This is therapy in the strict sense, treating the individual fetus as of value and worthy of concern. While this does not justify all therapeutic research, any more than it justifies every new and daring surgical procedure on adults, *it is a legitimate means of treating fetuses in general.* It has to be recognized however, that any innovative treatment may be relatively unsuccessful when first employed. Success rates improve gradually as experience is accumulated and modifications to procedures are undertaken. This is of the essence of any therapeutic research, and it will apply just as forcibly to the

treatment of fetuses as it does to the treatment of children and adults.

4. *Non-therapeutic research on live previable fetuses raises, as we have seen, a number of contentious issues.* Those with a high view of the status of the fetus are either opposed to all such research, or to most of such research. Differences among people of this persuasion are relatively minor compared with those who would allow considerable research on live previable fetuses. The gulf between these two schools of thought results from a preparedness to subordinate the interests of doomed fetuses to the good of medical science, or a refusal to accept this. Those who regard the fetus as an end in itself, with a dignity of its own, refuse by and large to treat it as a means to an end – however noble that end may be. This, I believe, concurs with a Christian perspective, and constitutes the major objection to unfettered or large-scale non-therapeutic fetal research. Additional reasons against such research are the wide-scale implications of this research for our approach to other human subjects and to human life as a whole.

Is it still possible, however, to approve of any non-therapeutic research on live previable fetuses, admitting that any research would be very limited in scope? Research in the uterus in anticipation of an abortion is unacceptable, on the sole ground of limiting the mother's freedom to change her mind about proceeding with the abortion. This, by itself, constitutes a major limitation on the freedom of action of the mother, and this is to regard the mother as less than a full human person. Since this is unethical in Christian terms, no other considerations need be taken into account in rejecting this type of research.

In the case of non-therapeutic research during or following an abortion of a live previable fetus, it has to be conceded that these fetuses would not be available for research if there were no abortions. Nevertheless, should it be argued that since abortions are being carried out in society (and this does not in any way justify the abortions themselves), obtaining valuable information from these doomed fetuses is the lesser of two evils? In this, there may be similarities to research using dead fetuses. Strong as this argument may be, live previable fetuses are a step away from the inevitability of death, representing as they do a life that is not ended although it is in the process of being ended by abortion. The research in this instance is an integral part of the abortion procedure, even though it is the responsibility of a different group of doctors from those undertaking the abortion. It is difficult to see how the logic of the abortion can be separated from the logic of the research. If this is so, the legitimacy of the research cannot be separated from the legitimacy of the abortion. If the grounds for the latter are considered inadequate, the fetus cannot be used in a research procedure – however laudable the goals.

This leaves little room for non-therapeutic research on previable fetuses for those who object to most or all abortions. But is there *any* room for this research where the abortion is considered legitimate or where no induced abortion is involved? It is at this point that the question of proxy consent becomes relevant. If this is accepted, some very limited research will prove acceptable on the grounds that this is what the fetus would have agreed to for the good of others. If it is not accepted, no research will be permitted.

Whichever position attracts us, it is probably true to say that in practical terms the difference between the positions is negligible. This is particularly true since McCormick makes the additional stipulation that the fetus must be exposed to no discernible risk or discomfort. In practice, neither position allows any non-therapeutic research of note on live previable fetuses. This is a conservative stance, and yet as far as I can see it is the only one that will protect the interests of fetuses as a group and also, in the long term, of other groups of dependent and fragile humans.

Research on Human Embryos

I have devoted a considerable amount of space to fetal research, since I felt this was necessary to clear the ground and to prepare the way for an ethical analysis of research on the human embryo. Inevitably, the questions which will occupy most of our attention are, yet again, the medical benefits of these procedures and the status of the human embryo. Hence the queries I have just raised with regard to fetal research apply, with some modification, to embryo research.

Both types of research have become realities because of prior human intervention in the reproductive process. The intervention in the case of fetal research is abortion; in the case of embryo research it is IVF and the production of spare embryos. In neither case however, does the research follow inevitably from the other procedure, although without the other procedure there could be no research of the types we are envisaging.

The debate, therefore, revolves not around the embryo *per se* but around the preimplantation embryo outside the human body, an embryo that has been expressly produced by technical means. In looking at embryo research we are concerned with embryos produced by IVF but not transferred to a woman's uterus for subsequent development. This is just one of a number of fates open to an IVF embryo, and it is not an inevitable fate. The question confronting us is how we can begin to assess whether this is an acceptable fate, and what rationale there is for such research.

General Considerations
Embryos such as these can be produced in a number of ways. They may be:

(a) superfluous to the needs of a couple in a clinical IVF programme ('spare' embryos);
(b) produced in the laboratory (using donated ovum and sperm) with the sole intention of employing them in a research programme;
(c) the by-product of another research programme aimed at studying, for example, the fertilizing capacity of human ova or sperm.

At present, most embryos used for research purposes are probably superfluous to clinical needs, although this may not remain the case.

The research imperative stems from the potential value of these preimplantation human embryos in the furtherance of a wide range of scientific and clinical objectives.[15] Research, which can be immediately envisaged, includes analysis of the structure and function of embryos, the process of fertilization, the reasons why chromosomal abnormalities arise, the basis of genetic disease, gene function, and transplantation issues. In broader terms, the following grounds for considering research on the early human embryo have been advocated: investigation of natural embryo wastage, investigation of embryo wastage in IVF programmes, early diagnosis of congenital disease, assessment of embryotoxic and teratogenic agents, research into the behaviour of cancer cells, investigation of fetal metabolic disorders, and the use of specific fetal tissue implants.

Although interest is currently focused on preimplantation embryos (existing guidelines only allow the use of these embryos), an inevitable extension of current studies would include the use of postimplantation embryos. Such studies would allow analysis of many aspects of tissue and organ maturation, and would allow the culture of individual types of embryonic tissue such as nervous tissue. Such cultures may prove helpful in unravelling the intricacies of tissue and cell differentiation, which may have important clinical applications involving the use of cultured fetal organs and tissue as replacements for defective organs and tissue in children and adults.

In order to focus the debate I would like to underline two points, which cannot be ignored by those implacably opposed to any form of research on human embryos. The first is that research is essential before IVF procedures can be introduced. The introduction of IVF procedures necessitates the development of methods for successfully culturing embryos. These have to be grown to establish standards of culture compatible with the introduction of a clinical programme for alleviating infertility. Even when pregnancies have been established, some embryos still need to be grown to ensure that conditions remain suitable for IVF procedures.

Data needing to be obtained in this way include the appropriate pH, osmotic pressure, and protein requirements for early embryonic development. Embryos of other species, for example, mouse and hamster embryos, do not require precisely the same conditions as human embryos. Hence, some human embryos have to be 'sacrificed', in order that other human embryos will have an opportunity to develop and mature to term.

The second point is that research of this nature has to be carried out if the present very high wastage rate caused by spontaneous abortions is to be combated. The reason for this is that more than 50% of spontaneously aborted fetuses during the first trimester of pregnancy have a chromosomal anomaly (see chapter 4). Chromosomally imbalanced abortuses have been identified after IVF, and examination of such abortuses would appear to provide one way of attacking this problem. In more general terms, knowledge could be gained by examining chromosomes at various stages throughout fertilization and embryonic growth *in vitro.*

Robert Edwards, the physiologist responsible for many of the technical developments behind IVF, has been involved in the ethical debate surrounding the use of human embryos for research purposes since the 1960s (see Chapter 2). He has consistently been an ardent advocate of this research, and a few quotations from his writings will help to place the rationale for research in perspective. In an address to the Pontifical Academy of Science [16] he wrote:

> What, then, is the justification of the research on these minute human embryos which are not sentient, and are virtually undifferentiated? I can only offer the balance between the sheer necessity of acquiring knowledge and the value placed on embryos before any of their senses or the central nervous system are differentiated.

The consequences of this position are recognized by Edwards who acknowledges that this 'stance confers very few rights, if any, on the early embryo'. Not surprisingly then, he concludes: 'I believe that the need for knowledge is greater than the respect to be accorded to an early embryo.' Edwards is prepared to accept the logic of this position, namely, that once the need for research on a *few* embryos is acknowledged, this opens the floodgates to research on *many* embryos: 'Once one embryo is studied, then there is no limit to the number that can be studied for almost any purpose.'

According to an editorial in the British journal *Nature* [17], the guidelines suggested by the Royal Society are based 'on the proposition that an early embryo is not a living thing, in the sense of being potentially autonomously self-replicating, but rather a kind of passing parasite, dependent on a uterus for full development'. For those with this point of view there appears to be no problem, except to decide when during embryonic development this state of affairs changes. And therein lies the problem. Consistency would suggest that there be no limitations whatsoever to research on the early embryo. If this is the case, and if we are faced with a movable upper age limit to research, we shall soon find that there are less restrictions on research on the human embryo and fetus than on laboratory animals.

The possibility of research on embryos is, not surprisingly, proving extremely contentious. For some, the human status of these embryos precludes their use in research under any circumstances. For others, the potential medical and scientific benefits for ameliorating mental and physical suffering are so great that they justify unlimited research using human embryos.

For those in the first group, research is morally wrong because the embryos – no matter how young – are human, with a potential for full human personhood.[18] To some in this group, the human embryo (both pre- and postimplantation) should be accorded the same status as a child or adult. This moral principle is considered to outweigh any of the possible medical benefits of the research. For those in the second group, it is morally wrong not to do everything possible to alleviate human suffering, whether this is the suffering of infertility or of a genetic or chromosomal disorder, such as Down's syndrome. Allied with this is the view that the early human embryo is not a person, since it is relatively undifferentiated and also is incapable of further development without implantation in a human uterine environment.

Those in the first group disapprove of any research at all on the human embryo. It is forbidden territory. Those in the second group however, go to the other extreme and see no necessity of imposing any upper limit on the age at which embryos can be used for research purposes. Since the human embryo, in their eyes, is little more than a useful tool in the furtherance of scientific and medical advance, they do not wish to restrict the nature of the research procedures. They also advocate the production of human embryos specifically for experimental studies.

Between these two extremes there is a medley of intermediate positions. Most reports issued by governmental and medical bodies have adopted an intermediate position, although with a clear bias towards the legitimacy of some research on the embryo. The Warnock Committee,[19] for instance, agreed that the human embryo should be afforded some protection in law, and should not be frivolously or unnecessarily used in research. Nevertheless, a majority of the Committee considered that the need for advances in the treatment of infertility and for increased medical knowledge outweighed this protection. The special status of the human embryo should not, according to this Committee, preclude research as long as the research is subject to stringent controls and monitoring.

Having committed itself to embryo research, the Warnock Committee argued for a 14 days time-limit on research. The reason for this limit (which has acquired almost mystical significance in debates on research using human embryos) was that the primitive streak, which forms at about 15 days after fertilization (see chapter 4), marks the beginning of individual development of the embryo. The significance of this stemmed from the Committee's view that each embryo is a potential human being. This also led to the Committee's stipulation that no embryo used for research should be transferred subsequently to a woman's uterus for further development.

The origin of the embryos used for experimental purposes caused the Warnock Committee considerable consternation. Although divided on the issue, it came down in favour of using embryos from all sources, including those generated specifically for research purposes. The reason, once again, was the potential scientific value of the research. Interestingly though, the Committee felt that the routine testing of drugs on human embryos was unacceptable. The reason appeared to be principally because of the large numbers of embryos required. Even here however, it was prepared to allow such testing on a 'very small scale'.

Strictures such as these imposed by the Warnock Committee clearly reflect the uneasy tension experienced by those seeking a half-way house on human embryo research. The logic of the position is unfettered research, even if many in society are not prepared to accept the stark outlines of such logic.

Ethical Assessment
Any assessment of research using human embryos inevitably forces us to weigh the value we place upon the human embryo against the value we place upon the benefits to medical science, and therefore to humanity, of advances in medical knowledge and therapeutic expertise. This is an invidious choice because it involves balancing an evil against a good. Does the *evil* of using human embryos as a means to an end outweigh the *good* that will accrue to all of us, or does the reverse hold? Some would argue that using human embryos in this way is not an evil; but if this is the case, at what point during development does it become evil?

Once the human, or potentially human, characteristics of the embryo are taken into account, pure research on living human embryos raises profound ethical considerations. This is because experiments on living embryos can only be carried out by denying their possible viability and their potential significance as human beings. The fundamental issue, from which there can be no escape, is whether respect should be shown to human embryos in view of their potential for full personhood, or whether they should be treated as non-human experimental material.

This is the basic ethical choice underlying research on human embryos. Once they are regarded as nothing more than dispensable experimental material, no logically-consistent limits can be placed on the whole range of feasible IVF applications. Although most of those involved in current IVF infertility research may not wish to go beyond the bounds of infertility, only ethically-determined limits will prevent this happening. And these limits, whatever they may be, will stem from an assessment of the value of embryonic and fetal material.

In practical terms, we are faced with the challenge of whether research on human embryonic material should continue. If in the light of the potential of this material for full humanness, we decide that such research should not continue, there will be repercussions. Any limitation on laboratory IVF research will inhibit the expansion of our knowledge of reproductive embryonic development.

I want to elaborate some general ethical considerations that seem to me to be relevant in tackling this matter.

(a) *Relationship between research on IVF-produced embryos and on fetuses.* I want to suggest that, when considering IVF research, a distinction [20] should be made between:

(i)   living fetuses facing abortion
(ii) living aborted fetuses used in research; and
(iii) embryos produced for the express purpose of being used in a research programme.

The fetuses in (i) are unwanted, regardless of the reason for this. In (ii) the research is conducted on the available products of abortions which were not undertaken for the sake of research. The procedure outlined in (iii), however, has as its aim the deliberate creation, and ultimately deliberate destruction of embryonic material. This would appear to place this type of laboratory IVF in a class of its own.

A more ambiguous case is that of spare embryos of clinical IVF. These have not been produced for the express purpose of research, and so do not fall into category (iii). Their situation is akin to that of (ii), except that they have been deliberately produced in a laboratory, whereas the aborted fetuses in that category have not. The problem here is whether it is better to allow these spare embryos to die, or to use them with the aim of increasing knowledge about fertilization and early embryonic development.

My assessment of this analysis is that, in ethical terms, there is an important distinction to be made between embryos which are superfluous to the needs of a clinical programme and those produced specifically for research purposes. Although this may be a theoretical distinction at present, I do not believe it will remain so for long. Research on genuine spare embryos may be akin to that on previable fetuses (see next section), and whatever conditions govern the fetal research may also govern the embryo research. However, research on human embryos produced as experimental tools introduces a new dimension to biological research.

(b) *Status of IVF embryos.* The debate about research on human embryos revolves not around the embryo *per se*, but around the preimplantation embryo outside the human body, an embryo that has been expressly produced by technical means. It has to be asked therefore, whether this makes any difference in discussing what is or is not allowable with respect to such an embryo.

As I have already discussed, a fertilized ovum, or an embryo, normally has the potential to develop into a new human person in every sense of that term. This is a potential we need to take very seriously. However, for an IVF-produced embryo to realize this potential, a positive act is required, namely, transferring it to a woman's uterus. An IVF-produced embryo outside the human body will never develop much further, at least, not until ecto-genesis becomes a reality. Hence, in this important respect, a major distinction should be made between an IVF embryo and an embryo *in utero*. The question we are confronted with is whether this distinction has any ethical consequences.[21]

Although some or all IVF embryos may be compared to a previable fetus (see previous section), there is one major difference between the two. The previable fetus is on the way to becoming a viable fetus; all that is required are the normal processes of gestation. Any interruption of these, by spontaneous or induced abortion, is an intrusion into the outworking of normal biological processes. In contrast, the IVF embryo lacks the appropriate environment to become a fetus, even a previable one in the narrow sense of that term (let alone a viable one). In this sense, it is not like a previable fetus since – if left to itself – it can never become viable.

In the light of this unique status of the IVF embryo, let me highlight three possible responses to it. First, IVF embryos do not merit special protection (even if *in utero* embryos do merit such protection), since they lack the potential for developing any further as human beings. Second, and in response to this, it may be argued that since this situation has been brought about by human intervention, the ethical choice regarding the use of IVF embryos is determined by the ethical nature of this human action and not by the biological limitations of IVF embryos. The creation of such embryos, with no intention of giving them the opportunity of developing further as human beings (as in (iii) in the previous section), is a fundamental denial of the potential of these embryos for full personhood and overrules their limited scope for further development. On the other hand, IVF embryos which are the spare embryos from an IVF programme are in a different category and are not, on these particular grounds, excluded from being used in research.

This brings us to the third possibility – the acceptance, in the case of spare embryos, of the distinction between IVF embryos and embryos *in utero*. And so, in their case, we have to ask whether this distinction allows them to be used in research programmes? Taken in isolation from other considerations, this may be so. Nevertheless, if this distinction is accepted as legitimizing research on IVF embryos, it would allow any research to be carried out on these embryos and would also constitute strong grounds for maintaining embryos outside the uterus for as long as possible. In other words, it says far more about our technological capabilities than about the status and worth of human embryos.

(c) *Therapeutic and non-therapeutic research on embryos.* There are a number of distinct forms of research, and these need to be distinguished. For instance, the information obtained may be relevant to the *individual embryo* on which the research is being carried out. An example is gene therapy, and the intended result is that that embryo will be given an opportunity to develop into a mature individual with an improved genetic constitution. A second possibility is that the information may be relevant to *embryos in general*, as in research aimed at decreasing the incidence of, or treating, infertility. This may involve the selection of a normal embryo from among a few embryos, in order that that one embryo will be allowed to develop to term. Alternatively, it may require the sacrifice of many present embryos so that embryos in future will benefit. A third category includes research of potential benefit to *non-embryos*, that is, to medicine in general. In this case the work on embryos may be of value in the transplantation of organs or tissues, or in understanding the growth of carcinoma cells. This non-therapeutic type of research makes use of particular embryos, in order to provide information of general medical usefulness.

Therapeutic research, of benefit to one particular embryo or possibly to embryos in general, poses less ethical problems than does non-therapeutic research, although the research parameters would be limited. Unfortunately, in the present state of knowledge, it is difficult to know what the precise nature of such research will be, while the dividing line between research of benefit to the embryo in question and embyros in general may sometimes be extremely unclear. This is especially so when a particular line of research is in its infancy. Nevertheless, there would appear to be value in the distinction between therapeutic and non-therapeutic research.

(d) *IVF, spontaneous abortion, and research.* IVF as a treatment for infertility had a background of years of research with animal and human embryos. It would not therefore, be at its present level of development without some research on human embryos. Likewise, the best hope of improving its success rate lies in further work on oocyte maturation, conditions of fertilization, and embryonic growth. Further, many of the ethical and legal dilemmas of embryo storage will be circumvented as a consequence of being capable of storing oocytes (see chapter 1). Whatever research is conducted on animal material will need to be tested on human oocytes before new procedures are applied clinically.

In other words, it is not possible to dispense completely with all forms of research in this area if reproductive technology in any guise is to continue. This is because research must accompany the elaboration of any new technique. This applies to IVF as it does to every new medical procedure. Nevertheless, society is under no obligation to allow unfettered experimentation on research subjects, let alone unconsenting human embryos. This brings me back to the concept of therapeutic research, and whether it is relevant here.

An area of even greater ambivalence for those with a high view of the status of the human embryo is the possible impact of this type of research on an understanding of the causes of many spontaneous abortions and stillbirths. Many of these are due to errors in division during meiosis and subsequent errors in tissue organization. The high incidence of major chromosome abnormalities in pre-implantation embryos may account to some extent for the high rate of embryonic loss after fertilization *in vitro* or *in vivo*. Work in this area may lead to increased appreciation of the causes of congenital malformations, such as spina bifida, and methods of preventing it.

This is a major conundrum. Means of combating the enormously high wastage rate of embryos and fetuses would be a positive good both clinically and ethically. And yet, can the destruction of other embryos be justified in attaining this 'good'? Is there any difference between technically-produced 'unwanted' embryos and naturally-produced 'wanted' embryos? We are back at the status we place on human embryos. Are all embryos equal in God's sight? Or do they acquire their value from the value *we* place upon them?

Yet another therapeutic area in the general sense is the identification, prevention and possible treatment of genetic disorders. The removal of individual cells (blastomeres) from the early embryo, and their genetic assessment before reimplantation in the uterus (Epilogue), could prevent the reimplantation of embryos carrying disabling genes. Specific gene probes for fetal sexing, phenylalanine hydroxylase, and alpha and beta globin, have already been applied on samples of chorionic villus. Such approaches would indeed constitute therapeutic research in the most specific sense, although this will have to be preceded by much research which will not benefit the particular embryo in question. And so, yet again, the conflict between present limitations and future possibilities is apparent.

(e) *Ambivalence of embryo research.* This discussion has left us with a number of loose ends, each one a problem area in its own right. The conclusions I reached previously were that research on dead fetuses is acceptable, whereas viable fetuses are to be protected under all circumstances. Therapeutic research on live previable fetuses has, as its goal, the welfare of the individual fetuses, and hence is to be encouraged. By contrast, non-therapeutic research on live previable fetuses, the feasibility of which is dependent upon the availability of fetuses emanating from abortions, raises a host of ethical dilemmas. The combined effect of these is to militate against the acceptability of this research under most circumstances.

The question of the deliberate production of embryos for use in research programmes has already been shown to have no parallel in any other medical research. It sets out to produce organisms with the potential for full personhood and yet which will only have the opportunity to be objects and never ends in themselves. It is on these grounds that I reject the production of embryos for the express purpose of being nothing more than experimental tools. My view of the human embryo precludes me from approving the deliberate production of embryos for research purposes. I do not consider there is justification for treating embryos as

nothing more than a means to an end. This is a major
negative in assessing this research, and its implications for
the research are enormous. If human embryos, no matter
how early in development they may be, are produced with
the express purpose of simply providing scientific information, that information has already taken precedence over
the significance of human existence. And that is not a
prospect we, as Christians or as societies, should relish.

I have argued that the use of spare embryos in research
is, with one major proviso, approximately equivalent to the
use of previable fetuses. If this is so, do the same arguments
apply, and do they weigh against the acceptability of non-
therapeutic research employing spare embryos? The major
difference is the absence of an abortion, so that there is no
association between the intended research and the question of abortion. The embryos in this case are the unre-
quired by-products of an attempt to create new human life,
not an expression of the destruction of unwanted human
life. Nevertheless, they are still 'unwanted' and it is their
'unwantedness' that makes them the objects of research
endeavours. In the end, therefore, if we argue against the
general use of live previable fetuses in non-therapeutic
research, we shall also have to argue against the general
availability of spare embryos in non-therapeutic research
programmes.

We still have to ask whether preimplantation embryos
outside the human body should be looked upon *as though*
they were equivalent to embryos or fetuses within the
uterus of a woman. They are incapable of further development as long as they remain in the laboratory (at least in
terms of current technical capabilities), and in this sense
may be compared to naturally fertilized embryos that cannot develop further within a woman's uterus because of
hormonal or other deficiencies. These naturally fertilized
embryos will be spontaneously aborted, and hence will die.
So too will IVF embryos, unless something is done to them.

Does this mean that they can be used in research programmes, simply because they are about to die? I have
already argued that the imminence of death does not provide a rationale for research, unless one believes that
human embyros or fetuses (or children or adults, for that
matter) can be treated as objects rather than as beings

having a value derived from God.

This argument against using IVF embryos as research objects is strengthened by their origin – deliberate human creation in the laboratory. This is true for spare embryos as much as for embryos produced with research in view. The creation of human embryos in this manner should bestow upon them a greater degree of protection, not a lesser degree.

I consider, therefore, that there are ample grounds for opposing most – if not all – non-therapeutic research using human embryos. But what about therapeutic research? In the case of research aimed at improving the future quality of life of the embryos in question, including various forms of gene therapy, there would seem to be no objections – at least in principle. The embryos are regarded as of sufficient value to justify concern over their welfare. This is akin to therapeutic research using older fetuses, children or adults. Assuming that proxy consent is accepted, all groups are being viewed in much the same way – as beings of value and dignity in the sight of God.

The ambivalence of research surfaces when the objects of concern are embryos in general, rather than the specific individual embryos on whom the research is being carried out. This, strictly speaking, is non-therapeutic research. It is at this interface that one has to consider research aimed at improving IVF techniques and at assessing the causes of spontaneous abortions, as well as more general research aimed at curbing infertility.

The question confronting us at this point is whether we can equate each individual embryo (whether inside the uterus or in the laboratory) with an individual fetus or child or adult. There is no way at present that more than 40% or so of these embryos (regardless of the wastage due to induced abortion) can develop any further. This situation will not change until major strides are made in our understanding of the causes of the genetic and chromosomal abnormalities giving rise to spontaneous abortions. What course of action, then, will stem from a high view of human embryos as beings created in God's image – a refusal to carry out any research aimed at combating spontaneous abortions, or research using *some* human embryos in an attempt to minimize the astronomically high wastage of embryos caused by chromosomal abnormalities? Which course of action will be the more conducive to an emphasis on the dignity and value of human life?

As I see it, both courses of action are fraught with danger. Both are a bewildering mixture of good and evil. Either way, we shall be choosing what we consider to be the lesser of two evils. The wastage of embryonic human life through spontaneous abortion is an affront to all who would bestow dignity on the embryonic stage of human existence. By the same token, unfettered research on countless millions of human embryos, however noble its goal, may well have detrimental effects on society's attitudes towards human life in general.

My own very tentative conclusion is to regard the use of some spare embryos for very well-defined and restricted research into infertility problems and chromosomal abnormalities as an illustration of therapeutic, rather than non-therapeutic, research. It is accepting that embryos in general may have to be employed to solve major problems regarding the welfare of embryos in particular. This is not an easy conclusion to reach, and it is an extremely tentative one. Nevertheless, it may well have the potential of bestowing dignity upon embryonic humans and of recognizing their value as a sub-set of human existence.

This possibility will undoubtedly prove exceedingly contentious, and a great deal of work is required in delineating the nature and boundaries of any such research. Before rejecting it out of hand however, it will have to be shown that an anti-research ethic is more conducive to an elevation of human dignity than the proposal put forward here. It is still my hope that as soon as feasible it will be possible to develop a research design which, within reasonable limits, will provide each embryo with an opportunity to develop into a baby. This applies to embryos naturally conceived, as well as to embryos artificially conceived and in research programmes.

8

Certainties and Quandaries

Christians and Technology

The positions I have adopted in the preceding chapters open the door to the use of selected technological procedures in reproduction. This, however, is not a new phenomenon. Rather, it is a continuation of a process that has been with us for many years and which, until recently, has been welcomed as much by Christians as by anyone else. Moreover, the use of technology in this area of medicine has been instrumental in decreasing dramatically the prenatal and postnatal mortality rates. While advanced technology is not alone in achieving this decrease, and while we should not rely excessively upon it, it would be foolhardy to downgrade it completely in our desire to turn our back on technology. One has only to think of the variety of ways in which fetal development and growth can be monitored, the role of Caesarian section in difficult deliveries, and the value in some instances of the hormonal induction of labour. Similar examples of the benefits of technology can be found after birth, with the contribution of immunization, oral rehydration therapy, and a plethora of examples of paediatric surgery from the routine to the heroic. All these developments have been carried out, in developed countries, within the context of the control of infectious diseases, such as diarrhoea and dysentery, pulmonary infections, communicable diseases, and malaria. While public health measures have proved of crucial importance in the control of these conditions, they would have been far less effective in the absence of sophisticated pharmaceutical products.

While it is easy to denounce technology, especially biomedical technology, this attitude needs to be analysed in the light of the above considerations. In the Asia-Pacific region, the only countries with an infant mortality rate of less than 20 per 1,000 live births are the more affluent countries with good standards of preventative medicine and an adequate technological base. These include Australia, Hong Kong, Japan, New Zealand, and Singapore. The rate increases to about 50 per 1,000 live births in countries such as Malaysia, South Korea, and Thailand, to between 50 and 100 in Burma, Indonesia, and Papua New Guinea, and to between 100 and 200 in countries such as Bangladesh, Afghanistan, and Kampuchea. These figures do not take into account antenatal mortality rates, nor childhood diseases which kill up to five million children and leave another five million mentally or physically disabled each year in this region.

In our desire to jump on the anti-technology bandwagon, it would be advisable to consider the consequences of such a move for human well-being. This should be a particularly pertinent consideration for those with a high view of the dignity of individuals. What is required is a balance between the drive for improving the quality of health care and the danger of succumbing to an all-alluring technological set of values. This is a tension with which we have to live. To reject this tension, and the decisions it entails, is to accept a series of consequences that are avoidable – including an increase in antenatal and postnatal mortality and morbidity rates. Anti-technology sentiments have a price tag in terms of human suffering and loss. The question confronting us is whether this price tag can be justified theologically by those who uphold the value of fetal life.

It may be argued that the technology to which I have been referring is of a different nature to that responsible for IVF and its offshoots. But though there are differences, they are more apparent than real. The aim of all these forms of technology is to improve the quality of human life (in its broadest sense). They are all illustrations of biomedical technology. If we wish to reject technology *per se*, all technological aspects of modern medicine have to be rejected, plus, I would contend, all technological aspects of modern life – both biological and physical. On the other hand, if we do not wish to reject technology as a whole, then each application of technology has to be examined on its merits and decisions have to be taken in each case. This is precisely what I have attempted to do in this book, and it is what I did in *Brave New People*. The easy way out of onerous decisions is to wipe one's hands of the whole technological enterprise. If this is done, however, it will require a serious Christian rationale and it will also have to be carried out in a consistent fashion.[1]

The use of technology to alleviate the pain of infertility has come in for considerable criticism in some quarters. Much of this criticism appears to be based on the belief that infertility is not an illness, in that neither the husband nor wife is ill in the sense that they are incapacitated in their own lives as individuals. In a sense this is true; their life together as a couple, however, is incapacitated. For those who place considerable stress on the importance of marriage and the family, and on the quality of relationships within marriage, this incapacity cannot be ignored. Since its basis is generally a physical one (for example, blockage of the woman's uterine tubes or a deficiency of sperm in the male), it is difficult to see how this has nothing to do with medicine.

It may be objected that there are more pressing medical problems, or it may be argued that the medical therapy should be directed at the source of the problem, namely the blocked tubes, rather than at the embryo.[2] Both objections are serious ones, and both should be taken into consideration. These objections are however irrelevant to the more general question of whether we should or should not approve of any technological excursions into reproduction, since the microsurgical repair of damaged uterine tubes is an example of very sophisticated technology. In a similar fashion, any attempts at understanding and, in the future possibly rectifying, the causes of infertility in the male will be experimental scientific ones; and hence, once again, technological in nature.

A common fallacy is to attempt to confine medical treatment to life-and-death situations. Once medical therapy is used in other situations, such as the alleviation of infertility, it is condemned as straying outside the boundaries of legitimate medicine. It is surprising when this criticism comes from Christians, who should be emphasizing the wholeness of human existence rather than the biological dimensions alone. While it would be dangerous to bestow upon the medical profession a priestly function as well as a healing one, health is more than simply physical well-being. A married couple who are physically well in most aspects of their lives, but who are infertile, cannot be regarded as being 'whole' as a couple (in a narrow medical sense). They are as much in need of assistance (physical, psychological and spiritual) as is the person who can benefit from a total hip replacement, a cardiac pacemaker, a pair of spectacles, or a set of dentures. The aim of each of these artifices is to improve the overall quality of a person's life, although in only one of these examples is the condition a life-endangering one. Each of the artifices is also a product of technology, and yet the ethical objections to these procedures have been remarkably few. The same could be said of plastic surgery following burns, or (in part) of intestinal surgery to alleviate severe weight problems. Here again, the aim of the medical treatment is to improve a person's self-image, an important facet in that person's wholeness as a human individual.

Unless all procedures such as these are to be condemned, it is inconsistent to separate out for condemnation medicine's involvement in the reproductive area. The developments in reproductive technology are a natural extension, some would say an inevitable extension, of developments throughout the rest of medicine. It may even be argued that they fit into the long line of developments stemming back to the beginnings of modern science, with its Christian influence and its desire to overcome the rampant forces of disease.

A further misconception starts from the premise that suffering, emptiness and yearning are important facets of our lives as human beings. Our ability to deal with loss may prove an immensely rewarding experience, and may enrich us as human beings. I fully concur with these sentiments, which we ignore at our peril. Nevertheless, when confronted with infertility, these are never to be our immediate responses, just as they are not our responses in other instances of illness.

Initially, infertility is to be investigated as we would investigate any other symptoms, whether a persistent pain, a tumour, or a haemorrhage. Our immediate reaction to these, or other symptoms, is not the enriching nature of suffering but the possibility of diagnosing the cause of the symptoms and deciding whether appropriate treatment is available. In this, our approach is to be exactly the same as it would be for a duodenal ulcer, cancer of the lung, a broken leg, or failing eyesight. If medical treatment can cure the illness in question, or simply alleviate the worst of the symptoms, it should be employed. Similarly with infertility – if medical treatment can overcome the cause of the infertility, by unblocking a blocked uterine tube, by treating a pelvic inflammatory disease in the woman, by putting together the relatively immobile sperm of the husband and the wife's ovum (as in AIH), or by IVF, this is the course of action to be seriously considered.

It is always possible that medical treatment will fail, or that it will only prove partially successful. It is then that the Christian is called upon to face the prospect of loss and thwarted hopes. This is the point at which we have to face up to handicap, the prospect of an early death, a lonely future, or a married life without children of our own. There are times when we have to accept that further treatment may prove futile or may well be accompanied by more hazards than the illness itself. And so it is with infertility. A time may arrive when the tests and monthly monitoring should come to an end, and when procedures galore should cease. When the hope of a child has finally vanished, then is the time for accepting the limitations of one's marriage, and for appreciating the riches of what together you have in one another even in the absence of children.

To inflict such a deep bereavement of hope upon a couple, against their wishes and without adequate use of what medical technology may be able to offer, is a dimension of cruelty we would not dare inflict upon cancer sufferers. To be sure, infertile couples will differ immensely in the lengths to which they will want to go in seeking medical help. It is for them to gauge the depths of their needs, and it is for them to assess the ethical acceptability or otherwise of the services made available by society. The task of Christian onlookers is to help both the infertile and society work out what reproductive technological facilities should be made available. It is also our task to support the infertile, and to help them place their infertility in the context of their lives as a whole; to give them hope as human beings, even when the hope of producing their own biological offspring has disappeared.

Christians and Public Policy
Infertility affects all levels of society, and it pervades the lives of all types of people. It affects Christians as much as non-

Christians, and non-Christians as much as Christians. Whatever conclusions we arrive at, therefore, will have widespread
repercussions.

In the preceding chapters I have spoken primarily to Christians, although it will have become obvious that, at the level of
detail, many of the arguments are not explicitly biblical ones. I
do not believe there are such arguments when debating the
pros and cons of IVF or the propriety of carrying out research
on the tissues of a dead human fetus. The arguments I have
employed therefore, will appeal to those outside the Christian
community who accept many of the same basic premises on
these matters as I accept. Having said this, however, we still
need to ask whether one would expect to find any differences
between what one might describe as Christian conduct in the
reproductive domain, and the conduct to be allowed or perhaps
merely tolerated within society at large. Indeed, is there such a
definable entity as 'Christian conduct' in these matters? Can it
even be said that some forms of conduct in these areas are
pleasing to God, whereas others are displeasing to him?
Further, what attitudes will be beneficial to society?

My position on many of the issues I have discussed will raise
problems for some Christian readers. I should, perhaps, have
totally rejected AID, IVF, surrogacy, and all forms of research
on human embryos and fetuses. To many of my brothers and
sisters in Christ, any technological inroad into the reproductive process is anathema to our standing as human beings. I
shall not retrace the steps of my arguments here, except to say
that I fail to find any injunctions in the Bible against a *responsible* use of *certain* of these procedures under *certain* circumstances.

I have already indicated the general framework within
which I believe Christians should operate in these matters.
There will not be unanimity of viewpoints among Christians,
and there is no reason why there should be. Christian couples
confronted by infertility will also reach a medley of conclusions
about the procedures they do or do not wish to pursue. Nevertheless, the basis on which Christians build their expectations
and from which they derive their attitudes should have much
in common.

But what about the expectations of others within society,
with different presuppositions and different goals? Do Christians have anything to say to them, and therefore to society in

general, about the manner in which the reproductive technologies might be employed? Is it possible to have any point of contact between Christian perceptions and those of our neighbours within society?

In an attempt to suggest ways in which Christian perceptions may influence social thinking on the reproductive technologies, the following recommendations are put forward *as a basis for discussion*. None of these recommendations is meant to be definitive. Indeed, in some instances they are exceedingly tentative. Their purpose is to focus the discussion, by suggesting ways in which the positions I adopt may be worked out in society. I have no doubt that some may prove unworkable in practice, and they certainly require far more thought and open discussion than they have received up to now.

Recommendations, such as the ones I am proposing, simply provide a framework within which I believe society might operate. They constitute limitations for society. *Under no circumstances do they encourage individuals to go in the direction of AID, IVF, or surrogacy.* It is for individuals to weigh up the issues for themselves, and in the light of this assessment, make a responsible decision regarding the direction they wish to take. This applies equally to Christians and others.

In order to clarify even further the nature of these recommendations, let me make the following points:

1. The recommendations represent a compromise between what I would advocate to and for Christians, and what I think the societies in which we live in the West may be prepared to accept.
2. The proposals put forward in these recommendations are an attempt to place limits on procedures already in existence or soon to be introduced.
3. Simply because I am prepared to accept the existence of a procedure or social arrangement should not be taken as implying my approval of that procedure or arrangement. I may however, be prepared to tolerate it because of my concern for the welfare and future life of any resulting children. This applies in particular to heterosexual couples living in a stable *de facto* relationship. It also applies to AID. What is uppermost in my recommendations is not the legitimacy or otherwise of *de facto* relationships or of AID, but the good of the children who result from these arrange-

ments. Whatever we may think of the arrangements in their own right, the children are made in God's image and are in need of society's protection and support.

4. Many of the procedures covered by these recommendations touch on ethically grey areas. My personal predisposition is frequently more conservative than the recommendations, so that any advice I might give to a Christian couple would probably be relatively conservative.

5. It would be quite unfair to interpret these recommendations as demonstrating that I approve of anything that is technologically possible. One has only to contrast the conservative nature of these recommendations with the very radical nature of those of utilitarians (see chapter 2) to appreciate the major safeguards built into my recommendations.

6. It should be self-evident that I am not committed to any particular ideologies of right or left. I have made no attempt to put forward recommendations that will please those committed to any well-formulated 'political' cause, however worthy that cause may be. My aim, however imperfectly it may be executed, is to transcend any ideological baggage and to allow Jesus Christ to be the decisive influence in the stand I take on issues of public policy. In dealing with society I have to accept much that I would not personally advocate. What I have attempted to do is to delineate the boundaries of the reproductive technologies, pointing to those that will enhance, rather than detract from, the humanness of all involved.

7. In searching for a satisfactory family environment in which artificially conceived children are to be brought up, my own position as a Christian is that this should be by a married couple within a conventional family setting. This is the norm, which should as far as possible be adhered to within society. The difficulty however, is that vast numbers of naturally conceived children are not brought up in such a setting. With regard to public policy therefore, it will be difficult, if not impossible, to ensure that this norm is expressed in legislative terms.

The dimensions of the problem with naturally conceived children can be illustrated from American figures.[3] In 1982 there were 2,495,000 marriages (10.8/1000 population) and 1,180,000 divorces (5.1/1000 population). Inevitably therefore, an exceedingly high number of children are involved in families undergoing separation and divorce, and therefore a change of social parentage. These figures for just one year are typical of every year in recent times.

Another illustration of the lack of the norm in children-parent relationships is provided by the number of children born to single women. In 1980 in the United States 665,700 children were born to single women, this number accounting for 18.4% of all births. While it is not known how many of these women were living in stable relationships, these figures do at least provide some indication of the scale of family settings deviating from the norm. American figures in 1982 showed that 3,851,000 children had ever been born in the United States to 13,780,000 single women (279 children/1000 single women).

These figures do not justify laxity of standards when dealing with artificially conceived children, but they should remind us of the enormous number of naturally conceived children being reared in single-parent families, or in families in which the social father (or mother) is not the biological father (or mother). We need to assess what is an adequate environment in which children can be brought up successfully, asking in particular what relationships are essential for this. My own response, along with that of many others[4] is that a warm stable relationship between heterosexual partners is required. To put a child into a family without this as the basic ingredient, is to do a grave disservice to that child. This is of concern whether the child has been naturally or artificially conceived. This is not to say that single-parent families may not cope remarkably successfully. They frequently do. But it is not the norm, or even close to the norm.

Christians will wish to stress that the partners are married. It is right that this should be stressed, and yet in the context of society as a whole they may have to accept less. What then becomes critical is that the child will have the opportunity to develop as a balanced individual in a stable, loving and stimulating environment. Hence my emphasis on the long-term commitment of the parents to each other and to the child.

Recommendations for Society

AID

1. AID should not be regarded as a medical procedure devoid of moral overtones. While it is true that it appears to be widely accepted within many communities, its acceptance has occurred surreptiously and at a time when there was little ethical debate about medical matters. Such acceptance should not be used as an argument in favour of the wholesale acceptance of gamete donation, regardless of the circumstances and of whether sperm or ovum donation is involved.

2. AID should only be carried out by registered medical practitioners, in authorized clinics. Only in this way can the procedure be adequately monitored.

3. All parties involved in AID should receive counselling – the donor as well as both members of the recipient couple. The medical staff should also be made aware of the ethical dimensions of the procedure.

4. Donors should be married, and should have had at least one child of their own. This would in effect, be equivalent to genetic screening of the donor. The donor's wife should have given her approval for the donation.

5. AID, on the grounds of infertility, should not be undertaken until all the appropriate medical investigations of the causes of the infertility have been carried out. AIH and IVF (if available) should also have been attempted if considered appropriate on medical grounds.

6. AID may be offered to couples where, for genetic reasons (for example, Huntington's chorea), it is inadvisable for the husband to father a child.

7. AID should only be made available to married couples, or to heterosexual couples living in a stable *de facto* relationship.[5] This stipulation is made since the child is of crucial concern in AID, and his or her rearing is of paramount importance. Many consider that this is aided by the relationships ideally found in a stable family environment encompassing at least male and female social parents.[6] While such an environment can never be assured (and is frequently not attained in a 'natural' family), the involvement of society necessitated by any form of artificial reproduction puts responsibilities onto society not found in

'natural' reproduction.

8. The AID child should have the opportunity, on reaching his or her late teens, of obtaining basic information about certain physical characteristics of the donor. Such 'non-identifying' information can only be made available if adequate medical records are kept by the AID clinic. This should be made mandatory in all clinics, and donors should not be able to veto the imparting of such information to the offspring of AID. The AID child should not be able to use such information to trace the donor.

9. In an attempt to minimize the secrecy and deceit so often associated with AID, the law should be changed absolving the donor of any responsibility for the child, and recognizing the social father as the father for all legal purposes.

10. Donors should not be paid for their donation, other than nominal travelling and inconvenience expenses. If the donation were to be made a commercial transaction, it would suggest that the donation was not a medical procedure but one with overtones of social engineering. It may also mean that AID would, at some stage in the future, be available only to those who could afford it. This would be unjust, and would also be a move towards acceptance of the view that babies can be bought.

IVF – Simple Case

1. IVF should be made available to married couples or heterosexual couples in stable *de facto* relationships; preference should be given to those couples who have not had previous children by 'natural' means.

2. IVF clinics should be set up in authorized institutions in the main centres of countries. Monitoring of the procedures used, the success rate obtained, and the children born using IVF, should be mandatory.

3. The standard form of IVF developed in IVF clinics should only resort to hormonal stimulation of the woman's ovaries, when this is part of a programme for the freezing of oocytes.

4. All IVF programmes should incorporate counselling for those being assessed for their inclusion in a programme, as well as for those on a programme. If a pregnancy is not achieved after three treatment cycles, treatment should cease, and counselling and direction should be given as appropriate.

5. IVF programmes should occupy an integral place in the infertility services offered by hospitals. They should therefore, be viewed in conjunction with other procedures such as AIH, AID, microsurgical approaches to tubal blockage, and surgical treatment of male infertility.
6. Considerable attention needs to be given to the financial implications of the development of IVF programmes. It has to be decided how extensive the programmes are to be, and how many programmes are to be developed in a country. These financial implications need to be assessed alongside others: the money required for (a) research into various aspects of IVF programmes, for example, further research into the freezing of oocytes, and improvement of the efficiency of microsurgical approaches to the alleviation of certain forms of infertility; (b) the development of public health measures aimed at lowering the incidence of infertility in the community, for example, infertility resulting from pelvic inflammatory disease, abortion at an early age, and prematurely-undertaken sterilization procedures.

IVF – Spare Embryos

1. My preference is for IVF programmes without the production of an excess number of embryros and without embryo freezing. However, I concede that many will not agree and will argue strongly for the availability of embryo freezing facilities. If such facilities are to be allowed, they should not be regarded as obligatory in all IVF clinics. The rationale for this recommendation is that frozen embryos will in the future not be required in straightforward IVF programmes (the simple case). Spare embryos will be required only in the case of couples who have given prior agreement to their use for donation and/or research procedures (this statement does not signify my own agreement with either of these procedures).
2. IVF clinics should be of two types: those carrying out exclusively clinical procedures to alleviate infertility problems in married or *de facto* couples, and those concerned with donations (if permitted) and research (if permitted). Should these latter two procedures be allowed, such clinics will require freezing facilities.

   The ready availability of freezing facilities in all (or most) IVF clinics will, in all probability, increase demands for the indiscriminate use of human embryos. This is a fear many people within the community have, and it is a legitimate one. For those who have a high view of the pre-implantation embryo (including myself), one means of safeguarding the interests of the human embryo is to impose stringent limits on what procedures can be carried out on it. A practical outworking of this is to limit the institutions where spare embryos are available.

3. Decisions regarding the use to which frozen embryos are put should be the prerogative of the couples producing them, or of the clinics' administrators when this is not possible. At the time of embryo freezing the couple should have been fully informed of the options available (these, in principle, are discarding such embryos, donating them to another couple, using them for research purposes) and should have signed a consent form declaring their wishes, if the stored embryo(s) are not transferred to the female partner's uterus. If a couple is unwilling to accept any of these options, they should be advised not to proceed with embryo freezing.

4. Embryos should be retained in a frozen state for a maximum of 10 years, or less if the couple wishes to dispose of them earlier.

IVF – Gamete Donations

All the recommendations regarding AID (except 4) apply to both ovum and embryo donations. The following are additional considerations:

1. The collection of a donor's ova should not entail any risks to the donor herself, for example, she should not, under normal circumstances, be operated upon for the sole purpose of collecting ova to be donated to another woman.

2. Ova should only be used for donation purposes with the consent of the donor (and her husband, if she is married).

3. The donation of ova should not be undertaken unless a satisfactory degree of anonymity for the donor can be assured.

4. The only *embryos* which should be employed for donation purposes are those that are surplus to the needs of a couple in an IVF programme. Embryos should never be specifically produced for donation purposes using the gametes of donors.

5. Embryos should only be used for donation purposes with the consent of the donating couple.

6. Where consent has been given for embryo donation, the biological parents relinquish all future rights to that embryo. The recipients of the donor embryo, following adequate counselling and signing of appropriate consent forms, should have all the rights attributed to parents who conceive by natural means. The child resulting from embryo donation should have all the rights and privileges attributed to children conceived by natural means. The child resulting from embryo transfer should have no rights of access, inheritance or legal action on the biological parents, and in turn the biological parents have no such rights to the child resulting from their embryo donation.

Surrogate Motherhood

1. Surrogacy is an extreme measure which, at present, is surrounded by a host of unknowns. It should be approached, therefore, with the greatest of caution, and society should be extremely careful before appearing to legitimize it.
2. Two forms of surrogacy should be recognized; the traditional form, and IVF-dependent surrogacy. These two forms should be treated separately in law, since they raise different ethical issues.
3. While many may wish to ban surrogacy arrangements, the ease with which the traditional form of surrogacy can be undertaken (especially when carried out informally or between relations) may make this unenforceable. Nevertheless, traditional surrogacy should not be encouraged, and payment of surrogate mothers and lawyers (and others) associated with these arrangements should be prohibited.
4. IVF-dependent surrogacy should not be permitted within IVF programmes.
5. Measures should be taken to prevent the exploitation of infertile couples and (potential) surrogate mothers in any proposed surrogacy arrangements within society. Measures will also have to be taken to protect the interests of children born as a result of surrogacy arrangements.

Research on Human Embryos

1. The use of human embryos for research purposes should not be permitted as a routine part of IVF programmes. The authorization of clinics to carry out IVF procedures should not include the authorization of research programmes using human embryos.

2. The production of human embryos from donated ova and sperm specifically for research uses should not be permitted under any circumstances.
3. My categorical preference is for no research on spare embryos. However, if some research is permitted, especially in the context of testing and improving the efficiency of IVF procedures, regulations are required. If this is the case, no research should be permitted until a decision has been taken concerning the nature of the research procedures to be approved. This should be undertaken by an officially appointed body composed of medical and lay personnel. If research on human embryos is permitted, this should not be interpreted as permission to carry out unspecified research (for definitions of research and experimentation, see chapter 7).
4. Considerable attention should be given to formulating criteria for distinguishing between therapeutic research (aimed at benefiting the embryo in question and embryos in general) and non-therapeutic research (of benefit to medicine in general) using human embryos. Only therapeutic research should be permitted, this should only be in authorized research laboratories, and consent must have been given by the originating couple for the use of embryos in a therapeutic research programme.
5. Before any therapeutic research using human embryos is allowed, those applying to do the research should prove to the appropriate authorities that they have experience in research employing animal embryos and that they have exhausted the possibilities using animal models. Therapeutic research using human embryos should only be permitted in a few centres throughout any country. This will enable stringent controls to be established and maintained.
6. Research into fertilization, the early stages of embryonic development, embryonic wastage, and infertility, using experimental animals, should be actively encouraged and adequately financed.

Reflections on Christian Attitudes
The nature of the topics discussed in this book cannot help but polarize viewpoints. This is especially the case with Christians, who expect, or at least hope for, uniformity of opinion within their ranks. All too readily they equate ambiguity on

social issues with a lack of clarity on theological matters. In my discussion of the reproductive technologies I have accepted that there are many unsettled issues. Indeed, I believe that opinions may be modified as time passes and as technological developments change. This is not to be decried, since our current understanding in many areas is incomplete. We see 'as through a glass darkly'; there is much we fail to comprehend, and we are unsure how to apply some theological principles, or even on occasions to know which theological principles are the most appropriate to apply to particular situations.

Unnerving as much of this is, we do have guideposts, as I have attempted to indicate. We do not however, have infallible rules. This should come as no surprise to us, since serious discussion of these issues has only been undertaken within the past 15–20 years. For many groups, discussion commenced only 2–3 years ago. To expect mature debate in such a short period is quite unrealistic, and to expect definitive resolution to these matters after such a brief time is even more unrealistic.

1. Accepting Uncertainties

Implicit within many of the ideas I have expressed in these pages has been the theme of uncertainty. There is much about which we are not sure; there are many possibilities about which we have reservations and stipulations. It is unnerving to have to live with such vast question marks and such profound queries. And yet I believe we have to contend with a population of unknowns, about which it would be foolhardy to express categorical assertions and dogmatic statements.

The reproductive technologies will not allow us to stray far from one crucial topic, and that is *fertilization*. We have already encountered some of the uncertainties surrounding fertilization, one consequence of which has been to convert what was once a joyful event into an idol. Now that we have shed so much of our ignorance of fertilization, and now that the mystique has largely disappeared, we are left with an event that we desperately long to control. Unfortunately, we are not quite able to do this, and instead we are left with frustration and conflict.

For one group of people, those who are desperately longing for a child, fertilization has been elevated to the status of an idol. It is the one thing they want more than anything, and for some, virtually anything may be sacrificed in order to attain it. Hence the willingness to cross previously uncrossable marriage boundaries. Paradoxically, this is not the only group in this position. At the other end of the spectrum those who appear to place more value on embryonic life than on any other form of human life have also made it an idol. For them, once new human life has been conceived, nothing whatsoever should come between that nascent life and its realization in the birth of a child. All the weight of the 'sanctity of human life' has to be borne by the event of fertilization, so that idol status has, in effect, been bestowed upon fertilization.

Perhaps I can illustrate this by reference to *contraception*. Let us imagine four couples, A, B, C and D. Not one of them wishes to conceive. Couple A decide not to have intercourse; thereby preventing a possible future child from coming into existence. Couple B have intercourse; since they are using an oral contraceptive, fertilization does not occur, and no child results. Couple C have intercourse, and the wife is using an IUCD; fertilization does occur, but the embryo is prevented from implanting; no child results. Couple D have intercourse, but no contraceptive is being employed since they are infertile and have no reason to expect to conceive; fertilization however, occurs on this occasion; a child is not wanted on account of the wife's chronic ill-health; a first trimester abortion is carried out, and no child results.

These four couples pose immense challenges to our ethical decision-making, and demonstrate clearly the stress we place on fertilization. The intention of all four couples is the same – none of them wishes to conceive and bring a new human being into existence. The result in all four cases is the same, and yet in two of them fertilization occurs. Are couples C and D acting unethically, or is there no difference between all four couples?

A second illustration refers to couples E, F, G, H and I. In this case the couples wish to conceive. Couple E are fertile; they have intercourse and fertilization occurs. Each time they want to conceive they know they will be successful within two to three months. Couple F are fertile but there are certain sexual problems requiring counselling. With help however, they overcome these problems and are able to conceive. With couple G the male partner has an infertility problem. However, the use of AIH helps to circumvent this problem, and fertilization occurs using AIH. In the case of couple H there is an infertility problem on the female side. This is solved by micro-surgery on her uterine tubes, and fertilization subsequently occurs. A similar problem exists with couple I; surgery is unsuccessful in this instance, although fertilization is brought about using IVF.

In each of these cases the couple wish to have a child of their own, derived from their own genetic materials. They do not want to introduce a third party into their marriage relation-ship. Each of them is successful, although different avenues are used. Each of them would, ideally, have wanted a child in the simplest, easiest and most natural fashion – just like couple E – and yet they are unable to do so. The question is: have couples F to I acted less ethically than couple E? Is there any distinction between the actions of couples F and G, both of whom have received therapy and yet only couple G have had artificial assistance in the reproductive process itself? Is there any distinction between couples H and I, both of whom have the same problem (blockage in the female partner's uterine tubes) and resort to the same initial treatment (microsurgery to repair the blocked tubes); and yet couple I had to go further and employed IVF?

Yet again, there is ethical uncertainty. The goal of all five couples is the same – the production of a child from their own bodies, a child who is the outcome of their marital love. In none of these instances has there been any abrogation of the mar-riage bond or any desire to do so. In each case the desire of the couple has been to raise a family of their own, to care for and to bring up any resulting children within the confines of the love and warmth of a couple committed to each other and also to others for whom they have responsibility. Any differences between these couples stem from the extent of their fertility, and the intrusion of therapy into the reproductive process.

A third set of illustrations concerns couples J, K, L and M in an IVF programme. Couple J conceive using the simplest form of IVF, with the husband's sperm and the wife's ovum; no freezing of embryos is involved. In the case of couple K six embryos are produced. Two are transferred to the wife's uterus on each of three successive months; she becomes pregnant on the third attempt. Although four embryos were initially frozen, none remains at the end of the treatment period. With couple L six embryos are again produced; in this case however, the wife becomes pregnant on the first treatment, leaving four spare embryos. All these are used a couple of years later to provide the couple with a second child, so that no spare embryos remain. In the case of couple M six embryos are produced and pregnancy occurs after four have been used. The two spare embryos are not required by this couple, and are discarded. Once again, there are ethical uncertainties which have nothing to do with transgressing the bounds of the marital relationship. They do however, raise once more the question of the artificial assistance of reproduction, and the production of an excess number of embryos, their freezing, and their fate.

These illustrations are not intended to justify any of the particular courses of action outlined. Nevertheless, they highlight some of the uncertainties surrounding the event of fertilization. Once it is idolized, it raises a further series of dilemmas, the ramifications of which may be much greater than anticipated. These include a reassessment of the legitimacy of contraception (both natural and artificial), the conflict that may arise between giving 'life' to the preimplantation embryo and the legitimacy of embryo donation (prenatal adoption), and the competing claims of the preimplantation embryo, the later fetus, and postnatal human life. These dilemmas are the direct result of treating fertilization as an idol.

The idolization of fertilization therefore, does not eliminate conflict and uncertainty. In fact, it increases both conflict and uncertainty. The nature of the uncertainties has, however, been changed, and the repercussions are enormous for almost every facet of reproductive bioethics, and even for our views of marriage and the family.

2. *Establishing Certainties*

Although I have outlined some of the principles basic to Christian attitudes in previous chapters, it is just as well to remind ourselves of some positive features in a Christian response. This is surely warranted, since so much of what we have been dealing with has been contentious and uncertain.

In Christian terms, the nature, purpose and dignity of human persons are derived from God and from his purposes for us as individuals and when acting in community. Our perspective therefore, can never be limited to biological horizons, however important these are. This dual perspective, provided by God and science, is crucial to any appreciation of the new reproductive technologies. They need to be seen within a framework provided by Christian understanding, but at the same time we dare not despise their roots in biology and their potential for alleviating some aspects of the human predicament.

A particular Christian contribution to the debate over the manufacturing of humans is that, since we as Christians have experienced God dealing with us in grace, mercy and love, we are to deal with others in the same way. We are to commit ourselves to the service of others, because God in Christ has committed himself to the self-sacrificial service of mankind. Against this background it would be totally unjustified for us to treat others – even (some would say, especially) embryos, fetuses or children – as mere means to an end. While this does not provide us with automatic solutions to some notoriously difficult bioethical issues, it does provide built-in constraints on actions we may otherwise take.

From this it follows that our aim as Christians should be to provide conditions that will enable each human being to discover and to attain his or her full potential. Idealistic as this is, even a few tentative steps in this direction have radical implications for our approach to human beings. They govern the actions of the doctor, the patient, and the community; they have medico-biological, psychological, social, and spiritual repercussions; and they affect the embryo, fetus, child and adult, the fertile as well as the infertile, those longing for a child of their own and those seeking to help them as doctors, counsellors, donors or surrogates.

This holistic view of human potential is reflected in a Christian understanding of health, with its emphasis on fulfilment and well-being as well as on physical 'normality'. To live a truly human life is to relate satisfactorily with one's neighbours, family, associates and peers; it is also to relate to God in loving trust and in dependence upon him; it includes the capacity to accept hardship, suffering, loss and emptiness, although it also ushers in commitment, drive and determination.

These competing sides of the human longing for health can be summed up in a conclusion reached by Donald MacKay,[7] namely, that 'we need a distinction between contentment with the unalterable, and complacency with the alterable'. MacKay continues 'If our lives were purely self-centred it could be argued that lingering in a defective but remediable condition is our own affair. But if our primary obligation is to serve and glorify God, and if an innocuous remedy were at hand that would increase our effectiveness to that end, complacency on our part would be clearly culpable.' To flee from the world of reproductive technology, because we are afraid of some of the possible consequences, is to admit to a lack of faith in the God who has bestowed these myriad powers upon us. It is to be complacent with that which is capable of being altered and improved; such an attitude is an illustration of faithlessness rather than of piety.

We should not idly contrast Christianity and technology, or holiness and health. A Christian framework incorporates technology (when necessary), just as there are intimate links between health – as a general state of wholeness, fulfilment and well-being – and holiness. The quality of human life is, therefore, important, as long as it is not narrowed down to biological and physical dimensions alone. Relationships and a meaningful interplay between one human and another and between humans and God are crucial, complementing as they do the drive for improvements in biological and psychological quality.

The overarching arena in which these dimensions of human life are to be played out, as far as reproduction is concerned, is that of marriage and the family. These are central to all discussions of human fertilization and sexuality, with their overtones of loving commitment, and self-giving relationships. It is within this context that we learn and express love for our neighbour, ourselves and God, whether we be husband/wife, mother/father, son/daughter, grandson/granddaughter, uncle/aunt, or adopted son/adopted daughter.

Marriage and the family provide not only the bounds of reproductive activities, but also the realm in which we learn that personal well-being is only part of the human story. We also learn the value of community, of giving and sharing, of helping and being helped. We learn that we are part of a much larger whole, involving other human beings like ourselves, with their needs and desires, their hopes and expectations, their strengths and frailties.

Christians are called to see Christ in their neighbour; in the weak and helpless, in the poor and downtrodden, in the vulnerable and exploited. It is within this framework that we are to approach the new reproductive technologies, and hence to view the infertile couple, the infertile husband or wife, the donors of semen or embryos, the surrogate mother, the couple prepared to use a surrogate mother, the unwanted child, the dispossessed fetus, and the spare embryo. We will not suddenly be confronted with an infallible solution to any dilemma, but we will begin to see the human factors in an otherwise impersonal wasteland.

3. *Advice to a Christian Couple*
The great danger in an area of conundrums is to give up serious thinking and analysis, and opt instead for a simple solution, namely, go wholeheartedly in the direction of biomedical technology or reject whatever biomedical technology has to offer. For Christians this temptation is just as great as for anyone else. How do we weigh up the pros and cons of infertility and childlessness, and how is a decision to be made regarding the nature and extent of the treatment to be sought?

The following hints are provided by way of guidelines for those in this situation.

(a) However important it is to have children of one's own, this is less important in the long run than obedience to the call of God, whatever form that may take. A marriage without children is no less of a marriage for being childless,[8] although this is not the way for most couples, including many infertile ones.

(b) We are to seek God's help and directives in the matter of infertility and childlessness. This is of as much concern to him as any other aspect of our lives. God loves the infertile as much as the fertile. With him there is no distinction. The issue is a spiritual one, as much as a physical and psychological one; to fail to trust in God's care will lead ultimately to spiritual depression and hopelessness.

(c) As Christians we are to realize that we are a part of a community of God's people. We are to seek out people therefore, with whom we can (hopefully) discuss these matters, and who will provide support and encouragement regardless of what decision we take.

(d) In order for the previous guideline to be of any practical value, it is imperative that Christians as a whole are informed about infertility and the new reproductive technologies. It is also imperative that they approach these technologies within a Christian framework, and that they are able to provide spiritual as well as practical guidance. What is essential is sympathetic understanding and wise counsel, realizing that different Christians may well come to different conclusions in the use of some of these techniques.

(e) Alongside the assistance of other Christians, the infertile couple need to be thoroughly informed themselves about the possibilities open to them. The ambivalent nature of all these technologies demands of those facing them a detailed knowledge of the technical data. While this may be very difficult for those without an adequate background in reproductive biology, they still need to acquire this knowledge – with the assistance of experts in the field, both Christian and non-Christian. None of these techniques is without its drawbacks, and so none should be embarked upon lightly. At the same time however, childlessness is not without *its* drawbacks either, and the couple need to appreciate this side of the infertility dilemma as well.

(f) The couple need to realize that the *final* decision will be theirs. While they should be supported in this by other Christians, it is they (especially the wife) who will have to endure tests galore, endless procedures, and perhaps repeated frustrations. They need to know themselves well enough to decide whether their resources are sufficient to see them through the confusing maze of hospital appointments. Do they want a child so badly that they are prepared for all they will have to endure? What other sacrifices will they have to make towards this end? Will these sacrifices have spiritual consequences – for good or bad? Alternatively, at what point will they be prepared to accept a life together without a child of their own?

(g) The couple will also need to weigh up the justification of doing everything possible to attain a child of their own, against the role they could play by adopting a child – especially perhaps a child not wanted by others, because of a medical problem or for racial reasons. Have they considered that the adoption of such a child (or children) would be a service they could render as Christians? Perhaps they feel they would be unable to cope with a handicapped or disadvantaged child. If so, is this an adequate reason for failing to respond to a child in need?

(h) The couple will need to consider the consequences of their decision for any others implicated in the techniques adopted. This applies to the medical staff undertaking the techniques, a donor or donor couple, a surrogate mother, and the resulting child. If the technique may result in embryos for which the couple themselves could, conceivably, have no use, they need to have thought through their own position on what should be the fate of those embryos. They are as responsible for those embryos as they are for embryos they hope will give them a child of their own. These considerations demonstrate that the consequences of our actions are never confined to ourselves alone, and for Christians the impact they may have on others are as important as the impact they will have on us. With this in mind, a couple may sometimes conclude that the untoward effects of a technique on others outweigh the possibly beneficial effects for them, and so they may decide to forego using the technique on these grounds.

(i) Ideally, a couple will need to agree on whatever course of action they decide on. This may be difficult to attain, and yet it is imperative if one of the artificial reproductive technologies is to be embarked upon. The demands of the procedures may well prove too much for a couple, if there is initial hesitancy on the part of one of them. A couple should be able to discuss even the most intimate details of the procedure openly and honestly; they should be able to pray together about it, and they should be able to discuss the pros and cons of the technique with close friends and confidants.

(j) In the final analysis we are in the hands of a sovereign God. He has a plan for our lives as his people, even if we do not understand it or if we are actively rebelling against it. Infertility seems to be a very unfair and a profoundly unjust condition from which to suffer. We should never underestimate this, and some infertile couples will have to work through their feelings at length. Finally, however, we all need to come to God in a spirit of positive commitment to him, seeking his ways for us, with or without children. There are no simple, rule-of-thumb solutions. To be childless is no more spiritual than to have children; to have children naturally is no more spiritual than to have them artificially; to have one's own genetic children is no more spiritual than to have adopted children; to have adopted healthy children is no more spiritual than to have adopted handicapped children.

We are persons entrusted with making responsible decisions as people made in the image and likeness of God. We have Jesus Christ as our master and example, and we are to live lives of service to others just as he did. We have the Spirit of the risen Christ to guide and direct us, and we are to listen to his guidance and to obey his dictates as set out by the biblical writers.

There are no simple solutions to the complex problems posed by infertility and the myriad responses to it now available to us, and yet the infertile couple is not alone. The God whom we worship understands the frailty and brokenness of our humanity, and he is with us as we respond in faith and trust. Having thought through the issues, having understood them to the best of our ability, having consulted others, having prayed about the dilemmas and having committed them to our heavenly Father, we have the assurance that he will be alongside us to strengthen and support us as we move forward in whatever ways we have concluded are pleasing to him and appropriate for us.

Epilogue

This book has been about techniques that are part of our present world. There is also, however, the realm of what we may call the 'future present', the new procedures that are very much of the future and yet are either present reality or promise to be so very shortly. While these techniques may not be as revolutionary as IVF, they either have to be seen in the light of it or they are direct extensions of it. While it is not my intention to analyse these procedures, a brief description of them may be helpful to demonstrate issues that will confront the general public in the near future.

1. Chorion Biopsy

At present amniocentesis is the major technique available for obtaining a sample of fetal cells and hence for detecting chromosomal abnormalities, such as Down's syndrome, and various other conditions, such as neural tube defects. The major drawback of this procedure is that, since it cannot be carried out until a sufficient quantity of amniotic fluid is present at around 14–18 weeks of gestation, therapeutic abortion – if carried out – will be a mid-trimester abortion between 18 and 23 weeks.[1]

A new technique, which may replace amniocentesis, is that of chorion biopsy (chorion villus sampling). This involves the removal through the cervix of tissue from the chorion, one of the membranes surrounding the fetus.[2] This can be undertaken at eight to ten weeks gestation; the biopsy material can be used for identification of the chromosomes and for analysis of the DNA. In this way it will probably prove possible to diagnose chromosomal disorders, such as that responsible for Down's syndrome, and to detect the genetic defects underlying conditions such as Duchenne muscular dystrophy, cystic fibrosis, haemophilia, sickle cell anaemia, thalassaemia and phenylketonuria.

This technique was developed in Europe in the late 1960s and, apparently, has been used by the Chinese since 1970 to determine fetal sex and to assist in family planning. In Europe, Australasia and North America it is currently undergoing extensive trials, and has been used on at least 10,000 occasions since 1983. One of its drawbacks at present is the increased risk of spontaneous abortion following it. This is put at 2% to 5%,[3] compared with 0.5% to 1.5% following amniocentesis.

The major advantages of chorion biopsy over amniocentesis are the early stage of pregnancy when it can be carried out, together with the speed with which the results of the procedure are available – within days or even hours. This is in stark contrast to the two weeks or so for the results of amniocentesis.

The value of these differences is that, if an abortion is indicated, chorion biopsy enables it to be carried out much earlier than with the currently available amniocentesis. This is of relevance if fetal handicap is detected or if the fetus is of the 'wrong' sex in the case of a sex-linked condition. While this will not eliminate any of the ethical dilemmas associated with therapeutic abortion, it will probably decrease some of the psychological sequelae that follow late abortions necessitated by the results of amniocentesis (see chapter 5). This is a matter of considerable importance for those who have decided to undergo a therapeutic abortion of an otherwise 'wanted' baby. Such sequelae should not be decried by those opposed to abortions under all circumstances, no matter how strong their disagreement with abortion on the ground of suspected or proven fetal handicap. By the same token, the availability of chorion biopsy will not make abortion any more acceptable in ethical terms. The ethical issue has to be decided on totally different grounds (see chapter 5).

Chorion biopsy may well have other contributions to make, besides that of simply detecting fetal sex or fetal abnormalities. It is becoming increasingly likely that it will form the basis of the treatment of fetal disorders. For example, experimental work in progress at present is aimed at treating a fetus suffering from a genetic defect affecting its ability to produce normal blood cells. This is being tackled by injecting into the bloodstream of the fetus tiny bone-marrow grafts taken from a healthy donor without this particular genetic defect.

The importance of chorion biopsy stems from the very early diagnosis it makes possible. Foreign material is not rejected until 18 weeks gestation, and so the hope is that the grafted bone marrow will provide a significant proportion of healthy red cells and thereby effectively cure the disease.

2. IVF – Related Techniques

The collection of a woman's ova prior to IVF is routinely carried out using a laparoscope, which is a telescope-like instrument that has to be inserted through the woman's abdominal wall. An alternative procedure being introduced in some IVF programmes is to use ultrasound. This enables the doctor to visualize the ovary and the path of the needle inserted to collect ova from ovarian follicles on a cathode ray tube screen. The enormous advantage of this technique is that it can be carried out under local anaesthesia, and can therefore be performed as an outpatient procedure. This could make IVF a far more amenable and less taxing undertaking for the woman.

Quite a different procedure is that of removing sperm from a man's testis or some other part of his reproductive system, and then fertilizing one of his wife's ova using IVF. This technique has been employed where the husband of a couple has undergone a vasectomy. Attempts to reverse the vasectomy have failed, and so, although the man is capable of producing healthy sperm, he has incomplete vas deferens. IVF is required for the fertilization process, rather than artificial insemination, since sperm obtained from deep inside the reproductive system are still in an immature state and are usually obtained in very small quantities. This approach to infertility is still in an experimental stage, and even when developed much further will probably only be used on a limited scale. This is because it necessitates a general anaesthetic for the man, and involves the collection of immature sperm thereby decreasing the chances of successful fertilization.

An even more dramatic development, reported first in 1984, is illustrated by a number of women who have become pregnant despite a lack of ovaries or of ovarian function.[4] In these instances donor ova were fertilized by the husband's sperm via IVF, prior to be being implanted in the woman's uterus. In order to maintain the pregnancy, the hormones oestrogen and progesterone are administered before insertion of the embryo and up to the fifth month of pregnancy. These hormones are normally produced by the ovaries, and their use in these cases is necessary to create an artificial menstrual cycle. This approach could prove relevant for women who have had their ovaries removed, and also for those born without ovaries.

A process which does not involve IVF, but which is akin to some aspects of it, is gamete intrafallopian transfer treatment (GIFT). In this, the woman receives hormonal treatment to stimulate ovulation and produce several ova. Some of these are then placed, together with a concentrated amount of her husband's sperm, into her fallopian (uterine) tubes. Fertilization, and subsequent development, occur normally.

3. Embryonic Biopsy
This is a more futuristic and also a more radical technique than any of those discussed up to this point. The aim of embryonic biopsy would be to take the diagnostic possibilities opened up by amniocentesis and chorion biopsy very much further than could ever be envisaged with these – even with chorion biopsy. Embryonic biopsy opens up the following scenario. After IVF, the embryo would be allowed to divide into four or eight cells. One cell would then be removed and examined for genetic and chromosomal abnormalities. While this was being carried out, the remainder of the embryo would be frozen, until it was known whether the biopsy revealed any abnormality. If it was decided to proceed with the development of this particular embryo, the frozen embryo (that is, the remaining three cells of a four-celled embryo) would be thawed and transferred to the mother's uterus.

The basis of embryonic biopsy is that the early embryo is capable of developing into a whole individual in the absence of one cell. The advantage of this technique as a diagnostic procedure is that, if an abnormality is detected and it is decided not to implant that embryo, it does not involve abortion in the conventional sense since the mother is not yet pregnant. The disadvantage of the technique in current terms is that it involves IVF, with all the attendant difficulties of IVF. Nevertheless, embryonic biopsy may one day revolutionize diagnostic approaches.

The possibilities opened up by this procedure are that, if and when genetic therapy becomes a reality, the cell(s) provided by embryonic biopsy will be amenable for treatment. Following gene manipulation, the treated cell(s) will be placed in the mother's uterus for subsequent normal gestation.

4. Trans-species Fertilization

Fertilization of this type is currently undertaken in the investigation of male subfertility. Human sperm is used to fertilize hamster eggs treated in a certain way, the basis of the test being that the occurrence of fertilization indicates good fertility prospects for the couple. These tests do not require the fertilized egg to develop beyond the two cell stage. Development could, however, be allowed to proceed further, on the grounds that a more mature embryo may be of value in diagnostic or research procedures. These are all examples of trans-species fertilization, resulting in each case in a hybrid embryo.

5. Mass Production and Culture of Human Embryonic Material

It is theoretically possible to produce a large bank of human embryos, for the testing of drugs and other substances. Should this be permitted, it may provide an alternative to the use of animals in many drug-testing regimes.

Another approach would be to culture human cell lines. The cells would be disaggregated and grown in tissue culture media. In this way they will produce more of the same kind of cells. Unlike human embryonic cells, they will not develop into a complex human organism. While this is a clear-cut distinction, the situation is not always this simple, for example, there are close similarities between carcinoma cell lines and embryonic cells. In mice, malignant carcinoma cells have been compacted with normal embryos to produce chimaeric progeny showing no signs of malignancy. While this type of research is far from clinical reality, it helps to reiterate the ambiguity and doubt surrounding some aspects of early human development. This, however, is a theme that will have to await further discussion at some future time.

Glossary

The definition of some of the following terms is controversial. Where this is the case, the definition employed is not to be taken as representing my own opinion.

abortus. Fetus weighing less than 500g at time of expulsion from the uterus, with no chance of survival.

amniocentesis. Procedure to obtain small quantity of amniotic fluid from around the developing fetus; carried out at around 14–18 weeks of gestation.

amniotic cavity. A cavity containing amniotic fluid, in which the embryo/fetus is suspended. The amniotic fluid is a clear, watery fluid, produced partly by the amniotic cells but derived primarily from maternal blood; it serves as a protective cushion for the embryo/fetus.

anencephaly. Absence of the vault of the skull, with the cerebral hemispheres of the brain completely missing, or reduced to small masses attached to the base of the skull.

artificial insemination. Introduction of semen into the vagina or cervix by artificial means; the semen may come from the woman's husband (AIH) or from a man other than the woman's husband – a donor (AID).

azoospermia. Lack of spermatozoa in the semen.

biological parents. The man and woman who provide the sperm and ovum, and therefore the embryo, from which a new human being develops.

biopsy. The removal and

(microscopic) examination of tissue from the living body; performed to establish precise diagnosis.

blastocyst. Name given to embryo at 4–5 days of gestation; formed from morula after latter reaches the cavity of the uterus; consists of sphere of cells, with a fluid-filled cavity.

blastomeres. Cells formed by cleavage (division) of fertilized ovum.

cell. A minute protoplasmic mass, consisting of a nucleus surrounded by cytoplasm, and enclosed within a cell membrane.

cerebellum. Brain region concerned with the coordination of movements.

cerebral cortex. The outer margin of the cerebral hemispheres consisting of the bulk of neurons found in the cerebral hemispheres; subdivided into functionally distinct regions such as motor and sensory cortices, and the visual cortex.

cerebral hemispheres. The right and left hemispheres form the largest part of the human brain: implicated in many functions, including motor and sensory functions, vision, hearing, speech, and 'higher' functions such as the maintenance of motivation, the ability to form stable plans and intentions, and the general regulation of behaviour.

child. The human young, from infancy to puberty.

chorion. Outermost membrane around embryo; develops villi two weeks after fertilization; gives rise to the placenta, which persists until birth.

chromosome. Structure in the nucleus of the cell containing a linear thread of DNA; genes are located on it; transmits genetic information. Each somatic (body) cell has 46 chromosomes, including the two sex chromosomes (XX, female; XY male).

cleavage. The segmentation of the fertilized ovum into zygote, then morula etc, containing an increasing number of blastomeres.

cloning. Asexual reproduction, in which the nucleus (and chromosomes) of an ovum is replaced with the nucleus of a somatic (body) cell of an adult. This fertilizes the ovum, without the involvement of sperm.

conception. Fertilization of the ovum; sometimes equated with implantation.

conceptus. The products of conception, that is, embryo (or fetus) plus surrounding membranes.

congenital defect. Birth defect; a structural or chemical imperfection present at birth.

consequentialism. The philosophical viewpoint which judges the rightness or wrongness of proposed courses of action on the basis of the goodness or badness of their likely outcomes. This is taken as the sole criterion of right and wrong.

dementia. Mental deterioration.

dendrites. One of the two types of processes of neurons; comprise most of the receptive surface of neurons.

ectoderm. Germ layer that gives rise to the nervous system and also to the epidermis of the skin.

ectogenesis. Development of the embryo, and later the fetus, in an 'artificial womb' throughout the whole of its gestation.

ectopic pregnancy. Development of the embryo outside the uterus.

EEG. Electroencephalogram (graph); the electrical activity ('brain waves') within the cerebral hemispheres of the brain; recordings are taken on the surface of the head.

embryo. The human conceptus from fertilization until the beginning of the eighth week of gestation.

experimentation. A procedure done in order to discover or demonstrate some fact or general truth; usually involves comparison of control and modified (experimental) groups.

fallopian tubes. Equivalent to the uterine tubes, which pass between the ovaries and the cavity of the uterus; fertilization takes place in them.

fecundity. Ability to produce offspring rapidly and in large numbers. In demographic terms, the physiological ability to reproduce (as opposed to fertility).

female pronucleus. Nucleus of fully matured ovum at fertilization; liberates its chromosomes to meet with those derived from male pronucleus.

fertility. The capacity to conceive or induce conception.

fertilization. The act of rendering gametes fertile or capable of further development; begins with contact between spermatozoon and ovum, leading to their fusion, which stimulates the completion of ovum maturation with release of the second polar body. Male and female pronuclei then form and may merge. The diploid number of chromosomes is restored. The process of fertilization leads to the formation of a zygote, and ends with the initiation of cleavage.

fetal death. Death prior to the complete expulsion from the mother of the products of fertilization. *Early* fetal death signifies death of a fetus of less than 20 weeks gestation; *intermediate* fetal death is between 20 and 28 weeks gestation; *late* fetal death (stillbirth) is over 28 weeks gestation.

fetal wastage. Extent of fetal death due to natural causes.

fetus. The human conceptus from the beginning of the eighth week of gestation until separation from the mother at birth.

gamete. The mature male or female sex cell.

gene. The biological unit of heredity; each gene is found at a definite position (locus) on a particular chromosome.

gestation. The period of development from the time of fertilization of the ovum until birth.

gonad. Male or female sex gland; testis or ovary respectively.

hormones. Chemical substances produced in the body by an organ or endocrine gland, and then transmitted via the blood stream to a target organ (*e.g.* ovary) on which their effect is exerted.

human being. A subject of experiences and actions embodied in an organism of the species *Homo sapiens.* In Christian terms, a being made 'in the image of God'.

Huntington's chorea. Hereditary disease characterized by jerky movements and mental deterioration terminating in dementia; onset is generally in the 40s, and death follows within 15 years.

hysterotomy. Incision of the uterus.

implantation. Embedding of the blastocyst in the endometrial lining of the uterus; commences 6–7 days after fertilization, and is completed by 14 days after fertilization.

infancy. Period from end of neonatal period (one month of age) to 12 months of age.

infant. In medical terminology this refers to a child between the ages of one and 12 months of age. This is a far more specific usage of the term than the general one of a child during the earliest part of life.

infertility. Inability of a couple to conceive after 12 months of normal sexual practice without contraception.

in vitro. Within a glass (in a petri dish or test-tube); in an artificial environment, outside the body.

in vivo. Within the living body.

karyotype. Chromosomal constitution of the nucleus of a cell.

laparoscopy. Examination of the interior of the abdomen by means of a laparoscope (an instrument through which abdominal organs, such as the ovary, can be seen). The laparoscope is passed through a small incision made in the anterior abdominal wall.

male pronucleus. The nuclear material of the head of the spermatozoon after it has penetrated the ovum and fertilization has taken place.

media. In the context of IVF, where chemical substances are used to support the growth of cells in tissue culture preparations in the laboratory.

meiosis. Cell division occurring during maturation of the sex cells, by which each daughter nucleus receives half the number of chromosomes characteristic of the body cells.

mesoderm. Middle layer of the three primary germ layers of the embryo; gives rise to connective tissue, bone, cartilage, muscle, blood vessels, kidney etc.

miscarriage. Spontaneous abortion.

morula. Embryo at 3 days of gestation, consisting of solid sphere of 16 or so cells (blastomeres); found in uterine tube.

myelin. The fatty substance forming a sheath around larger nerve fibres.

neonatal. First four weeks after birth.

neural tube. One of the earliest forerunners of the central nervous system in the embryo; present during the third and fourth weeks of gestation.

neuroglia (glia). The supporting cells of the central nervous system; supply nutrients etc. to the neurons; one type has a role in myelin formation.

neurons (nerve cells). The conducting cells of the nervous system; their processes are known as axons and dendrites, the axons (with the sheaths) forming nerve fibres.

neuropores. The openings at each end of the neural tube; they close between days 24 and 26 of gestation.

non-therapeutic research. Clinical research which has, as its primary goal, the acquisition of knowledge rather than the benefit of the patient (therapeutic research).

oocyte. Precursor of the ovum; *primary* oocyte is formed near time of the woman's birth; *secondary* oocyte is derived from primary oocyte many years later, shortly before ovulation.

oogenesis. Development of the ovum.

organ. A part of the body set aside to perform a special function or functions.

organogenesis. Formation of an organ by the assembly of tissues of different kinds.

ovary. The female sexual gland in which ova are formed.

ovulation. Liberation of the secondary oocyte from the ovary.

ovum. The mature female gamete (germ or sex cell).

perinatal death. Fetal deaths of 28 completed weeks of gestation and over (stillbirths), plus infant deaths under seven days of age.

person. Sometimes used as a synonym for *human being*, but increasingly used to mean a sentient being that has a concept of itself, and is capable of reflective, rational thought.

pharyngeal (branchial) arches. Structures which appear during the fourth and fifth weeks of gestation, and contribute to the formation of the head and neck.

placenta. Organ joining mother and embryo/fetus, for nourishment of embryo/ fetus.

polar bodies. Minute cells extruded from the oocyte during meiosis.

pontine flexure. A bend in the region of the hindbrain during the development of the brain at the fifth and sixth weeks of gestation.

pre-embryo. A term used by some writers to refer to the embryo prior to implantation (two weeks of gestation) or for the first eight weeks of development.

pregnancy wastage. Loss of an embryo or fetus during the period of gestation; it is the failure of a fertilized ovum to result in the birth of a living newborn (excluding factors such as induced abortion or use of contraception). Main cause is spontaneous abortion; other causes include fetal death, ectopic pregnancies, and prematurity.

preimplantation embryos. Embryos existing in the laboratory (or human body) prior to the time when they would normally become attached to the wall of the uterus. Generally taken to refer to embryos less than 14 days after fertilization.

premature infant. Infant born between 27 weeks gestation and full term; sometimes defined as weighing between 1,000 and 2,500g.

prenatal. Period prior to birth.

prenatal adoption. Term used to refer to embryo donation in an IVF programme.

previable fetus. A fetus lacking the capacity to sustain independent existence; defined as less than 28 weeks gestation (for further details, see 'viable fetus').

postnatal. Period after birth.

primitive streak. Important structure in early embryonic development; linear zone of cell migration from the ectoderm to form the embryonic mesoderm; clearly visible in the 15 to 16 day embryo.

reflex action. A response resulting from the passage of nerve impulses from a receptor (*e.g.* in the skin) to a muscle or gland; the neurons involved are in the spinal cord, and do not involve a conscious response (via the cerebral cortex) on the part of the person concerned.

reflex arc. The group of neurons involved in a reflex action; generally confined to one level of the spinal cord.

research. Scientific study of a subject, involving critical investigation in an endeavour to discover new data and understand the subject under investigation; may involve careful comparison of different groups of individuals or one group under different conditions. In some cases, *experimentation* may be carried out, but this is not an essential part of research.

semen. Secretion of the male reproductive organs; composed of spermatozoa in their nutrient plasma, plus secretions from various glands.

social parents. The man and woman who rear the child.

somites. Segmental cell

blocks formed from mesoderm.

somite period. Twentieth to thirtieth days of gestation, during which somites appear.

spermatozoa. The mature male gametes (germ or sex cells).

spontaneous abortion. An abortion (of an embryo or previable fetus) occurring naturally.

stillbirth. Death of a fetus over 28 weeks of gestation.

subfertility. Less than normal fertility.

sulci. Furrows on the surface of the brain.

superovulation. Acceleration of ovulation in a woman by hormonal treatment, in order to produce an excess number of ova in a cycle; used in IVF procedures.

synapse. The point of communication between two neurons, where a nerve impulse is transmitted from one neuron to the next.

syngamy. The union of two gametes to form a zygote in fertilization.

therapeutic research. Clinical research which is incidental to the primary aim of helping the patient, and from which the patient is likely to benefit.

tissue. An aggregation of similarly specialized cells

united in the performance of a particular function.

trophoblast. The cells on the outer aspect of the wall of the blastocyst; attaches the ovum to the uterine wall and supplies nutrition to the embryo. Chorion is derived from it.

uterus. Hollow muscular organ in the female body, in which the fertilized ovum normally becomes embedded, and in which the developing embryo and fetus is nourished.

utilitarianism. A philosophical term; a form of *consequentialism*, according to which the goodness or badness of happenings is guaged entirely on the overall benefit that is conferred on the affected parties.

viable fetus. A fetus having the capacity to survive and sustain independent existence. This refers to a fetus of 28 weeks or more gestation (the official figure in many countries), although in practice a fetus of little more than 20 weeks may be viable (depending on its weight and the medical facilities available to sustain it).

womb. Uterus.

zygote. The structure resulting from the fertilization of an ovum by

a sperm; initially consists of
a single cell before dividing
to form two- and four-cell
stages (after which it is
known as a morula).

Notes on Chapters

Chapter 1 – An Odyssey Through The New Reproductive Technologies
1. The terms *ovum* and *oocyte* have been used interchangeably throughout the text. The term *egg* has not been used, when referring to humans.
2. A technique for freezing ova has been developed at the Department of Obstetrics and Gynaecology, at the Flinders Medical Centre, Adelaide in Australia. It is thought that, with this technique, unfertilized ova can be stored for up to 10 years. At the time of writing (May 1986) one pregnancy had been achieved by the fertilization of thawed ova. The method involves culturing ova to maturity after extraction, and then trimming by microsurgery prior to freezing. See: C. Chen, 'Pregnancy after human oocyte cryopreservation', *Lancet*, i, 1986, pp. 884–886.
3. I have considered cloning at length in *Brave New People*, (Inter-Varsity Press, Leicester, and Eerdmans, Grand Rapids, 1984 and 1985), chapters 4 and 6. Modern developments have been summarized by Anne McLaren, 'Methods and success of nuclear transplantation in mammals', *Nature*, 309, 1984, pp. 671–672. Very recently, a form of cloning has been successfully carried out in sheep, in which 'enucleated' halves of unfertilized ova were fused with single blastomeres from 8-cell embryos. The resulting reconstituted embryos were placed in the oviducts of ewes, and three of the four transferred blastocysts developed into full-term lambs. See: S. M. Willadsen, 'Nuclear transplantation in sheep embryos', *Nature*, 320, 1986, pp. 63–65.
4. C. Grobstein, *From Chance to Purpose: An Appraisal of External Human Fertilization* (Addison-Wesley Publishing Co., Reading, Massachusetts, USA, 1981).
5. From a discussion of the various roles of mother and father, see R, Snowden, G. D. Mitchell and E. M. Snowden, *Artificial Reproduction: A Social Investigation* (Allen and Unwin, London, 1983).
6. P. Singer and D. Wells, *The Reproduction Revolution: New Ways of Making Babies* (Oxford University Press, Oxford, 1984).

Chapter 2 – Responses to the New Reproductive Technologies
1. P. Ramsey, *Fabricated Man* (Yale University Press, New Haven, 1970).
2. *Ibid.*, p. 113.

3. P. Ramsey, 'Shall we reproduce? 1. The medical ethics of *in vitro* fertilization', *Journal of the American Medical Association*, 220, 1972, pp. 1346–1350; 'Shall we reproduce? 2. Rejoinders and future forecast', *Journal of the American Medical Association*, 220, 1972, 1480–1485.

4. P. Ramsey, 'Manufacturing our offspring: weighing the risks', in T. A. Mappes and J. S. Zembaty (eds.) *Biomedical Ethics* (McGraw-Hill Book Company, New York, 1981), pp. 490–493.

5. L. Kass, 'Making babies – the new biology and the "old" morality', *Public Interest*, 26, 1972, 18–56; see also, 'New beginnings in life', in M. P. Hamilton (ed.) *The New Genetics and the Future of Man* (Eerdmans, Grand Rapids, 1972), pp. 15–63.

6. *Ibid.*

7. *Ibid.*

8. L. Kass, '"Making babies" revisited', *Public Interest*, 54, 1979, pp. 32–60.

9. *Ibid.*

10. R. A. McCormick, 'Genetic medicine: notes on the moral literature', in M. E. Marty and D. G. Peerman (eds.) *New Theology No. 10* (Macmillan, New York, 1973), pp. 55–84.

11. R. G. Edwards, 'Aspects of human reproduction', in W. Fuller (ed.) *The Biological Revolution* (Anchor Books, New York, 1972), pp. 128–144.

12. D. G. Jones, 'Making new men: a theology of modified man', *Journal of the American Scientific Affiliation*, 26, 1974, pp. 144–154.

13. B. Ramm, 'An ethical evaluation of biogenetic engineering', *Journal of the American Scientific Affiliation*, 26, 1974, pp. 137–143.

14. R. Edwards and P. Steptoe, *A Matter of Life* (Hutchinson, London, 1980).

15. Medical Research Council (UK), 'Research Related to Human Fertilization and Embryology', *British Medical Journal*, 285, 20 November 1982, p. 1480.

16. British Medical Association, 'Interim Report on Human In Vitro Fertilisation and Embryo Replacement and Transfer', *British Medical Journal*, 286, 14 May 1983, pp. 1594–1595.

17. *Report of the Committee of Inquiry into Human Fertilisation and Embryology* (Her Majesty's Stationery Office, London, 1984).

18. Victorian Government Committee to Consider the Social, Ethical and Legal Issues Arising from In Vitro Fertilization, *Interim Report* (September 1982).

19. Victorian Government Committee to Consider the Social, Ethical and Legal Issues Arising from In Vitro Fertilization, *Report on Donor Gametes in IVF* (August 1983).

20. Victorian Government Committee to Consider the Social Ethical and Legal Issues Arising from In Vitro Fertilization, *Report on the Disposition of Embryos Produced by In Vitro Fertilization* (August 1984).

21. *Infertility (Medical Procedures) Act 1984*, No. 10163 (Victorian Government Printing Office, Melbourne).

22. National Health and Medical Research Council, *Ethics in Medical Research Involving the Human Fetus and Human Fetal Tissue* (Australian Government Publishing Service, Canberra, 1983); Supplementary note 4: 'In vitro fertilization and embryo transfer'.

23. Ethics Advisory Board, US Department of Health, Education and Welfare, 'Report and Conclusions: HEW Support of Research Involving Human In Vitro Fertilization and Embryo Transfer, 4 May 1979', *Federal Register*, 18 June 1979, pp. 35033–35058.

24. Evangelical literature illustrates this point very clearly. *Decision Making in Medicine: The Practice of its Ethics*, edited by Gordon Scorer and Antony

Wing, and containing chapters by members of the Christian Medical Fellowship of UK (Edward Arnold, London, 1979; reprinted by Christian Medical Fellowship, London, 1985) contains a chapter on genetic advance, and one on the control of the beginning of life (contraception and sterilization; termination of pregnancy). IVF is not mentioned. In *Horizons of Science*, edited by Carl F. H. Henry (Harper and Row, New York, 1978), there are chapters on dilemmas in biomedical ethics, and on biological engineering. While each of these contains helpful general principles, no reference is made to either AID or IVF. *Baker's Dictionary of Christian Ethics*, edited by Carl F. H. Henry (Baker Book House, Grand Rapids, 1973), has articles on abortion, artificial insemination, birth control, genetics and infanticide. In this, it was ahead of its time, even if the only reference to reproductive technologies was to 'cloning' in the article on 'genetics'. One of the foremost attempts to treat this area seriously was made by Sir Norman Anderson in his 1975 London Lectures in Contemporary Christianity, *Issues of Life and Death* (Hodder and Stoughton, London, 1976). Although a non-biologist, Anderson made a thorough study of the literature up to that time, and was prepared to tackle questions of genetic engineering and artificial insemination, as well as birth control and abortion. In this, he relied heavily on the earlier masterly study of some of the pertinent theological dilemmas by G. R. Dunstan in *The Artifice of Ethics* (SCM Press, London, 1974). It is surprising that, even in the mid-1980s, John Stott in his comprehensive survey of *Issues Facing Christians Today* (Marshalls, Basingstoke, 1984), fails to deal with any of the reproductive technologies, although he devotes a chapter to abortion. Exceptions were provided by my own initial forays into bioethics, as demonstrated by the booklet *Genetic Engineering* (Grove Books, Nottingham, 1978), with its treatment of AID, IVF and cloning as well as of genetic issues. It is encouraging to note that *Christianity Today* is giving serious attention to biomedical issues. Recent examples are provided by Dennis Chamberland's article: 'Genetic engineering: promise and threat', 30 (2), 1986, pp. 22–28, and the Christianity Today Institute's symposium: 'Biomedical decision making: the blessings and curses of modern technology', 30 (5), 1986, pp. 25–40.
25. J. K. Anderson, *Genetic Engineering* (Zondervan, Grand Rapids, 1982).
26. D. Ch. Overduin and J. I. Fleming, *Life in a Test-Tube* (Lutheran Publishing House, Adelaide, 1982).
27. J. B. Nelson and J. A. S. Rohricht, *Human Medicine* (Augsburg, Minneapolis, 1984, revised and expanded edition).
28. P. D. Simmons, *Birth and Death: Bioethical Decision-Making* (Westminster Press, Philadelphia, 1983).
29. O. O'Donovan, *Begotten or Made?* (Clarendon Press, Oxford, 1984).
30. A. Nichols and T. Hogan (eds.) *Making Babies: The Test Tube and Christian Ethics* (Acorn Press, Canberra, 1984). Another useful Australian report is: L. Miller, *A Christian View on In Vitro Fertilisation* (Anglican Information Office, Sydney, 1985), produced by the Social Issues Committee for the Diocese of Sydney.
31. For a representative sample of responses within British society, see editorial comment in *Nature*, 310, 1984, p. 269; 312, 1984, p. 389; 313, 1985, pp. 417, 424; 314, 1985, p. 11; 315, 1985, p. 534; 320, 1986, p. 95. See also, H. J. Evans and A. McLaren, 'Unborn children (protection) bill', *Nature*, 314, 1985, pp. 127–128. This is but a very small sample of the responses made by numerous groups and individuals of all persuasions to the Warnock debate.

32. T. F. Torrance, *Test-Tube Babies* (Scottish Academic Press, Edinburgh, 1984).
33. O. R. Johnston, *Warnock: 'Weighed .... and Found Wanting'* (CARE Trust, London, n.d.). A similar position on most of the issues raised by CARE Trust is manifested by contributors to a symposium on the Warnock Report published in the journal *Ethics and Medicine*, 1 (2), 1985, pp. 1–12, the publication of Rutherford House, Edinburgh (a research centre with a Protestant and conservative theological position). The underlying principle is again that the embryo is a person, deserving of the greatest respect. Most contributors however, would appear to allow the use of AIH and IVF in the treatment of infertility, as long as there was no breaching of the marriage relationship. Respect for the embryo is spelled out by one of the contributors, Richard Higginson (pp. 10–12). He writes: 'A zygote that you and I once were is as much a person as what you or I are now; there is individual identity and continuity which has survived some very obvious changes in appearance.' He also argues that, even if one believes the acquisition of personhood occurs at a later stage in pregnancy: 'This should not lead one to think that the early embryo has no claims to protection up to that point ... For is not the embryo worthy of the greatest respect in view of that capacity which is so much prized into which he or she is growing every moment?' Another symposium emanating from British evangelical circles is that of the Biblical Creation Society and Evangelicals for Life: D. C. Watts (ed.) *Creation and the Christian Response to Warnock* (Biblical Creation Society, Rugby, 1985). In one of the essays, 'Image in embryo', Nigel Cameron (pp. 3–12) takes the Warnock Inquiry to task for by-passing the question of the nature of the embryo. He stresses the moral significance of the early embryonic stages of human life, using the incarnation of Jesus as his starting-point. He argues: 'For God to become man in embryo therefore requires that man in embryo already bear the image, and absolutely forbids the possibility that in the early stages of his biological life man can lack the divine image because lacking something which is its pre-requisite.'
34. Christian Medical Fellowship, 'Response to Warnock', *In the Service of Medicine*, 31 (2), 1985, pp. 1–2.
35. Compare: D. Short, 'Embryo experimentation – the case for a moratorium', *In the Service of Medicine*, 31 (2), 1985, pp. 2–3, with J. W. Dundee, 'In vitro fertilisation: an alternative viewpoint', *In the Service of Medicine*, 31 (3), 1985, pp. 3–4.
36. Board of Social Responsibility of the Church of Scotland, 'Response to report of the Committee of Inquiry into Human Fertilisation and Embryology (Warnock Report)', *1985 General Assembly of the Church of Scotland*, pp. 287–291. Reprinted in *Ethics and Medicine*, 1 (2), 1985, pp. 13–15.
37. Social Policy Committee, Board for Social Responsibility, *Human Fertilisation and Embryology* (Central Board of Finance of the Church of England, London, 1984).
38. Board for Social Responsibility (Working Party on Human Fertilisation and Embryology), *Personal Origins* (CIO Publishing, London, 1985). The Working Party consisted of Professor R. J. Berry, Dr. Mary Seller, Rev. Professor Keith Ward, Rev. Professor Oliver O'Donovan, and Prebendary John Gladwin.
39. *Ibid.*
40. H. O. Tiefel, 'Human in vitro fertilization: A conservative view', *Journal of the American Medical Association*, 247, 1982, pp. 3235–3242.

41. Report of a Working Party, Council for Science and Society, *Human Procreation: Ethical Aspects of the New Techniques* (Oxford University Press, Oxford, 1984). The introduction to the Report contains a helpful historical analysis of the Christian tradition concerning the value of embryonic life.

42. C. Grobstein, *From Chance to Purpose: An Appraisal of External Human Fertilization* (Addison-Wesley Publishing Co, Reading, Massachusetts, 1981).

43. Ethics Advisory Board, US Department of Health, Education and Welfare, *op. cit.*

44. C. Grobstein, 'External human fertilization', *Scientific American*, 240, 1979, pp. 33–43.

45. P. Singer and D. Wells, *The Reproduction Revolution: New Ways of Making Babies* (Oxford University Press, Oxford, 1984).

46. R. Arditti, R. Duelli Klein, and S. Minden, *Test-Tube Women: What Future for Motherhood?* (Pandora Press, London, 1984).

47. J. Raymond, 'Feminist ethics, ecology and vision', in *Test-tube Women: What Future for Motherhood?* pp. 427–437.

48. F. Hornstein, 'Children by donor insemination: A new choice for lesbians', in *Test-Tube Women: What Future for Motherhood?* pp. 373–381.

Chapter 3 – Perspectives on Human Life

1. For a far more extensive discussion of these approaches see: P. D. Simmons, *Birth and Death: Bioethical Decision-Making* (Westminster Press, Philadelphia, 1983).

2. M. Hill, 'IVF from a biblical perspective', in A. Nichols and T. Hogan (eds.) *Making Babies: The Test Tube and Christian Ethics* (Acorn Press, Canberra, 1984).

3. For a much fuller discussion, see L. Smedes, *Mere Morality: How Do We Make Decisions on the Things That Matter Most?* (Eerdmans, Grand Rapids, 1983).

4. An extended version of some aspects of the discussion in this section is to be found in the companion volume: *Brave New People: Ethical Issues at the Commencement of Life* (Inter-Varsity Press, Leicester, 1984; revised edition: Eerdmans, Grand Rapids, 1985). See also: G. Carey, *I Believe in Man* (Hodder and Stoughton, London, 1977); C. S. Evans, *Preserving the Person* (Inter-Varsity Press, Downers Grove and Leicester, 1977); D. Kidner, *Genesis* (Tyndale Press, London, 1967); E. L. Mascall, *The Importance of Being Human* (Oxford University Press, Oxford, 1959); H. Thielicke, *The Doctor as Judge of Who Shall Live and Who Shall Die* (Fortress Press, Philadelphia, 1976).

5. See discussion in my *Our Fragile Brains* (Inter-Varsity Press, Downers Grove and Leicester, 1981).

6. J. R. Nelson, *Human Life: A Biblical Perspective for Bioethics* (Fortress Press, Philadelphia, 1984).

7. D. Atkinson, 'The price of life', *Third Way*, November 1985, p. 13.

8. See my article: 'Malnutrition means people', *Interchange*, 20, 1976, pp. 223–234.

9. I am indebted to J. Robert Nelson's discussion of these and related points in *Human Life: A Biblical Perspective for Bioethics*.

10. An extended discussion of this point is found in *Brave New People*.

11. The making of choices such as these is a salutary reminder that there can be no escape from such decision-making, which frequently has to be undertaken on financial grounds. This occurs not only in the medical area, but

also in, for instance, the planning of road systems where costs and safety factors are integral facets of planning. These general considerations are relevant to the IVF debate, since one of the reasons sometimes given for rejecting IVF on moral grounds is that choices have to be made between one embryo and another. This is considered by some to be unethical, entailing as it does the choice of one 'human life' at the expense of another. Quite apart from the observation that this is a constant occurrence in natural fertilization, it is also placing demands on our ethical system that we do not make in other areas (such as most other medical areas).

12. O. O'Donovan, 'A neutered morality', *Third Way*, September 1984, p.27. O'Donovan's criticism of my book *Brave New People* describes my discussion of IVF as 'bland', suggesting that I have 'written under the constraints of social pressure', and so have 'not raised the most fundamental ethical issues'. He further suggests that my approach leads to a constant retreat, as I (and others like me) 'retract one after another of the criticisms [I] once dared to make, and repeat, more or less indifferently about anything under the sun, the same familiar refrain: "This, too, may be welcomed – if only we can use it responsibly!" These are fighting words, based as they are on a radical dichotomy between a technological culture (with its value-choices) and the gospel of Jesus Christ. O'Donovan appears to be saying that no technological procedure can be legitimate for a Christian, since technology is part-and-parcel of a technologically-inspired worldview and the social pressures in favour of accepting technological developments are irresistible. Before this premise can be accepted however, it needs to be demonstrated that acceptance of *individual* technological developments commits one inevitably to a technological *vision of the good*. I resolutely reject such a technological vision, and this is demonstrated by my *selective* acceptance of the various procedures encompassed by the new reproductive technologies. O'Donovan's stringent criticism of my rejection of AID and cloning, but acceptance of the simple case of IVF, ushers in an 'all-or-none' phenomenon – acceptance of every technological possibility or rejection of every such possibility. This is deceptively attractive in some areas but horrendously difficult to apply in others. I should also point out that my acceptance of IVF dates from 1974 (*Journal of the American Scientific Affiliation*, 26 pp.144–154) before it was a clinically feasible procedure. My assessment of it therefore, did not alter when it became a practical possibility. On O'Donovan's premise I should accept AID wholeheartedly, since it has been a readily available procedure for very many years.

O'Donovan severely criticizes what he describes as 'the sad story of Christian medicine in the last quarter century'. From this I can only conclude that he personally rejects most aspects of modern medicine. If this is not the case, it is essential that criteria are formulated for determining whether to accept or reject life-saving surgery on a neonate, radiotherapy to combat the spread of carcinoma secondaries, the use of a CAT scan to investigate the location of a brain tumour, or the use of tubal microsurgery in overcoming infertility. If the whole of the technological enterprise is to be rejected on Christian grounds, one also needs to ask what criteria are being developed to assess the theological and social legitimacy of microcomputers, word processors, automatic cameras, automobiles, jumbo jets and nuclear power plants. Social pressures in favour of these technological developments are just as strong as those in favour of IVF.

For further discussion on the relationship between biotechnology and bioethics see: M. Charlesworth, 'Biotechnology and bioethics: New ways of life and death', *Current Affairs Bulletin*, 61, 1984, pp. 4–24.

13. P. D. Simmons, *Birth and Death: Bioethical Decision-Making, vide supra.*
14. J. I. Packer, *Knowing God* (Hodder and Stoughton, London, 1973).
15. W. S. Mooneyham, Orphans. In C. F. H. Henry (ed.) *Baker's Dictionary of Christian Ethics* (Baker Book House, Grand Rapids, 1973), pp. 477–478. See also articles on adoption and children.
16. The human side of infertility and adoption, as well as the plight of unacceptable babies, is brought out in Joy Cooke's book: *Why Us Lord?* (Pickering Paperbacks, Basingstoke, 1985). Perhaps the most controversial and unsatisfactory aspect of this personal account of the trauma of infertility comes with the Cookes' rejection of a mentally retarded baby, suffering from galactosaemia, who was offered to them for adoption. While the pathos of this choice is self-evident, the rejection of the child is interpreted as God's will, for them. Since the author was strongly opposed to abortion one is left wondering what is God's will for those who have no choice about caring for a mentally retarded child. This incident also throws a great deal of light on contemporary attitudes (even on the part of some Christians who would resolutely deny such attitudes) emphasizing: adoption as a means of overcoming childlessness rather than caring for a child in desperate need of a loving family, the importance attached to an adequate 'quality of life' (defined in strictly biological terms), and the assumption that children are an essential part of marriage.
17. For this analysis I am greatly indebted to a paper by Michael Schluter and Roy Clements, entitled: 'Family policy in Old Testament Israel: Some lessons for British social policy in the 1980's', published by the Universities and Colleges Christian Fellowship (UCCF), Leicester, 1984.
18. Further aspects of the concept of the family are to be found in: F. J. Kline, 'Family'. In *Baker's Dictionary of Christian Ethics*, pp. 237–242; T. C. Mitchell and D. W. B. Robinson, 'Family, household', in J. D. Douglas, (ed.) *The Illustrated Bible Dictionary, Part 1* (Inter-Varsity Press, Leicester, 1980), pp. 500–502; J. I. Packer, M. C. Tenney and W. White (eds.), articles on 'Family relationships' and 'Birth and death' (*The Bible Almanac*, Nelson, Nashville, 1980), pp. 411–419 and pp. 440–449.
19. M. A. Inch, 'Concubinage', in *Baker's Dictionary of Christian Ethics*, p. 122.
20. D. J. Hesselgrave, 'Polygamy', in *Baker's Dictionary of Christian Ethics*, pp. 514–515.
21. J. H. Olthuis, 'Marriage', in *Baker's Dictionary of Christian Ethics*, pp. 407–409.
22. R. Snowden, G. D. Mitchell and E. M. Snowden, *Artificial Reproduction: A Social Investigation* (Allen and Unwin, London, 1983).

Chapter 4 – The Fetus, My Fellow Traveller

1. I was criticized by some reviewers of *Brave New People* for using the term 'fetus'. It was alleged that the use of this term rather than 'unborn baby' or 'unborn child' denotes a view of the unborn as less than human, and therefore as of less value than a human being. This is quite untrue, since I am using a strictly biological term with precise biological connotations. The term 'fetus', in my writings at least, has no ethical overtones. In exactly the same way, I refer to 'uterus' rather than 'womb', and to 'ovum' rather than 'egg', since in each instance the former term is the accurate technical one whereas the latter is a lay expression. I prefer 'fetus' to 'unborn baby', since it is technically the more correct expression.
    In connection with the concept of viability, it is useful to note that the

overall survival of infants with a birthweight of 1000–1500g is about 85%, while that of infants with a birthweight of 500–1000g is about 50%. Of the surviving infants, approximately 10–15% of the former group have either severe or mild handicap, and 20–30% in the latter group. See, for example: S. V. Crombie, B. A. Darlow, 'Neurodevelopmental outcome for infants of very low birthweight admitted to a regional neonatal unit, 1979–1983', *New Zealand Medical Journal*, 99, 1986, pp.223–226. See also: T. G. Powell, P. O. D. Pharoah, R. W. I. Cooke, 'Survival and morbidity in a geographically defined population of low birthweight infants', *Lancet*, i, 1986, pp.539–543.

2. The description here is principally based on that found in Marjorie A. England's book *A Colour Atlas of Life Before Birth: Normal Fetal Development* (Wolfe Medical Publication, London, 1983). The diagrams of fetal development are based on photographs appearing in England's book. Figure 2 is based on a photograph appearing in: J. E. Garcia, 'In vitro fertilization', in R. M. Wynn (ed.) *Obstetrics and Gynecology Annual, Volume 14* (Appleton-Century-Crofts, Norwalk, Connecticut, 1985), pp.45–72. More detailed descriptions of early developmental processes can be found in any standard text of embryology, for example, K. L. Moore, *The Developing Human* (Saunders, Philadelphia, 1973); T. W. Sadler, *Langman's Medical Embryology* (5th edition, Williams and Wilkins, Baltimore, 1985).

3. The data used here have been obtained from a variety of sources. These include standard texts such as: M. L. Barr and J. A. Kiernan, *The Human Nervous System* (4th edition, Harper and Row, Philadelphia, 1983); J. P. Schadé and D. H. Ford, *Basic Neurology* (Elsevier, Amsterdam, 1973); S. Reinis and J. M. Goldman, *The Development of the Brain: Biological and Functional Perspectives* (Charles C. Thomas, Illinois, 1980). Other sources used include: R. O'Rahilly, F. Muller, G. M. Hutchins and G. W. Moore, 'Computer ranking of the sequence of appearance of 100 features of the brain and related structures in staged human embryos during the first 5 weeks of development', *American Journal of Anatomy*, 171, 1984, pp.243–257; W. F. Windle, 'Development of neural elements in human embryos of four to seven weeks gestation', *Experimental Neurology, Supplement 5*, 1970, pp.44–83, T. Humphrey, 'The development of human fetal activity and its relation to postnatal behavior', in H. W. Reese and L. P. Lipsitt (eds.) *Advances in Child Development and Behavior, Volume 5* (Academic Press, New York, 1970); K. A. Kooi, R. A. Tucker and R. E. Marshall, *Fundamentals of Electroencephalography* (2nd edition, Harper and Row, New York, 1978), pp.60–65. See also references in M. Tooley, *Abortion and Infanticide* (Clarendon Press, Oxford, 1983), pp.347–407.

4. For further details, see the discussion in *Brave New People*.

5. See, for example, J. Stott, *Issues Facing Christians Today*, (Marshalls, Basingstoke, 1984); chapter on 'The Abortion Dilemma'. Also O. O'Donovan, *The Christian and the Unborn Child* (2nd. edition, Grove Books, Bramcote, Nottingham, 1975).

6. A criticism of the genetic uniqueness position is made by Lewis Smedes in *Mere Morality* (Eerdmans, Grand Rapids, 1983), pp.132–153.

7. O. O'Donovan, *The Christian and the Unborn Child*.

8. Complete hydatidiform moles have no amniotic sac with membranes, no embryonic formation, and no cord or evidence of fetal placental circulation. They have a diploid karyotype, mainly 46 XX, the chromosomes being paternally derived. Although moles are rare in Western countries (one in 2000 pregnancies), they are more frequent in countries, such as Japan and

the Philippines (one in 200 pregnancies) and in Senegal and the Ivory Coast (one in 400 pregnancies).

9. C. J. Roberts and C. R. Lowe, 'Where have all the conceptions gone?' *Lancet*, 1, 1975, pp.488–489. A. F. Zakharov, 'Reproductive loss in man: total and chromosomally determined', *Prevention of Physical and Mental Congenital Defects, Part C: Basic and Medical Science, Education, and Future Strategies* (Alan R. Liss, New York, 1985), pp.9–14; C. L. Erhardt, 'Pregnancy losses in New York City, 1960', *American Journal of Public Health*, 53, 1963, pp.1137–1152; F. E. French and J. M. Bierman, 'Probabilities of fetal mortality', *Public Health Reports*, 77, 1962, pp.835–847; S. Shapiro, F. W. Jones and P. M. Densen. 'A life table of pregnancy terminations and correlates of fetal loss'. *Millbank Memorial Fund Quarterly*, 20, 1962, pp.7–45.

10. F. D. Abramson, 'Spontaneous fetal death in man', *Social Biology*, 20, 1973, pp.375–403.

11. J. J. Schlesselman, 'How does one assess the risk of abnormalities from human in vitro fertilization?' *American Journal of Obstetrics and Gynecology*, 135, 1979, pp.135–148.

12. H. U. Lane (ed.) *The World Almanac and Book of Facts 1985* (Newspaper Enterprise Association for Doubleday, 1984), pp.778–785. See also: *National Data Book and Guide to Sources: Statistical Abstract of the United States* 1984, (104th edition, US Department of Commerce, Bureau of the Census), pp.61–77.

13. A. Boué and J. G. Boué, 'Chromosome abnormalities and abortion', in F. Fuchs (ed.) *The Physiology and Genetics of Reproduction, Volume 2*, (Plenum, New York, 1974), pp.317–339; J. G. Boué and A. Boué, 'Chromosomal anomalies in early spontaneous abortion', *Current Topics in Pathology*, 62, 1976, p.193.

14. E. D. Alberman and M. R. Creasy, 'Frequency of chromosomal abnormalities in miscarriages and perinatal deaths', *Journal of Medical Genetics*, 14, 1977, pp.313–315. See also the review by A. Boué, J. Boué and A. Gropp, 'Cytogenetics of pregnancy wastage', in H. Harris and K. Hirschhorn (eds) *Advances in Human Genetics, Volume 14* (Plenum Press, New York, 1985), pp.1–57.

15. H. Leridon, *Human Fertility: The Basic Components* (University of Chicago Press, Chicago, 1977).

16. J. J. Schlesselman, *op. cit.*

17. D. H. Carr, 'Detection and evaluation of pregnancy wastage', in J. G. Wilson and F. C. Fraser (eds.) *Handbook of Teratology, Volume 3. Comparative Maternal and Epidemiology Aspects* (Plenum Press, New York, 1977), pp.189–213.

18. T. Kushner, 'Having life versus being alive', *Journal of Medical Ethics*, 10, 1984, pp.5–8.

19. P. Singer and D. Wells, *The Reproduction Revolution: New Ways of Making Babies* (Oxford University Press, Oxford, 1984).

20. G. E. Chatrian, 'Electrophysiologic evaluation of brain death: a critical appraisal', in M. J. Aminoff (ed.) *Electrodiagnosis in Clinical Neurology* (Churchill Livingstone, New York, 1980). See also: President's Commission for the Study of Ethical Problems in Medicine and Biomedicine and Behavioral Research, *Defining Death* (US Government Printing Office, Washington DC, 1981) (guidelines in *Journal of the American Medical Association*, 246, pp.2184–2186). J. L. Bernat, C. M. Culver and B. Gert, 'Defining death in theory and practice', *The Hastings Center Report*, 12 (1), 1982, pp.5–9. C. Pallis 'Whole-brain death reconsidered – physiological

facts and philosophy', *Journal of Medical Ethics*, 9, 1983, pp. 32–37.

21. C. M. Anderson, F. Torres and A. Faoro, 'The EEG of the early premature', *Electroencephalography and Clinical Neurophysiology*, 60, 1985, pp. 95–105.

22. In a postmortem examination of seven anencephalic fetuses (duration of gestation 16–33 weeks), the cerebral hemispheres and midbrain were absent in all of them, while the hindbrain (pons, cerebellum and medulla) was also absent in four of them – the remaining three fetuses showing varying degrees of hindbrain aplasia. Even the cervical spinal cord was absent in three of the fetuses (G. H. A. Visser, R. N. Laurini, J. I. P. de Vries, D. J. Bekedam, H. F. R. Prechtl, 'Abnormal motor behaviour in anencephalic fetuses', *Early Human Development*, 12, 1985, pp. 173–182. In the same study it was shown that the movements of these fetuses even during the first half of pregnancy were abnormal. From this it also emerged that fetal movements can occur in the presence of only a few motor neurons.

23. R. G. Edwards, 'Test-tube babies: the ethical debate', *The Listener*, October 27, 1983, p. 19. Edwards has written: 'I would suggest that the period between day 12 and day 30 after fertilisation is a time to consider carefully, as the neural tissue appears and begins its early development. . . . At 30 days the forebrain begins to take its shape, and I would be increasingly reluctant to culture embryos as this stage approaches.'

24. B. Häring, *Medical Ethics* (St. Paul Publications, Slough, 1972). See also Board for Social Responsibility (Working Party on Human Fertilisation and Embryology), *Personal Origins* (CIO Publishing, London, 1985).

25. J. M. Goldenring, 'Development of the fetal brain', *New England Journal of Medicine*, 307, 1982 p. 564. A much fuller version of Goldenring's position is to be found in his article 'The brain-life theory: towards a consistent biological definition of humanness', *Journal of Medical Ethics*, 11, 1985, pp. 198–204. The time of eight weeks is based on his interpretation of the EEG activity in 8-week-old fetuses. He writes: 'I have chosen to use the eight-week point for this paper since there is no doubt at that point that an active brain by electrical and anatomic definition is clearly present . . . (since) we should prefer the 'integration of the brain as a whole' as the starting point for human beings.'

26. M. Tooley, *Abortion and Infanticide*.

Chapter 5 – The Fetus: Master or Servant?

1. G. Wenham and R. Winter, *Abortion: The Biblical and Medical Challenges* (CARE Trust, London, 1983).

2. This principle is sometimes used to argue against induced abortion, on the grounds that had Jesus been aborted his saving work as Messiah would have been annulled. While this may make a good debating point, it overlooks the many other factors which could have brought the life of Jesus to an end as a fetus or young child – spontaneous abortion, disease or the fury of Herod (Mt. 2: 13–18). What this argument overlooks is the sovereignty of God and his ability to fulfil his purposes in and through his Son.

3. G. Wenham and R. Winter, *op. cit.*

4. J. Stott, *Issues Facing Christians Today* (Marshalls, Basingstoke, 1984); in chapter on 'The Abortion Dilemma', pp. 280–300.

5. A very helpful discussion of biblical interpretation has been provided by Duncan Vere, 'Embryos and fetuses – inferences from Scripture', *In the Service of Medicine*, 31 (3), 1985, pp. 11–19. He distinguishes between *deduction* and *induction*. By deduction is meant inference from a generally

true statement to a particular case within the class to which the general truth applies, for example, it is not legitimate to deduce from Scripture that all embryos are persons. Induction is used to argue that the tenor of Scripture is profoundly conservative with respect to human life, so that all embryos should be regarded as fully human and should therefore be accorded the same respect as that owed to all persons. Vere concludes that only a very restricted kind of induction ('guarded' induction) is permissible, and that it is the sort of induction which is based upon personal knowledge of a reliable kind. In the light of this, Vere considers that the embryo/fetus merits more than general respect; it has God's care over it as the intended 'house' or 'tent' to be indwelt by a person. This principle has to be worked out when principles such as life conservation and mercy come into conflict.

6. Innumerable examples could be quoted of writers using Exodus 21: 22–25 in one way or another. Among those who argue for the equivalence of mother and fetus are: J. W. Montgomery, *Slaughter of the Innocents* (Cornerstone Books, Westchester, Illinois, 1981); J. Stott, *Issues Facing Christians Today*. Those who argue against this view, or place it in a broader historical framework are: P. D. Simmons, *Birth and Death: Bioethical Decision-Making* (Westminster Press, Philadelphia, 1983); G. R. Dunstan, in the Introduction to the Report of a Working Party of the Council for Science and Society, *Human Procreation* (Oxford University Press, Oxford, 1984), pp. 1–11.

7. T. F. Torrance, *Test-Tube Babies* (Scottish Academic Press, Edinburgh, 1984).

8. G. Wenham and R. Winter, *op. cit.*

9. O. O'Donovan, *Begotten or Made?* (Clarendon Press, Oxford, 1984). In this section I have maintained the term 'conception', rather than fertilization, since it is the term employed by many writers on personhood, including O'Donovan.

10. D. M. MacKay, 'The beginnings of personal life', *In the Service of Medicine*, 30 (2), 1984, pp. 9–13.

11. O. O'Donovan, *op. cit.*

12. The views of Oliver O'Donovan in this discussion are based on his book: *Begotten or Made?*, and on a chapter of his, 'Again: who is a person?', in J. H. Channer (ed.), *Abortion and the Sanctity of Human Life* (Paternoster Press, Exeter, 1985). Reference has also been made to his booklet, *The Christian and the Unborn Child* ([Grove Booklet on Ethics, No. 1, Second Edition], Grove Books, Bramcote, Nottingham, 1975).

13. J. Scott, *op. cit.*

14. This is expressed in a variety of ways, the end result of which is that the fetus is to be treated precisely as we would treat an adult. For instance, Francis Schaeffer and C. Everett Koop appear to argue that abortion is equivalent to infanticide, since all that makes up the adult is present once the ovum and sperm are united. *Whatever Happened to the Human Race?* (Revell, Old Tappan, New Jersey, 1979). Richard Winter adopts the same position, starting from the categorical assertion that 'the Bible teaches that a person begins at the time of fertilization of the ovum', *Abortion: The Biblical and Medical Challenges*, p. 9. See also a number of the contributions to: *Abortion and the Sanctity of Human Life* (n. 12 Supra.).

15. L. Smedes, *Mere Morality* (Eerdmans, Grand Rapids, 1983; Lion Publishing, Tring, Herts, 1983); see chapter on 'Respect for human life', and associated footnotes, pp. 107–164, and pp. 268–276.

16. D. M. MacKay, *op.cit.*

17. In his reply to this article of Donald MacKay's, Richard Winter reverses each of MacKay's statements of commitment. For instance, he writes: 'The evidence from Scripture, science and experience *requires* us to make a commitment to protect the developing embryo.' In 'The beginnings of personal life', *In the Service of Medicine*, 31 (2), 1985, pp. 20–23, Winter also argues for 'the possibility of a person existing before the advent of the "self-supervisory function".' MacKay, in replying to Winter, justified his approach by contending that 'the man who dares pronounce deductions in the name of God ... must shoulder the onus of proof, not those who remain unconvinced by his rhetoric.' *In the Service of Medicine*, 31 (2), 1985, pp. 23–24.

18. L. Smedes, *op. cit.*

19. J. Fletcher, *Humanhood: Essays in Biomedical Ethics* (Prometheus Books, New York, 1979).

20. See 'Declaration on abortion', in *Official Catholic Teachings: Love and Sexuality*, edited by O. M. Liebard, (McGrath, Wilmington, 1974), p. 490. See also Father Brian Johnstone's discussion of the official position: 'The moral status of the embryo', in *Test-tube Babies*, edited by W. Walters and P. Singer, Oxford University Press, Melbourne, 1982, pp. 54–55.

21. M. Charlesworth, 'Biotechnology and bioethics. New ways of life and death', *Current Affairs Bulletin*, 61 (5), 1984, pp. 4–24.

22. Examples of this position are provided by B. Johnstone, 'The moral status of the embryo', in *Test-tube Babies*; R. A. McCormick, *How Brave a New World: Dilemmas in Bioethics* (Doubleday, New York, 1981), p. 148; C. E. Curran, 'Abortion, law and morality in contemporary Catholic theology', *Jurist*, 33, 1973, pp. 162–183. John Mahoney in *Bioethics and Belief* (Sheed and Ward, London, 1984), writes that the official Vatican statement 'deliberately leaves aside at what moment in time the spiritual soul is infused. On this matter tradition is not unanimous and writers differ'.

23. See the summary provided by Max Charlesworth (n. 21, *Supra.*).

24. R. A. McCormick, *How Brave a New World*, pp. 147–148.

25. T. Iglesias, '*In vitro* fertilisation: the major issues', *Journal of Medical Ethics*, 10, 1984, pp. 32–37.

26. P. Singer and D. Wells, *The Reproduction Revolution: New Ways of Making Babies* (Oxford University Press, Oxford, 1984).

27. M. Tooley, *Abortion and Infanticide* (Clarendon Press, Oxford, 1983).

28. This point is made by Christian Hoff Sommers in a review article of Tooley's book: 'Tooley's immodest proposal', *The Hastings Center Report*, 15 (3), 1985, pp. 39–42.

29. The scientific data assembled by Tooley are impressive and his conclusions regarding the neurological and behavioural capacities of older fetuses and infants are very well documented. What is at issue are not these data, but his perspective on personhood.

30. C. H. Sommers, *op. cit.*, (n. 28, *Supra*).

31. E. A. Langerak, 'Abortion. Listening to the middle', *The Hastings Center Report*, 9 (5), 1979, pp. 24–28.

32. For further discussion of some of the issues raised here see *Brave New People*, and also my article: 'Abortion: an exercise in biomedical ethics', *Journal of the American Scientific Affiliation*, 33 (4), 1982, pp. 6–17.

33. E. A. Langerak, *op. cit.*

34. The potentiality principle is a general ethical principle. Within a Christian context I would want to emphasize that, throughout development, the fetus is treated not just with respect but also as a being of worth in the sight of God. It may be argued that we never reach our full potential, even

as adults. This is true. It is also true that, in neurobiological terms, an individual's brain continues to develop for many years after birth. Neither of these objections invalidates the potentiality principle, since the latter only applies to *prenatal* existence and to situations where prenatal and postnatal considerations come into conflict.

35. I have in mind the Warnock Committee Report. For an explanation of the Report, and especially of what the committee saw as the relation between law and morality, see Mary Warnock's *A Question of Life* (Basil Blackwell, Oxford, 1985). This includes a reprint of the Report.

36. H. O. Tiefel, 'Human in vitro fertilization', *Journal of the American Medical Association*, 247, 1982, pp. 3235–3242.

37. P. Ramsey, *The Ethics of Fetal Research* (Yale University Press, New Haven, 1975).

38. This is a general question, to which I believe there is no definitive answer. It may, however, be argued that the embryo which developed into Jesus was both God and man, in the way in which Jesus as a postnatal human was both God and man; therefore, this answers the question in a clear-cut manner – all embryos have God-like attributes. I would question whether it is legitimate to make this transition as readily as this, and whether we can use a unique event and a special person (the God-man about whom we know God the Father had very clearly-defined purposes) as the model for all embryos ever produced.

39. See my discussion of the relationship between our brains and ourselves in *Our Fragile Brains* (Inter-Varsity Press, Downers Grove and Leicester, 1981).

40. P. D. Simmons, *Birth and Death: Bioethical Decision-Making* (Westminster Press, Philadelphia, 1983).

41. C. J. Roberts and C. R. Lowe, 'Where have all the conceptions gone?' *Lancet*, 1, 1975, pp. 498–499.

42. T. F. Murphy, 'The moral significance of spontaneous abortion', *Journal of Medical Ethics*, 11, 1985, pp. 79–83.

43. *Ibid.*

44. H. O. Tiefel, 'The cost of fetal research: ethical considerations', *New England Journal of Medicine*, 294, 1976, pp. 85–90.

45. I accept that most who describe fetuses as innocent wish to draw attention to the fact that fetuses have done nothing for which they deserve to die; they do not intend to regard them in some utopian fashion. However, this use of the term innocent is theologically misleading, since there are many other groups within society who are innocent in this sense, and yet are killed during, for instance, wars. When it is known that certain actions in a modern war are almost bound to kill 'innocent' people (let alone innocent fetuses), or inflict genetic damage on fetuses from radiation in a nuclear conflict, does this knowledge render such actions unethical? It would appear that, for those who regard fetuses as 'innocent', a consistent answer must be in the affirmative.

46. In making this statement I am not suggesting that the effects of the fall can be reversed by genetic engineering. This is not possible since any genetic engineering that may be carried out will be the product of 'fallen' human minds.

Chapter 6 – Freedom to Bring Life into Existence?

1. For a helpful historical perspective on attitudes towards AID in the United Kingdom, see the following reports: Report of a Commission Appointed by His Grace the Archbishop of Canterbury, *Artificial Human Insemination*

(Society for the Propagation of Christian Knowledge, London, 1948); Feversham Committee, *Report of the Departmental Committee on Human Artificial Insemination* (Cmnd. 1105, Her Majesty's Stationery Office, London, 1960); Peel Committee, 'Report of the panel on human artificial insemination', *British Medical Journal*, 2, 1973, suppl. appendix V.

2. K. R. Daniels, 'The practice of artificial insemination of donor sperm in New Zealand', *New Zealand Medical Journal*, 98, 1985, pp. 235–239. For further references on AID see K. R. Daniels and J. R. Fairweather, *Artificial Insemination by Donor: A Bibliography* (Sociology Department, University of Canterbury, Working Paper Number 3, 1983).

3. Although my discussion of AID is confined to its use in the alleviation of infertility, it may also be used by couples where there is a risk of a serious genetic disease being transmitted to offspring by the husband. The best known illustration of this is Huntington's chorea. The choices facing the couple in this instance are: having a child (male) with a high probability of suffering from this very serious disease; aborting a male fetus; remaining childless; having a child by AID. Whichever course of action is taken, the ethical dilemmas faced by the couple are enormous.

4. Many of the social aspects of AID are discussed by R. Snowden and G. D. Mitchell in *The Artificial Family: A Consideration of Artificial Insemination by Donor* (George Allen and Unwin, London, 1981).

5. R. Snowden, G. D. Mitchell and E. M. Snowden, *Artificial Reproduction: A Social Investigation* (George Allen and Unwin, London, 1983). Further examples of follow-up studies on AID families are provided by: J. C. Czyba and M. Chevret, 'Psychological reactions of couples to artificial insemination with donor sperm', *International Journal of Fertility*, 24, 1979, pp. 240–245, R. S. Ledward, E. M. Symonds and S. Eynon, 'Social and environmental factors as criteria for success in artificial insemination by donor (AID)', *Journal of Biosocial Science*, 14, 1982, pp. 263–275. For further examples, see the *Bibliography* by K. R. Daniels and J. R. Fairweather.

6. It is interesting to compare the attitudes on AID found in a variety of reports by Christian bodies. These range from acceptance (i), through grave doubt coupled with an attempt to control its usage in society since it is widely accepted (ii), to total rejection (iii). Examples of these three attitudes are represented respectively by the following British organizations: (i) The Board for Social Responsibility of the General Synod of the Church of England, *Personal Origins* (CIO Publishing, London, 1985), (ii) A Working Party under the Auspices of The Free Church Federal Council, London, 1982; (iii) CARE Trust, *Warnock 'Weighed . . . . and Found Wanting'* (CARE Trust, London, n.d.).

7. *Personal Origins* (see n.6).

8. D. Ison, *Artificial Insemination by Donor* (Grove Books, Bramcote, Nottingham, 1983).

9. This point has been developed at length by Leon Kass in a number of his writings. See, in particular; 'Making babies – the new biology and the "old" morality', *Public Interest*, 26, 1972, pp. 18–56; '"Making babies" revisited', *Public Interest*, 54, 1979, pp. 32–60.

10. R. Snowden and G. D. Mitchell, *The Artificial Family*.

11. *Ibid.*

12. For an insight into lesbian and feminist attitudes towards AID, see the chapters by Francie Hornstein, 'Children by donor insemination: a new choice for lesbians' and Renate Duelli Klein 'Doing it ourselves: self insemination' in: *Test-Tube Women*, edited by R. Arditti, R. D. Klein and

S. Minden, Pandora Press, London, 1984. An ethicist's justification of a physician assisting a lesbian couple with AID is put forward by John C. Fletcher, 'Artificial insemination in lesbians', *Archives of Internal Medicine*, 145, 1985, pp. 419–420.

13. See, for instance, G. R. Dunstan, 'Ethical aspects of donor insemination', *Journal of Medical Ethics*, 1, 1975, pp. 42–44.

14. P. Ramsey, *Fabricated Man* (Yale University Press, New Haven, 1970); P. Ramsey, 'Shall we reproduce? I. The medical ethics of *in vitro* fertilization', *Journal of the American Medical Association*, 220, 1972, pp. 1346–1350; P. Ramsey, 'Shall we reproduce? II. Rejoinders and future forecast', *Journal of the American Medical Association*, 220, 1972, pp. 1480–1485; L. Kass, 'Making babies – the new biology and the "old" morality', *Public Interest*, 26, 1972, pp. 18–56.

15. See my article, 'IVF and the wider ethical debate of genetic engineering'. In A. Nichols and T. Hogan (eds.), *Making Babies: The Test Tube and Christian Ethics* (Acorn Press, Canberra, 1984), pp. 93–101.

16. No attempt has been made in this book to review any of the technical aspects of IVF. For an overview of many facets of IVF see: Centre for Human Bioethics, *Developments in Human Reproduction* (Resource Kit No. 1, Monash University, Clayton, Victoria, Australia, 1984). At the time of writing (May 1986), over 1,000 IVF babies had been born in Australia. A similar number of IVF babies had been born in the UK, 500 of which had started life at the Bourn Hall centre, in Cambridge (T. Richards, 'IVF update', *British Medical Journal*, 292, 1986, pp. 1156–1157). Twenty-five centres are operating in Britain, of which only one is operated by the National Health Service. Treatment in Britain costs between £1,000 and £2,500 per treatment cycle. The cost in salaries and running expenses for a unit treating five patients a week is about £100,000. Waiting lists in Britain are approximately four years. The Voluntary Licensing Authority for Human In Vitro Fertilisation and Embryology was set up in March 1985, and reported in April 1986. Success rates for IVF vary considerably from one centre to another. Data from 200 IVF centres worldwide, with a cumulative experience of 11,000 pregnancies, are: when one embryo is replaced the chances of a pregnancy are 9.5%, with two embryos they are 15%, with three embryos 19%, and with four embryos 25%. When three to four embryos are replaced, the multiple pregnancy rate is 14–24%.

17. Considerable research has been carried out in Australia on the outcome of IVF, as well as on areas such as community attitudes towards IVF. In a review of 244 pregnancies resulting from IVF reported to a national register in Australia, it was found that early pregnancy losses were high, with 5% tubal ectopic pregnancies, 18% biochemical pregnancies, and an incidence of spontaneous abortion of 27%. Among pregnancies of at least 20 weeks gestation 22% were multiple. The incidence of preterm births was three times higher than in the general population. Low birth weight rates were also higher, although the sex ratio and the incidence of congenital malformations were similar to those in naturally conceived pregnancies. Australian In Vitro Fertilisation Collaborative Group, 'High incidence of preterm births and early losses in pregnancy after in vitro fertilisation', *British Medical Journal*, 291, 1985, pp. 1160–1163.

In a survey of community attitudes conducted in Victoria, Australia in July 1982 and April 1983, 74% approved of IVF in 1983 (compared with 67% in 1982); 56% approved of ovum donation, 43% approved of embryo freezing and 44% approved of embryo donation (compared with 70%, 63% and 58% respectively for childless married couples' approval). In all cases, disapproval rates were much lower than approval rates. M. Brumby, 'Australian community attitudes to in-vitro fertilization', *Medical Journal of Australia*, 2, 1983, pp. 650–653.

In a survey in Edinburgh directed at women in a family planning clinic, an ante-natal clinic, and an infertility clinic, 94% thought that IVF treatment should be allowed in the UK with 90% considering that it should be available on the NHS. In regard to embryo research, 74% would permit research on a 3-day embryo and 67% on a 14-day embryo if the research had as its goal the improvement of IVF treatment. Equivalent figures for research directed at avoiding the birth of babies with defects were 81% and 77% respectively. Of this sample, 24% thought that a 3-day embryo should be given the same legal rights and protection as a human person; 9% considered that the UK Parliament should pass a law forbidding all research on human embryos (63% thought it should not). 79% agreed with ovum donation. E. M. Alder and coworkers, 'Attitudes of women of reproductive age to in vitro fertilisation and embryo research', *Journal of Biosocial Science*, 18, 1986, pp. 155–167.

18. The ethical literature on IVF has burgeoned to such an extent over the past few years, that it is impossible even to begin to keep track of it. Apart from the books and articles quoted elsewhere, the following are a few articles in the general ethical literature representing a range of positions: J. Harris, '*In vitro* fertilization: the ethical issues', *The Philosophical Quarterly*, 33, 1983, pp. 217–237; M. Warnock, '*In vitro* fertilization: the ethical issues (II)', *The Philosophical Quarterly*, 33, 1983, pp. 238–249; P. Singer and D. Wells, '*In vitro* fertilisation: the major issues', *Journal of Medical Ethics*, 9, 1983, pp. 192–195; G. D. Mitchell '*In vitro* fertilisation: the major issues – a comment', *Journal of Medical Ethics*, 9, 1983, pp. 196–199, T. Iglesias, '*In vitro* fertilisation: the major issues', *Journal of Medical Ethics*, 10, 1984, pp. 32–37. Two examples of approaches to social policy in relation to IVF are: S. Elias, G. J. Annas, 'Social policy considerations on noncoital reproduction', *Journal of the American Medical Association*, 255, 1986, pp. 62–68; B. K. Rothman, 'The products of conception: the social context of reproductive choices', *Journal of Medical Ethics*, 11, 1985, pp. 188–192.

19. O. O'Donovan, *Begotten or Made?* (Clarendon Press, Oxford, 1984).

20. M. Charlesworth, 'Biotechnology and bioethics: New ways of life and death', *Current Affairs Bulletin*, 61, 1984, pp. 4–24.

21. C. Grobstein, 'External human fertilization', *Scientific American*, 240, 1979, pp. 33–43.

22. J. F. Kerin and C. D. Matthews, Submission to the Legislative Council Select Committee on Artificial Insemination by Donor, In Vitro Fertilization and Embryo Transfer Procedures in South Australia. Up to August 1984 the results of cryopreservation at the Queen Victoria Medical Centre/ Epworth Hospital in Melbourne were as follows: since the beginning of 1982 more than 300 embryos had been frozen. Since January 1982, 130 embryos had been thawed, and 45 had been transferred. In 1983 there were three established pregnancies, of which one miscarried at 24 weeks. As at August 1984, there had been one successful birth, with four continuing pregnancies. For a discussion of some of the ethical issues raised by the freezing of embryos, see: D. T. Ozar, 'The case against thawing unused frozen embryos', *The Hastings Center Report*, 15 (4), 1985, pp. 7–12.

23. Arguments in favour of surrogacy are presented by Peter Singer and Deane Wells in *The Reproduction Revolution: New Ways of Making Babies* (Oxford University Press, Oxford, 1984), pp. 107–130. See also the series of chapters on surrogacy in D. Ganos, R. E. Lipson, G. Warren and B. J. Weill

(eds.), *Difficult Decisions in Medical Ethics: Volume 4*, (Alan R. Liss, New York, 1983), pp. 137–164.

24. For a useful summary of competing claims in relation to surrogacy (and also other new reproductive techniques) see: *New Birth Technologies: An Issues Paper on AID, IVF, and Surrogate Motherhood* (Law Reform Division, Department of Justice, Wellington, New Zealand, 1985). Arguments against surrogacy are presented in one form or another in all Christian assessments of the new reproductive technologies (see notes on Chapter 2 for references).

25. See Mary Warnock's comments on this in 'Legal Surrogacy – not for love or money?', *The Listener*, 24 January 1985, pp. 2–4.

Chapter 7 – Freedom to Manipulate Human Life?

1. L. Walters, 'Ethical issues in experimentation on the human fetus', *Journal of Religious Ethics*, 2, 1974, pp. 33–54.

2. A survey of the literature up to 1975 is found in L. Walters, 'Ethical and public policy issues in fetal research', in 'The National Commission for the Protection of Human Subjects of Biomedical and Behavioral Research', *Appendix: Research on the Fetus* (US Department of Health, Education and Welfare (DHEW), Washington DC, 1975).

3. Report of the Advisory Group (Peel Committee Report), *The Use of Fetuses and Fetal Material for Research* (Her Majesty's Stationery Office, London, 1972).

4. The National Commission for the Protection of Human Subjects of Biomedical and Behavioral Research, *Research on the Fetus* (DHEW, Washington DC, 1975).

5. National Health and Medical Research Council, 'Ethics in Medical Research Involving the Human Fetus and Human Fetal Tissue', *Medical Journal of Australia*, May 12 1984, pp. 610–620.

6. Report of the Advisory Group (Peel Committee Report).

7. L. Walters, *op. cit.*

8. See note 2, *Supra.*

9. P. Ramsey, *The Ethics of Fetal Research* (Yale University Press, New Haven, 1975).

10. R. A. McCormick, *How Brave a New World?* (SCM Press, London, 1981). See also his contribution, 'Experimentation on the fetus: policy proposals', in: Report of The National Commission for the Protection of Human Subjects of Biomedical and Behavioral Research, *Appendix: Research on the Fetus*. I have retained the term 'experimentation' throughout the section on his views, since this is the term he employs. However, the term 'research' – in the general sense in which I am using it – may be more appropriate.

11. For a conservative stance, see also H. O. Tiefel, 'The cost of fetal research: ethical considerations', *New England Journal of Medicine*, 294, 1976, pp. 85–90.

12. W. Gaylin and M. Lappé, 'Fetal politics', *Atlantic Monthly*, May 1975.

13. M. Lappé, 'Balancing obligations to the living human fetus with the needs for experimentation', in: The National Commission for the Protection of Human Subjects of Biomedical and Behavioral Research, *Appendix: Research on the Fetus*.

14. W. Gaylin and M. Lappé, *op. cit.*

15. For an outline of some of the research possibilities using the human embryo, refer to: R. G. Edwards, 'The case for studing human embryos and their constituent tissues *in vitro*', in R. G. Edwards and J. M. Purdy (eds.),

Human Conception In Vitro (Academic Press, London, 1982), pp. 371–388.
R. G. Edwards, 'The ethical, scientific and medical implications of human conception in vitro', *Pontificiae Academiae Scientiarum Scripta Varia*, 51, 1984, pp. 193–249. J. F. Kerin and C. D. Matthews, submission to the Legislative Council Select Committee on Artificial Insemination By Donor, In Vitro Fertilization and Embryo Transfer Procedures in South Australia.

16. R. G. Edwards, 'The ethical, scientific and medical implications of human conception in vitro', *Pontificiae Academiae Scientiarum Scripta Varia*, 51, 1984, pp. 193–249.

17. Editorial, *Nature*, 302, 1983, pp. 735–736.

18. For a review of the competing ethical positions on embryo research, see L. Walters, 'Human in vitro fertilization: a review of the ethical literature', *The Hastings Center Report*, 9, 1979, pp. 23–43. See also many of the reports and books discussed in Chapter 2.

19. *Report of the Committee of Inquiry into Human Fertilisation and Embryology* (Her Majesty's Stationery Office, London, 1984).

20. L. R. Kass, '"Making babies" revisited', *Public Interest*, 54, 1979, pp. 32–60.

21. Leon Kass in the article referred to in n. 20 contrasts the blastocyst and the 12 week abortus. He suggests that the blastocyst in the laboratory is *pre-viable* in that it is capable of *becoming* or *being made* viable, whereas the abortus is not-at-all viable. As a result, he compares the early embryo *in vitro* to the early embryo *in vivo*, and that the early embryo should be treated as a pre-viable fetus.

Chapter 8 – Certainties and Quandaries

1. For further discussion of this issue see footnote 12 in Chapter 3 and the ethical assessment of the simple case of IVF in Chapter 6.

2. Many critics of IVF and related techniques opt for tubal microsurgery (surgical reconstruction of the woman's uterine tubes) as a means of overcoming infertility caused by blockage of the uterine tubes. Tubal microsurgery is an attractive option in that it does not focus attention on the embryos (as does IVF); however, it too has drawbacks on account of its technological nature. The incidence of ectopic tubal pregnancy following microsurgery ranges from 4 to 29%, depending on the type of tubal surgery undertaken (compared to 6% in an IVF programme). Such a high rate of ectopic pregnancies means that a high percentage of embryos has to be removed (aborted). Little is known about the physical and chemical environment within the repaired tube (which may have considerable implications for embryonic development), while there has been no long-term follow-up of children born after tubal surgery. It should also be noted that tubal microsurgery was introduced without a background of much research on animals nor of study of animal embryos following this procedure. See: C. Wood, B. Downing, 'In-vitro fertilization and tubal microsurgery – their status compared', *British Journal of Obstetrics and Gynaecology*, 93, 1986, pp. 3–5.

3. *National Data Book and Guide to Sources* (Statistical Abstract of the United States 1984, 104th edition, US Department of Commerce, Bureau of the Census, pp. 61–77.

4. R. Snowden and G. D. Mitchell, *The Artificial Family* (George Allen and Unwin, London, 1981).

5. In making this statement I am not advocating *de facto* relationships. Since they exist in society, and since societies accept such relationships, infertile

couples in a *de facto* relationship have to be assessed for their suitability to have a child by AID or IVF. My contention is that, if their commitment to one another is a loving and stable one, there is no reason – in society's terms – to deny them the opportunity of having a child of their own. In moral terms, I consider that such a relationship is sub-Christian and is not to be encouraged.

The co-existence of an ideal practice and of one which is less-than-the-ideal is well illustrated by marriage and divorce respectively. Christians in general accept divorce as a social reality, even when they disagree with it on theological grounds. Divorcees are accepted, as are those who have re-married, even though certain churches impose various restrictions on them.

6. R. Snowden and G. D. Mitchell, *op. cit.*
7. D. M. MacKay, Biblical perspectives on human engineering. In C. W. Ellison (ed.) *Modifying Man: Implications and Ethics* (University Press of America, Washington DC, 1977), pp. 67–90.
8. W. Trobisch, *I Married You* (Inter-Varsity Press, Leicester, 1971).

Epilogue

1. Amniocentesis and its moral implications are discussed in *Brave New People* – Chapter 3.
2. For further details on chorion biopsy see: J. C. Anderson, R. J. Trent, A. Boogert, A. Smith, R. P. Shearman, 'Ultrasound guided chorion biopsy in antenatal diagnosis of genetic disorders', *Australian and New Zealand Journal of Obstetrics and Gynaecology*, 25, 1985; pp. 29–33, M. Lappé, 'The predictive power of the new genetics', *The Hastings Center Report*, 14 (5), 1984, pp. 18–21. Chorion biopsy can also be carried out during the second and third trimesters of pregnancy, see: K. H. Nicolaides, P. W. Soothill, C. H. Rodeck, R. C. Warren, 'Why confine chorionic villus (placental) biopsy to the first trimester?', *Lancet*, 1, 1986, pp. 543–544.
3. M. Clarke, 'Fetal diagnosis trial', *Nature*, 315, 1985, p. 269.
4. Two reports of pregnancies occurring in women with primary ovarian failure are: P. Lutjen, A. Trounson, J. Leeton, J. Findlay, C. Wood, P. Renou, 'The establishment and maintenance of pregnancy using *in vitro* fertilization and embryo donation in a patient with primary ovarian failure', *Nature*, 307, 1984, pp. 174–175, also D. Navot, N. Laufer, J. Kopolovic, R. Rabinowitz, A. Birkenfeld, A. Lewin, M. Granat, E. J. Margolioth, J. G. Schenker, 'Artificially induced endometrial cycles and establishment of pregnancies in the absence of ovaries', *New England Journal of Medicine*, 314, 1986, pp. 806–811.

Addendum

The rapidity with which events are moving in the areas covered by this book means that some aspects of the debate are out of date by the time of publication. A brief addendum (written in December 1986) is hardly sufficient to counteract this trend. Nevertheless, it may help in some small measure.

1. Studies on IVF
These are now numerous. Some further examples are: M. C. Andrews and others, 'An analysis of the obstetric outcome of 125 consecutive pregnancies conceived in vitro and resulting in 100 deliveries', *American Journal of Obstetrics and Gynecology*, 154, 1986, pp. 848–854; G. T. Kovacs and others, 'In vitro fertilization and embryo transfer', *Medical Journal of Australia*, 144, 1986, pp. 682–683; G. Sher and others, 'In vitro fertilization and embryo transfer: two-year experience', *Obstetrics and Gynecology*, 67, 1986, pp. 309–315; and J. Testart and others, 'Relationships between embryo transfer results and ovarian response and in vitro fertilization rate: analysis of 186 human pregnancies', *Fertility and Sterility*, 45, 1986, pp. 237–243.

2. Studies of infertile couples
An interesting study of the motives of infertile couples for wanting a child concluded that the central motive is that a child is an ultimate expression of love between a man and a woman. See: A. Lalos and others, 'The wish to have a child: a pilot-study of infertile couples', *Acta Psychiatrica Scandinavia*, 72, 1985, pp. 476–481.

3. GIFT technique (p. 268)
This is rapidly becoming a readily available means of overcoming infertility where the woman's uterine tubes are patent. It is a variation of IVF, and is very similar to natural conception. Those eligible for the GIFT programme may suffer from: oligospermia (reduced sperm counts), endometriosis, or unexplained infertility. It involves: a) tests to assess patency of the uterine tubes (including a laparoscopy); b) hormonal stimulation, so that the woman produces a number of ova per cycle; c) collection of ova by laparoscopy (and/or an ultrasound collection technique), and introduction of the ova (often two) and

prepared sperm into the ovarian end of each tube. Excess ova may be inseminated and frozen for later use, donated for research, donated to an ovum-donation programme, or disposed of. The risks associated with the GIFT procedure are multiple pregnancy and ectopic pregnancy. The success rate is of the order of 45%. Quite clearly, the ethical issues raised by this technique are much the same as those associated with the simple case of IVF (depending on the use that is or is not made of excess embryos).

4. Infertility Medical Procedures Act

One of the consequences of this Act in the state of Victoria in Australia, when it came into force in August 1986, was to bring to a halt most research using human embryos. This was because it carries penalties of up to four years' imprisonment for those undertaking procedures entailing the destruction of, or damage to, living human embryos. Implicit within the Act is the stipulation that a human embryo, once fertilized, must be allowed to develop to maturity (although observations on spare embryos may be allowed). However, it appears that some research may be able to resume, since the Victorian Standing Review and Advisory Committee on Infertility has decided that 'cells' do not achieve embryo status until 20 hours after fertilization (when the male and female genetic material fuses). This allows research into issues such as the effects of freezing on ova, since the major way of assessing this is to attempt to fertilize them. The obvious question to ask is whether this particular redefinition of an embryo is justified scientifically. It also raises the query of whether a *scientific* redefinition can, by its very nature, solve an *ethical* problem. If not, further manipulation of scientific concepts will be required in future to enable more extensive research in this area.

5. CARE Trust (pp. 42, 43)

In an up-date of its original booklet on the Warnock Committee Report (p. 282), *Wanted Human Embryos Dead or Alive?* (CARE Trust, London, 1986), the major points of the original are re-iterated. Although it does not denounce either AIH or IVF within marriage, it comments that 'Some Christians are firmer in their beliefs that all artificial reproductive techniques deviate from God's creation pattern and purpose. They would add that there is no shame in infertility and that it even has certain advantages'.

6. Christian perspectives on infertility

Relatively little popular Christian literature deals with infertility. Joy Cooke's contribution was mentioned on p. 285. Another contribution is that of Martha Stout, *Without Child* (Zondervan, Grand Rapids, Michigan, 1985). This is a practical guide for couples faced with infertility problems.

Index of Scripture References and Names

Genesis
1:26   48, 63, 68
1:27   63, 68, 80
1:28   68, 81
2:7   63
2:8, 24, 25   80, 88, 91
2:16, 17   68
2:18ff   90
2:19   68
3:6   70
3:20   81
3:22   71
4:1   126
5:1   68
9:1–7   68, 71
15:3, 4   82
16:1–16   6, 82, 83, 90, 126
21:10   90
21:14   90
25:23   127
29:31, 32   126
30:1–23   6, 82, 126
38   81

Exodus
18:21   73
21:12   130
21:22–25   129–131, 133, 289
22:22   84

Leviticus
19:15   72

Numbers
33:54–56   88

Deuteronomy
10:18   84
21:15ff   90
25:5–10   81, 88
26:12   84

Joshua
13–19:   88

Judges
13:7   127
19:1–3   90

Ruth
4:13   126

1 Samuel
1:5–18   81, 90
2:1   81

2 Samuel
9:13   90

1 Kings
9:1–8   90
12:24   88

Job
10:8–12   125, 127
10:18, 19   128
31:13–15   126

Psalms
8:6–8   68
22:9, 10   126
51:5   127, 166
68:5, 6   84
82:3   84
127:3   90
139:13–16   126, 127, 128, 142

Ecclesiastes
11:5   128

Isaiah
1:17   84
46:3   127
49:1   126

Jeremiah
1:5   126, 127
22:13–17   73

Amos
2:6, 7   72
3:9, 10   72
4:5   72
5:7–20   72

Micah
5:2   89

Habakkuk
2:9–11   73

Malachi
3:5   84

Matthew
1   *89*
1:20   *127*
2:6   *89*
5:43   *73*
6:25   *67*
10:39   *67*
12:13–18   *288*
16:25–26   *67*
19:3–9   *90*
22:37   *67*
22:40   *73*

Mark
6:3–5   *89*
7:8–13   *89*
8:35–36   *67*
10:1–12   *90*
12:28–34   *67, 73*
12:44   *66*

Luke
1:41–44   *48, 126, 133*
2:12, 16   *133*
3   *89*
6:27–31   *73*
9:24–25   *67*
10:25–28   *67, 73*
15:12–30   *66*
18:15   *133*
18:20   *89*

John
9:1–5   *38, 81*
10:10   *67*

Romans
1:30   *89*
8:14, 15   *84*
12:20   *73*

1 Corinthians
6:16   *90*

6:19, 20   *74*
7:1   *90*
11:7   *68*

Galatians
4:1ff   *89*
4:4–7   *84*
4:22–27   *82*
6:10   *89*

Ephesians
1:4   *127*
1:5   *84*
4:13ff   *89*
5:22–23   *90*

Colossians
3:10   *68*

1 Timothy
1:9   *89*
2:2   *66*
3:2   *90*

2 Timothy
1:9   *127*
3:2   *89*

James
1:27   *84*
3:9   *68*
4:17   *73*

1 Peter
4:2   *67*

1 John
2:16   *67*
3:16–18   *73*
4:7   *38*

Abram, *6, 7, 81–83*
Abraham, *88*
Adam, *68, 70*
Amos, *72*
Bethlehem (clan-city of), *89*
Bilhah, *6*
Dan (tribe of), *88*
David, *126, 127*
Elizabeth, *126*
Esau, *127*
Eve, *70, 81*
Hagar, *6, 7, 82, 83*
Hannah, *81*
Ishmael, *6, 83*
Israel (nation of), *88, 90*
Jacob, *6, 81, 88, 127*
Jeremiah, *72, 126, 127*
Jesus *69, 73, 89, 127, 131–133*
Job, *127, 128*
John, *73*
John the Baptist, *133*
Joseph, *127*
Judah (tribe of), *88, 89*
Leah, *6*
Mary, *126, 127, 131, 133*
Onan, *81*
Paul, *74, 89, 127*
Rachel, *6*
Rebekah, *127*
Samson, *127*
Sarai, *6, 7, 81, 82*
Tamar, *81*
Zilpah, *6*

Index of Names

This index does not include biblical names, nor does it refer to names found in the chapter notes.

Anderson, J. Kirby, *34, 35*
Atkinson, David, *71*
Board of Social Responsibility of Church of Scotland, *44, 45*
Board for Social Responsibility of the General Synod of the Church of England, *46–48*
British Medical Association (BMA) guidelines, *27*
Christian Action Research and Education (CARE) Trust, *42, 43, 45*
Christian Medical Fellowship (CMF), *43, 44*
Church of England Working Party on AID, *174*
Clements, Roy, *88*
Council for Science and Society, *50, 51*
Curran, Charles, *145*
Department of Health, Education and Welfare (DHEW), Ethics Advisory Board, *33, 34, 51*
Dunstan, G. R., *178*
Edwards, Robert, *24–26, 228*
Fleming, John, *35, 36*
Fletcher, Joseph, *145*
Gaylin, Willard, *222*
Grobstein, Clifford, *51, 52, 192*
Häring, Bernard, *34*
Iglesias, Teresa, *146*
Infertility (Medical Procedures) Act 1984, *32*
Ison, David, *174*
Joyce, Robert E., *146*
Kass, Leon, *23, 24*
Lappe, Marc, *222*
MacKay, Donald, *136, 142–144, 162, 259*
McCormick, Richard, *23, 34, 145, 220, 221, 225*
Medical Research Council (MRC) guidelines, *26*
Mitchell, G. D., *171, 176, 177*
National Health and Medical Research Council (NH & MRC), *32, 33*
Nelson, James B., *36, 37*
Nelson, J. Robert, *66*
O'Donovan, Oliver, *38, 39, 136–140, 143, 151*
Overduin, Daniel, *35, 36*
Packer, James, *84*
Peel Committee Report, *215*
Pontifical Academy of Science, *228*
Rahner, Karl, *145*
Ramm, Bernard, *25*
Ramsey, Paul, *21–23, 34, 157, 219–221*
Rohricht, Jo Anne Smith, *36, 37*
Royal College of Obstetricians and Gynaecologists (RCOG) guidelines, *26*
Royal Society guidelines, *26, 228*
Schlesselman, James, *116*
Schluter, Michael, *88*
Simmons, Paul D., *37, 38, 81*
Singer, Peter, *52–56, 147–149*
Smedes, Lewis, *140, 144*
Snowden, Robert, *91, 171, 176, 177*
Social Responsibilities Commission of the Anglican Church of Australia, *39*
Steptoe, Patrick, *25*
Stott, John, *128, 139, 140, 143*
Tiefel, Hans, *49*
Tooley, Michael, *149–151, 162*
Torrance, Thomas, *40–42, 131*
Waller Committee Reports, *31, 32*
Waller, Louis, *30*
Walters, LeRoy, *216*
Warnock Committee Report, *27–30, 50, 229, 230*; responses to, *40–48*
Warnock, Mary, *27*
Wells, Deane, *52–56, 147–149*
Wenham, Gordon, *127, 128, 133*

Subject Index

This index does not include any reference to terms that occur in the glossary, or in notes on chapters.

Abortion, 24, 34, 39, 44, 55, 56, 60, 80, 86, 129, 130, 132, 138, 140, 144, 149, 155, 161, 163–165, 215, 237, 266; and fetal research, 211–217, 220–224, 231; and potentiality principle, 154; induced, 76, 117, 159, 160, 166, 212, 219; liberal practices of, 86, 166; spontaneous, 76, 116, 117, 158, 159–162, 166, 186, 219, 233, 235, 236

Adoption, 5, 6, 10, 12, 35, 39, 40, 83–87, 92, 93, 171, 175, 179, 191, 195–200, 205, 262; prenatal, 10, 12, 182, 195, 197, 198, 199

Adultery, 3, 4, 60, 62, 92, 173

agape, 62

Amniocentesis, 56, 265, 266

Anencephaly, 122, 138

Artificial insemination, 9, 13, 17, 39

Artificial Insemination by Donor (AID), 4, 8, 11, 28, 33, 36–47, 50, 92, 168–181, 190, 194–196, 199–201; and lesbians, 51, 56, 57, 178, 179; anonymity of donor, 170, 171, 178, 179, 201; arguments against, 169, 170; arguments for, 169; as adultery, 170, 174; Christian views of, 174, 177, 179; recommendations for society, 249, 250; secrecy surrounding, 170, 171, 176–179, 198, 200

Artificial Insemination by Husband (AIH), 8, 28, 36, 42, 43, 45, 168, 184

Bible, guidelines provided by, 63; in bioethics, 59, 60; source of moral principles, 60, 61, 63; source of moral rules, 60, 61

bios, 66, 75

Blastocyst(s), 24, 25, 96, 137

Blastomeres, 96, 112, 236

Brain, and consciousness, 148; 'birth' (life), 108, 118–124, 136, 143, 162; cerebral hemispheres (cortex) of, 104–111, 145, 150; characteristics of human, 111; 'death', 118, 119, 139; development of, 97, 101–112, 122, 135, 155, 162; EEG pattern of, 106, 107, 120–122

Brave New People, ix, x, 242

brephos, 133

Child-bearing, 9; in Jewish society, 82

Child-rearing, 9

Children, artificially conceived, 247, 248; born to single women, 248; desire for, 79, 80, 86; gift from God, 81; handicapped, 90, 223, 262, 264; naturally conceived, 247

Chorion biopsy, 265–267

Cloning (asexual reproduction), 16, 17, 27, 33, 36, 42, 148

Conception, 9, 17, 50, 87, 113, 126, 137, 184, 188, 199; artificial, 87, 184; moment of, 136, 139; personal identity at, 133, 139

Contraception, 26, 150, 184, 188, 190, 256

Ectogenesis, 15, 16, 55, 148

Embryo(s), 54, 94, 97, 98; as a non-person, 148, 163, 229; as a person, 146; as a 'thing', 148, 228; as human being, 48; as potential human person, 113, 146, 147, 229, 231, 233; biopsy of, 268, 269; destruction of, 41, 43; development of, 94–98, 145; disposal of, 32, 186; donation of, 10, 12, 15, 29, 46, 47, 57, 193–201; experiments on, 21, 26, 41; freezing of, 12, 29, 32, 39, 42, 182, 183, 193, 194; genotypes of, 114, 115; manipulation of, 2, 14, 21, 27, 41, 165, 192; preimplantation, 14,

52, 95, 193, 198, 226, 227, 229, 232, 237; presentient, 148; previable, 23; relationship to God of, 144; right of ownership of, 29; spare (surplus), 10, 12, 14, 27, 30, 32, 45, 181–183, 192–201, 226, 232, 233, 237, 238, 251, 252, 258; status of, 29, 42–44, 46, 48, 49, 54, 130, 145, 147, 155, 162, 163, 181, 186, 194, 199, 200, 229, 235; storage of, 29, 32, 33, 42, 45; treated as means to an end, 41, 164, 165, 259

Embryo research, 14, 15, 23, 26, 29–33, 42, 45–47, 50, 54, 138, 148, 161, 193, 194, 208, 225–239, 269; ethical assessment of, 230–239; non-therapeutic, 234, 237–239; on IVF embryo, 232–234, 238; recommendations for society, 253, 254; therapeutic, 234, 236–239

Embryo transfer (ET), 18, 19, 27

Ethics, humanitarian, 25; Kantian, 59; of responsibility, 37; person-centred, 25; relational or response approach in, 61; rule, 35, 36; slippery slope argument in, 34; utilitarian, 25, 41, 52, 53, 56, 59, 147, 216, 221, 247; utopian, 25

Father, biological, 4, 5, 8, 13, 176, 178, 201; complete, 19; genetic, 19; nurturing, 19; social, 4, 5, 8, 13, 178

Family, 23–25, 28, 41–43, 46–48, 50, 62, 82, 83, 84, 86, 91, 175,

180, 183, 187, 191, 206, 242, 260; biblical perspective on, 87–91; church, 90; extended, 88–93, 205; God's, 84, 85; lesbian, 53; nuclear (conjugal), 86, 88, 89, 92, 93; single parent, 6, 7, 53; society's view of, 180; sociological perspectives on, 91, 92; 3G, 88; traditions of Israel, 129

Fertilization, 9, 26, 27, 42, 95, 100, 112–114, 126, 131, 160, 255, 256, 258; external human, 18; God's purposes before, 127; in laboratory, 10, 183, 187; interspecies, 26, 30, 41, 42, 269; moment of, 43, 52, 145; personhood at, 134, 140, 145, 160; products of, 115

Fetal research, 98–100, 209–225, 231; consent to, 218, 219; during abortion, 211, 212, 215, 224; ethical assessment of 219–225; following abortion, 211, 213, 215, 224, 231; in anticipation of an abortion, 211, 214, 224, 231; non-therapeutic, 212, 213, 216–221, 224, 225; on dead fetus, 215, 222, 223; proxy consent in, 220, 221, 225; therapeutic, 212–215, 221, 223

Fetus, 126, 127, 208; as part of human continuum, 164; as person, 134–142, 144–147, 156; as non-person, 147–151; as potential person, 151–154, 156, 162; become

a person, 200–205; biblical attitudes towards, 128; consent of, 22, 23, 181; damage (harm) to IVF, 21, 22, 181, 220; development of, 99, 100, 143; experimentation on, 41, 210–221; humanity of, 133, 156, 157; innocence of, 160, 165–167; inviolability of, 45, 129–133, 140, 159–166; previable, 95, 209, 211, 213, 215, 216, 218, 222, 224, 225, 233; protection of, 155, 157, 164, 166; status of, 130, 133, 143, 154, 155, 162, 163, 216, 217, 219, 221, 223, 224; value of, 164, 223; viable, 95, 209, 211, 213, 223

Fostering, 6, 39, 93, 191

Gametes, 3, 10, 26; disposal of, 29; donation of, 10, 28, 31, 37, 50, 53, 83, 173–175, 194–201, 252, 253

Genetic uniqueness, 74, 113–115, 134, 135, 140, 158, 159, 173

Human beings, as biological and spiritual beings, 66; as created beings, 63, 64; as end in themselves, 70; as God's creatures, 64, 65, 79; capacities of, 54; co-creators with God, 81; dignity of, 60, 61, 63, 69, 70, 153, 223, 224, 238, 241, 258; God-like attributes of, 68; God-relatedness of, 179; in the image of God, 41, 46, 67–70, 80, 157, 159, 188, 189, 205, 238, 247; inviolability of, 42, 77, 146; potential as, 77; value of, 74, 75, 135;

wholeness of, *74*
Human life, beginning of, *52, 129;* choices involving, *77, 132;* intrinsic value of, *67, 187;* on loan from God, *74;* potential of, *75;* precious to God, *69;* prenatal, *125–133;* quality of, *25, 75, 241, 243;* taking of, *60;* value of, *70, 76, 77, 140;* wastage of, *76;* wholeness in, *61*
Humanness, *66, 231*
Human responsibility, *25, 68, 75, 77–79, 190;* misuse of, *70, 71*
Human (technical) control, *2, 25, 65, 183, 188, 190, 191*
Identical twins, *16, 114, 115;* as persons, *14*
Implantation, *26, 94, 96, 113, 137, 192;* chromosomal abnormalities at, *118*
Incarnation of Jesus, *41, 70, 127, 128, 131*
Infanticide, *149, 150*
Infant mortality rate, *241*
Infertile couple, *22–24, 33, 34, 45, 47, 53, 63, 85, 179, 181, 190, 195, 207, 261–264*
Infertility, *2, 28, 37, 38, 42, 79, 81, 83, 181, 183, 190, 194, 229, 242;* and childlessness, *81–83, 85, 89, 180, 186, 191, 201, 207, 261;* and public policy, *244–248;* human dilemma of, *182;* treatment of, *22, 26, 29, 30, 33, 41, 43, 45, 229, 234, 242, 243, 244*
in vitro fertilization (IVF), *1, 2, 10–14, 18, 21–58, 181–207, 267, 268;* embryo donation in, *12, 22, 31, 45;* fate

of embryos in, *185;* GIFT in, *268;* hormonal stimulation in, *182;* ovum donation in, *11, 27–31, 33, 45;* pastoral care dimensions of, *40, 48;* programme, *31–33, 39, 63, 185, 193, 194, 196, 198, 207;* recommendations for society, *250–253;* simple case of, *10, 35, 36, 181–191, 250, 251;* sperm donation in, *11, 31;* technological nature of, *181, 187*
Jesus Christ, *243, 264;* as embryo, *133;* attitudes of, *61, 62, 69;* conception of, *132*
Justice, in human society, *72, 73*
Laparoscopy, *9, 10, 267*
Lavage, *9, 10, 12, 29;* embryo donation and, *10;* ovum donation and, *9, 11*
lex talionis, 130
Marriage, *23, 28, 36, 41–43, 45–48, 50, 91, 92, 169, 170, 191, 198, 207, 242, 257, 260, 261;* and AID, *172–178;* biblical view of, *35;* children in, *80, 91;* concubines and, *90;* levirite, *81, 88;* monogamous, *24, 90, 92, 184;* patriarchal pattern of, *81;* polygamous, *83, 90;* representational begetting in, *82*
Morula, *96*
Mother, biological, *3–5, 8, 11, 39, 87, 170;* carrying, *19, 20, 50, 197, 201;* genetic, *19, 20, 197, 201;* nurturing, *19, 20;* social, *4, 8, 11, 13, 197*
Myelin, *107, 109*
Natural law, *36*

Nervous system, early development of, *26, 104, 119, 136, 148*
Neurons (nerve cells), *106–111;* connections between (synapses), *107, 109–111*
Orphans, *7, 84, 85*
Ovum (ova), *1–3, 9, 11, 14, 16, 18, 19, 26, 36, 95, 112, 113, 115, 163, 267;* donation (donor) of, *10, 13, 14, 37, 47, 50, 53, 57, 194–196, 198;* freezing of, *183, 196*
Pain, *43, 106, 148*
Parent(s), biological, *3–5, 7, 8, 10, 15–17, 19, 23, 91, 92, 177, 179, 184, 198;* social parents, *3–5, 7–10, 15, 17, 19, 91, 177, 198;* step-, *4, 5, 93, 170*
Personhood, *52, 114, 136, 137, 139, 141, 142, 152, 153, 157, 205;* and brain birth, *123;* and developing brain, *148, 158;* beginning of, *118, 134;* biblical concept of, *80;* developmental (gradualist) school of, *134–136, 144;* genetic (conception) school of, *134, 135, 137, 146;* growth into, *144;* of embryo, *113, 146, 154, 156;* of fetus, *140, 143, 145–154, 158, 163, 217;* social consequences school of, *134, 135, 137*
Person(s), *33, 48, 52, 66, 68, 136, 137, 142, 204;* embryo as, *128;* New Testament concept of, *66;* potential, *149, 151–154, 156, 162, 192;* quasi-, *150*
Potentiality principle, *151–154, 159*
Preembryo, *52, 94, 95*

Pregnancy wastage, *115–118, 139, 159–162, 227;* chromosomal abnormalities in, *117, 118, 161, 162, 226, 227, 235, 238, 265, 268*
Preperson, *52, 137*
Primitive streak, *97, 230*
Procreation, *22, 23, 35–37, 42, 79–81, 91, 183, 190*
psuchē, 67, 75
Research, *24, 185, 209, 210*
Reproductive technologies (new), *6, 7, 17, 24, 34, 35, 40, 43, 47, 52, 56–58, 62, 87, 89, 93, 140, 144, 147, 154, 155, 206, 246, 247, 255, 260, 261;* non-therapeutic, *23, 50, 210;* therapeutic, *26, 165, 210*

Sanctity of human life, *35, 129*
Sperm, *3, 8, 9, 14, 36, 95, 112, 113, 163, 244, 267, 269;* donation (donor) of, *8, 10, 11, 13, 14, 27, 31, 37, 46, 50, 53, 198;* freezing of, *29;* penetration capacity of, *26*
Step-parent, *4, 5, 93, 170*
Surrogate mother(hood) [surrogacy], *8, 12–14, 16, 19, 20, 27, 29, 32, 33, 35, 36, 41, 42, 45, 53, 57, 81, 87, 192, 198, 201–207;* arguments against, *202, 203;* arguments in favour of, *202;* commercial, *29, 202, 206;* commissioning parent(s), *9, 201, 204, 205;* ethical assessment of, *204–*

207; full, *12, 13, 20, 55, 201, 206, 207;* legal requirements of, *55;* partial, *9, 12, 20, 55, 201, 202, 206;* recommendations for society, *253*
Technocracy, *76*
Technology, *35, 37, 47, 51, 69, 71, 76, 78, 181, 188, 207, 240–244, 260;* anti-, *39, 43, 188, 190, 241;* associated with conception, *39, 185;* choices implicit in, *78;* excesses of, *200;* misuse of biomedical, *71;* rejection of, *78, 188, 189*
Tuboplasty, *35, 242, 257*
zōē, 67, 75
Zygote, *96, 112, 137, 146;* as person, *146, 152, 159*